COLOR ATLAS OF
VETERINARY HISTOLOGY

WILLIAM J. BACHA, JR., Ph.D.
Professor of Zoology
Department of Biology
Rutgers University
Camden College of Arts and Sciences
Camden, New Jersey

Adjunct Professor
Department of Animal Biology
University of Pennsylvania
School of Veterinary Medicine
Philadelphia, Pennsylvania

LINDA M. WOOD, M.S., V.M.D.
Lecturer in Comparative Microscopic Anatomy
Department of Animal Biology
University of Pennsylvania
School of Veterinary Medicine
Philadelphia, Pennsylvania

Adjunct Professor of Biology
Department of Biology
Camden County College
Blackwood, New Jersey

COLOR
ATLAS
OF
VETERINARY
HISTOLOGY

LEA & FEBIGER

PHILADELPHIA ● LONDON

1 9 9 0

Lea & Febiger
200 Chesterfield Parkway
Malvern, PA 19355
U.S.A.
1-800-444-1785

Lea & Febiger (UK) Ltd.
145a Croydon Road
Beckenham, Kent BR3 3RB
U.K.

Chapter and page reprints may be purchased from Lea & Febiger in quantities of 100 or more.

Library of Congress Cataloging in Publication Data

Bacha, William J.
    Color atlas of veterinary histology / William J. Bacha, Jr., Linda
M. Wood.
        p.   cm.
    Incudes bibliographical references.
    ISBN 0-8121-1303-9
    1. Veterinary histology—Atlases.   I. Wood, Linda M.   II. Title.
    SF757.3.B33   1990   89-14516
    636.089'18—dc20   CIP

Printed in Hong Kong

Print number: 5 4 3 2 1

this book is dedicated
to
ALL THE ANIMALS

Although we have written this atlas primarily to fulfill a need of the student of veterinary medicine, we believe that clinicians, private practitioners, and researchers will find it a useful reference for normal tissues and organs. Currently, students rely heavily, if not exclusively, on atlases of human histology for guidance in the laboratory. There are, of course, similarities between organs and tissues of domestic animals and those of humans. There are also differences, however, and these are rarely encountered in atlases dealing specifically with human histology.

Our aim has been to compare the histologic structure of organs in a variety of domestic animals. We have used representative examples in instances where tissues and organs from different animals share a common structure. Wherever differences exist, we have tried to provide examples that are characteristic of a particular group of animals. Our selection of animals includes the dog, cat, horse, cow, sheep, goat, pig, and chicken because they are most frequently referenced in veterinary school curricula.

All photomicrographs and drawings are original. Some drawings were done freehand, while others were made with the aid of a camera lucida. Light microscopy and colored photomicrographs have been used exclusively. We have chosen color rather than black and white because of its correspondence to stained preparations. With the exception of the few histologic preparations loaned to us by generous donors or purchased from a dealer, slides were prepared by the authors. Fresh organ samples were obtained from a slaughterhouse or from animals that were euthanized for various reasons. With the exception of smear preparations (blood, bone marrow, and vaginal), mesenteric spreads, ground bone, and a single plastic section, slides were prepared using the paraffin method. All slides were stained with hematoxylin and eosin unless otherwise noted. Magnifications of photomicrographs are total magnifications (enlargement of photograph $\times$ objective $\times$ projector lens). Throughout the atlas, hollow structures, e.g., blood vessels, kidney tubules, alveoli, etc., are usually identified by labeling the lumen of the structure.

William J. Bacha, Jr.
Linda M. Wood

Camden, NJ

ACKNOWLEDGEMENTS

Help is often just around the corner. Dr. Henry Stempen, whose office was down the hall from ours at Rutgers University in Camden, New Jersey, stopped by one day and volunteered his artistic talents. We'd like to thank him for his excellent pen and ink drawings of various animal parts, which are somewhat removed from the fungi he usually draws. Our gratitude also to Ms. Kathleen Carr for her secretarial services. Special thanks are extended to Dr. Edward Zambraski, Ms. Kathleen O'Hagan, and Ms. Gail Thomas of Cook College, Rutgers University, for making fresh porcine material available to us; and to Dr. Barry Jesse and Dr. James Harner for supplying us with sheep parts.

Without the unqualified use of the facilities and equipment of the Biology Department of Rutgers, our tissue processing and photomicrography could not have been accomplished. Our special thanks to the Department for this courtesy.

This book would never have had a beginning were it not for the generosity of Dr. Leon Weiss, Department of Animal Biology, University of Pennsylvania School of Veterinary Medicine, who invited us to teach in the veterinary histology laboratory and kindly allowed us access to the slide collection and facilities of the Department. We would also like to express appreciation to the following individuals from the University of Pennsylvania School of Veterinary Medicine: Mr. Richard Aucamp and Mrs. Katherine Aucamp, who provided us with specimens, slides, advice, and assistance in a variety of other ways; Dr. Mark Haskins for kindly making available fresh canine and feline material; Dr. John Fyfe and Dr. Vicki Meyers-Wallen for supplying us with canine vaginal smears; Dr. and Mrs. Loren Evans and Dr. David McDevitt for lending us reference material; Dr. Peter Hand and Ms. Graziella Mann for providing material on the nervous system; and Dr. Helen Acland, Dr. Linda Bachin, Mr. James Bruce, Dr. Sherrill Davison, Ms. Dawn Dowling, Dr. Robert Dyer, Dr. Robert Eckroade, Dr. George Farnbach, Dr. David Freeman, Dr. Wendy Freeman, Dr. Alan Kelly, Mr. Joseph McGrane, and Dr. Mary Sommer for their time and consideration in helping us to obtain tissue specimens.

We are grateful to Dr. Carol Jacobson and the Department of Anatomy of the Iowa State University College of Veterinary Medicine for providing valuable slide preparations and text material.

Our gratitude is also extended to Hill's Pet Products, Topeka, Kansas, and Pitman-Moore, Inc., Washington Crossing, New Jersey, for their generous financial assistance.

Many thanks also to: Dr. Caroline Czarnecki of the University of Minnesota,

College of Veterinary Medicine, for providing copies of her informative laboratory guide; Dr. Deborah Ganster, Dr. James Lawhead, Dr. Virginia Pierce, Dr. Maria Salvaggio, Dr. Barbara Strock, and Dr. Cindi Ward for assisting us in obtaining tissue samples; Mr. Jeff Bringhurst, Bringhurst Brothers, Tansboro, New Jersey, for allowing us access to fresh large animal material; the Longenecker Hatchery, Elizabethtown, Pennsylvania, for providing chicken specimens; Ms. Susan Ulrich, Cornell University Press, for lending us a difficult-to-obtain reference; the helpful people at Optical Apparatus Company Inc., Ardmore, Pennsylvania, for supplies and for assistance with microscopic equipment; and to Mr. Charles Behl and Mr. James Durso of Webb and Company Inc., Cherry Hill, New Jersey, for their courteous service and helpful advice.

We are indebted to Mr. William J. Bacha, Sr. for building a super light box for us, and to Mr. Thomas H. Wood, Jr. for providing black and white prints of our photomicrographs, which saved us countless hours of drudgery in the darkroom.

Thanks also to family members Lola Wood, Tommy and Dawn, Jeanne and Pete, Sally and John, Alison and Steve, Anne, and Grandmom Wood (who we know will read the atlas from cover to cover) and to Brandi, Kevin, Darcy, and Ashley (who are not yet able to read but who will probably enjoy recoloring the pictures) for their support and for putting up with the grief we gave them as this project was put together. Our hats are off also to Snuff, Chew, Chapter Seat, Angel, Clyde, and all the other animals for their participation.

We are especially grateful to the following people at Lea & Febiger for their patience, understanding, friendliness, professional judgment, and advice: Mr. Christian Febiger Spahr, Jr., Mr. Sam Rondinelli, Ms. Dorothy Di Rienzi, and Ms. Jessica Martin. It was a pleasure to have such great assistance.

William J. Bacha, Jr.
Linda M. Wood

CONTENTS

GENERAL PRINCIPLES OF HISTOLOGY

PREPARATION OF HISTOLOGIC SECTIONS

A histologic section is a thin slice of tissue varying, usually, from 0.5 to 10 or more micrometers (μm) thick. In preparing such a section, a piece of tissue is either infiltrated with a supporting medium or frozen, and then cut with an instrument called a microtome. Sections obtained from tissue infiltrated with plastic can be as thin as 0.5 μm and show superior detail. Excellent preparations as thin as 2 or 3 μm can also be made from tissue infiltrated with paraffin-based embedding media. Sections are affixed to microscope slides and colored with one or more stains to increase the visibility of various cellular and intercellular components.

Schematically, Figure 1–1 outlines various steps involved in producing a stained histologic slide using the paraffin procedure. After being removed from an animal, a tissue or organ is cut into pieces. These pieces are placed into a fixative, such as buffered formalin or Bouin's, which, ideally, preserves normal morphology and facilitates further processing. After fixation, the specimen is dehydrated by transferring it through a series of alcohols of increasing concentrations to 100% alcohol. Next, it is placed into a substance such as xylene, which is miscible with both 100% alcohol and paraffin. This intermediate step (called clearing) is essential before infiltrating the dehydrated tissue with paraffin because alcohol and paraffin do not mix. During infiltration, melted paraffin completely replaces the

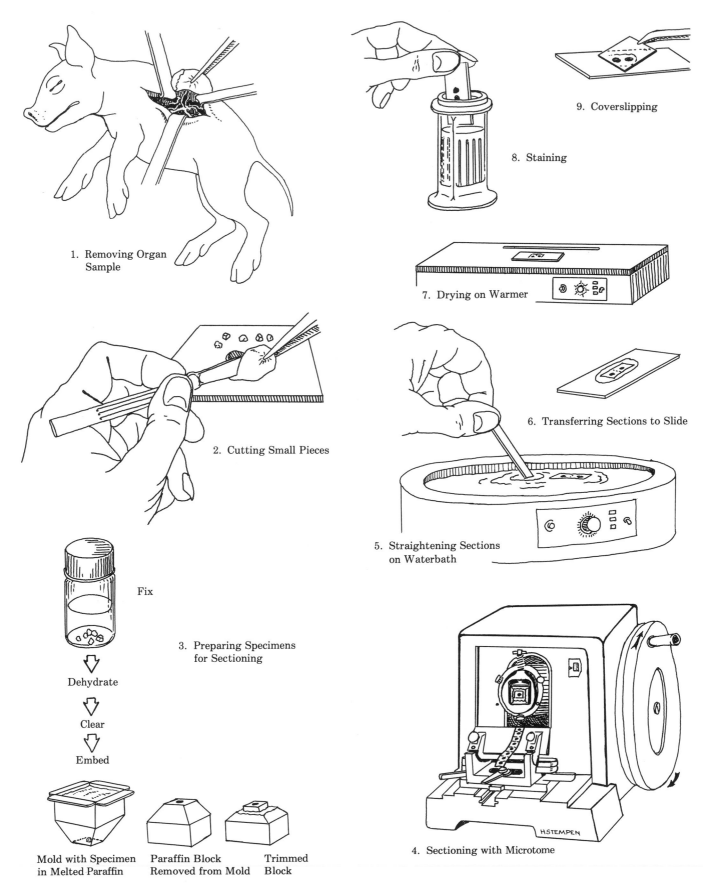

1. Removing Organ Sample

2. Cutting Small Pieces

3. Preparing Specimens for Sectioning

Fix

Dehydrate

Clear

Embed

Mold with Specimen in Melted Paraffin

Paraffin Block Removed from Mold

Trimmed Block

4. Sectioning with Microtome

5. Straightening Sections on Waterbath

6. Transferring Sections to Slide

7. Drying on Warmer

8. Staining

9. Coverslipping

HSTEMPEN

FIG. 1–1. *The various steps involved in producing a histologic slide using the paraffin method.*

xylene. This procedure is done in an oven at a temperature just above the melting point of the paraffin mixture. When infiltration is complete, the specimen is transferred to an embedding mold of fresh, melted paraffin, which is allowed to harden. The mold is eventually removed and excess paraffin is trimmed away.

The block of paraffin is then secured to the microtome and oriented appropriately with respect to the knife. With each revolution of the microtome handle, the specimen moves through the blade and a section of the desired thickness is produced. Each successive section adheres to the preceding one, forming a continuous ribbon. Subsequently, one or more sections are carefully separated from the ribbon and transferred to the surface of warm water in a waterbath. This softens the paraffin and flattens the section, eliminating wrinkles. The flattened section is floated onto a slide, which is then placed on a warming table. As the preparation dries, the section adheres to the surface of the slide.

Next, the paraffin is removed with xylene and the specimen is rehydrated. It is then stained, dehydrated, cleared (made transparent) with xylene, covered with a resinous mounting medium, and topped with a coverslip.

Various stains are available to the histologist. Hematoxylin and eosin (H&E) is a frequently used combination of stains. Hematoxylin imparts a purple color to substances, but must be linked to a metallic salt called a mordant before it can function effectively. This combination, called a lake, carries a positive charge and behaves as a basic (cationic) stain. The lake combines electrostatically with negatively charged radicals such as phosphate groups of nucleoproteins. Substances that become colored by a basic stain are said to be basophilic. Methylene blue, toluidine blue, and basic fuchsin are basic stains. Unlike hematoxylin, these stains have molecules that carry a positive charge of their own and do not require a mordant. Acidic (anionic) stains carry a negative charge and color cell or tissue components that bear positive charges. Eosin is an acid stain. It imparts an orange or red color to acidophilic substances. Other commonly used acid stains are orange G, phloxine, and aniline blue.

In addition to the widely used H&E staining procedure, numerous other stain combinations and techniques are available. Some are especially useful for identifying certain tissue elements. For example, trichrome procedures, such as Mallory's and Masson's, specifically stain collagenous fibers within connective tissue. Orcein and Weigert's resorcin fuchsin are stains used to color elastic fibers, providing a means of distinguishing them from other fibrous elements. Reticular fibers and nervous tissue components such as neurons, myelin, and cells of the neuroglia can be stained by procedures employing the use of silver. There are also special histochemical and immunohistochemical procedures that make possible the localization of various carbohydrates, lipids, and proteins found in tissue. Lastly, stains such as Wright's and Giemsa's (Romanovsky stains) are available for differentiating the various cells found in blood and bone marrow.

INTERPRETING SECTIONS

One must know the gross structure of an organ before a histologic section from it can be comprehended. It is also helpful to know how the section was cut, i.e., whether it was a cross section (x.s.), a longitudinal section (l.s.), or an oblique slice through the organ. Was the cut made through the entire organ or only through a portion of it? Frequently, prepared slides are labeled indicating the particular orientation of the section. This is not important in an asymmetric organ such as the spleen or liver because their appearance would be unaffected by the direction of the cut. Conversely, the small intestine is radially symmetric and its appearance is affected by the direction of the cut.

The three-dimensional structure of organs and their components must also be considered when examining a histologic preparation. Cells are three-dimensional objects differing in size and shape. For example, some are long and thin, some cuboidal, and others ovoid. They may have a random or specific arrangement within an organ. How they appear depends on their shape as well as how they were cut. Imagine how the spindle-shaped and tall columnar cells shown in Figure 1–2A would look if sectioned in various planes. Note that the nucleus may or may not be included in a particular cut through a cell.

The histologist examines multicellular structures having a wide variety of shapes. Some are hollow, some branch repeatedly, some open onto surfaces, etc. Figures 1–2B and C and 1–3 show a variety of three-dimensional structures and how they would appear if cut at different levels. Examine these carefully. They will help you to understand situations you will encounter on actual slides.

HELPFUL HINTS

Be sure that the lenses of your microscope are clean before you begin examining slides. Use a piece of lens paper or a soft, clean cloth, such as an old (but clean) linen handkerchief. If the lenses have been coated with oil or another substance, remove it using lens tissue

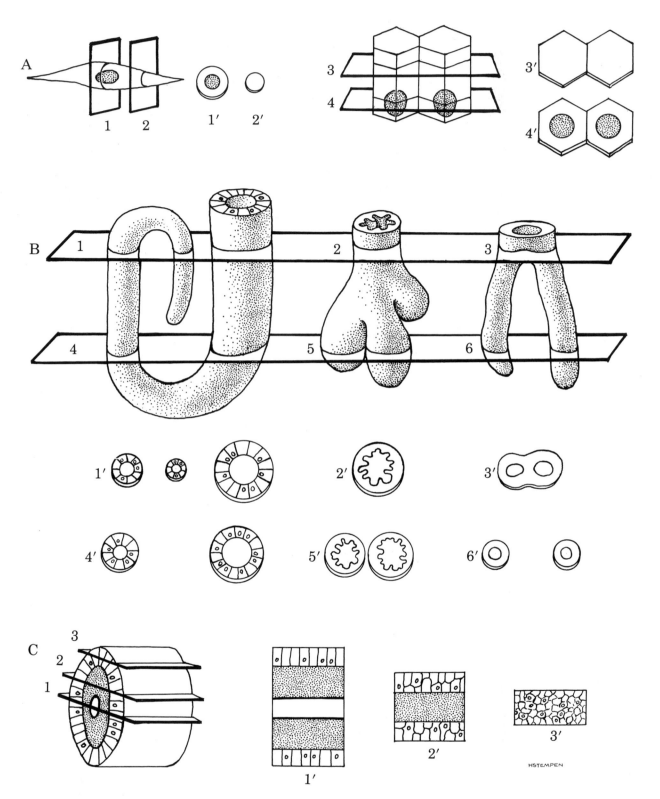

FIG. 1–2. A. Slices, indicated by numbered planes, taken through two different types of cells would appear as identified by the prime numbers. Only if the plane of the cut passes through the nucleus will the latter be seen. **B and C** illustrate planes of section taken from different levels in four separate multicellular objects. Note how the appearance of sections varies with the level of the cut.

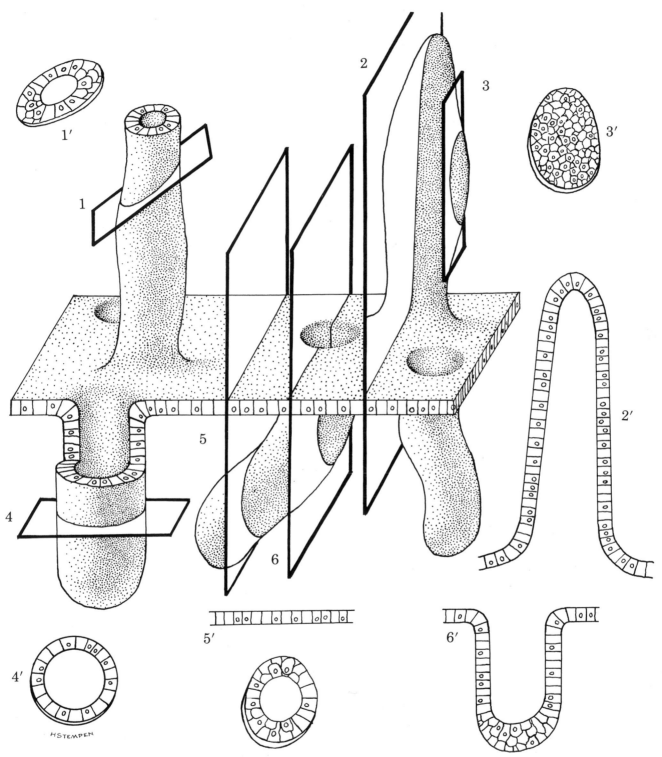

FIG. 1–3. The prime numbers illustrate sections resulting from transverse **(4)**, oblique **(1)**, and longitudinal **(2,3,5,6)** cuts made through a plate of cells bearing hollow projections (above plate) and invaginations (below plate). Plane 3 differs from the others because it passes only through the cellular wall of a projection, and not the lumen; therefore section 3' appears as a plate of cells rather than a hollow structure. You should also be aware that structures may often appear unrelated to a surface or another object, when in fact they are. Compare planes 5 and 6 with sections 5' and 6', where continuity of the invagination with the surface is evident only in 6 and 6'. When not apparent from a single section, such continuity, of course, would become evident only if an uninterrupted series of sections through the entire invagination were made and examined.

moistened sparingly with a glass cleaner such as Windex. Slides should also be cleaned using a soft, lint-free cloth or tissue moistened with glass cleaner.

Every microscope should have a pointer in the ocular. This is usually supplied by the manufacturer, but can be made from a short piece of hair. The latter is cemented into place inside the ocular with a dab of quick-drying glue or nail polish. Without a pointer, it is not possible to accurately indicate an object in the microscope field for another observer.

Before beginning a session at the microscope, make sure that the fine adjustment knob is near the middle of its range of rotation. If you do not, you may find that the knob is at the limit of its excursion when you are busily making observations. At that point, you must stop everything and correct it.

It is also a good habit to examine your slide with the unaided eye before placing it on the stage of your microscope. If you do so, you will gain information about the gross aspects of the specimen and be more likely to center it properly over the light source. Centering is especially important for small specimens that might otherwise be difficult to locate. Also, make sure that you put the slide on the stage with the coverglass uppermost. If the slide is upside down, you will not be able to focus on it with the high power lenses. Do not snicker; we have seen this happen often in the teaching laboratory!

It is always a good idea to start your observations using the lowest power objective available on your microscope. This is usually the 4X lens. The field of view will be large, enabling you to locate regions of special interest more easily. When you locate something you wish to examine at a higher magnification, center the object in the middle of the field of view. Then, when you change to a stronger lens, the object should be somewhere in the field.

Binocular microscopes often have at least one ocular that can be adjusted to accommodate your vision. It is important that you adjust this properly if you want to have a comfortable, headache-free session at the microscope. Assuming that your microscope is of the binocular type and that it has at least one adjustable ocular, you should first bring the specimen into focus with the ocular that is not adjustable by using the fine adjustment knob. When you have done this, focus the other eye using the adjustable ocular. Use of this procedure will ensure a proper focus for both eyes and prevent eye strain.

Bright, even lighting is absolutely essential to effective microscopy. The best way to achieve this is to use Köhler illumination. This can be obtained with any microscope that is equipped with both a condenser aperture diaphragm (the one in the condenser) and a field diaphragm (the one in the light source). If you have such an instrument, proceed as follows:

1. Center the light source, using the directions you received with the microscope.
2. Open both the field and aperture diaphragms fully.
3. Raise the condenser to its uppermost position.
4. Place a specimen on the stage and focus it with the 10X objective.
5. Close the field diaphragm so that its leaves are clearly imaged in the field of view.
6. Center the image of the diaphragm by manipulating the condenser centering screws, then open the condenser until its leaves disappear just beyond the edge of the field of view.
7. Remove an ocular and, while looking into the back aperture of the objective, close the aperture diaphragm completely and then open it until only approximately 25% of the radius of the field is covered circumferentially by the diaphragm.

You now have Köhler illumination. If you want to increase or decrease the light intensity, use the rheostat or neutral density filters, but do not adjust the condenser aperture diaphragm. If the aperture diaphragm is open to excess, the image will lack some contrast and be flooded with light. If it is closed too far, there will be a loss of resolution and increase in contrast. This increase in contrast is often confused with sharpness or high resolution; this is a common error in microscopy. All of the above adjustments (except for centering the light source) must be made each time a different objective is used.

If your microscope lacks a field diaphragm, you will not be able to obtain Köhler illumination. You can still acquire good and useful lighting, however. Place a specimen on the stage, open the aperture diaphragm fully, and adjust the light intensity with the rheostat so that it is comfortable for your eyes. Be sure that the condenser is raised to its highest position, or close to it, when you do this. Now, remove an ocular and look at the back aperture of the objective. Close the aperture diaphragm fully and then open it until only approximately 25% of the radius of the field is covered. This will provide proper lighting for most purposes. If you should need more or less illumination, make adjustments only with the rheostat or neutral density filter; do not use the aperture diaphragm.

To get the most from a specimen, you must avoid being a passive microscopist, that is, one who finds an object and then stares at it admiringly without making further adjustments of the focus. Get into the habit of focusing continuously with the fine adjustment as you peruse a slide, because even though a tissue section may be only a few micrometers thick, the depth of field of the higher power objectives may be less than the thickness of the specimen. Therefore, if you do not focus repeatedly as you examine a preparation, you will certainly miss seeing structural detail that might be important to your work.

You might like to return to a particular location on your slide preparation at a future time. Remembering landmarks in the vicinity of the object of interest will aid you in locating the object later. A more expedient way of relocating structures is by using verniers, which are mounted on both the X and Y axes of the mechanical stage. A vernier consists of two parallel, graduated, sliding scales, one long and one short. The smaller scale is 9 millimeters (mm) long and is divided into 10 subdivisions (0 to 10). The larger scale is several centimeters (cm) long and is graduated in millimeters, for example, 0 to 80 or 100 to 160. To relocate an object on a slide, you must first center it in the field. Once this has been done, you establish its location by reading each of the verniers (X and Y). For example, the 0 point on the small scale of the vernier on the X axis might be located somewhere between lines 42 and 43 on the larger scale. To determine its specific location, find the line on the small scale that coincides exactly with a line on the longer scale. Then count, on the smaller scale, the number of spaces between 0 and the point of coincidence. This number is your decimal point. In the example given (Fig. 1–4), the decimal is 0.6 and you should read 42.6 as the vernier value. Do the same for the other vernier (Y) and record the numbers for both. In the future, if you want to return to the same location, simply secure the slide to the mechanical stage and move the stage controls until the verniers are adjusted to the numbers you previously recorded. These manipulations will have returned the slide to its former position, and the object you are looking for should be somewhere within the microscope field.

By knowing the approximate diameter of a red blood cell in a section, you can estimate the size of other tissue components. You might find it useful to know, therefore, that in tissue sections prepared by the paraffin method, the average size of erythrocytes for each of the following animals is:

Goat — 2.4 μm diameter (smallest erythrocytes of the domestic mammals)
Dog — 4.9 μm diameter (largest erythrocytes of the domestic mammals)
Chicken — 9.4 μm long

Each average value is based on a total of 20 to 30 cells that were measured from five different slide preparations of tissues embedded in Paraplast X-TRA (Monoject Scientific, Division of Sherwood Medical, St. Louis, MO 63103).

ARTIFACTS

Folds, knife marks, stain precipitate, spaces (where none belong), shrinkage, and air bubbles are examples of commonly occurring imperfections seen in slide preparations. They were introduced during processing and are called artifacts. Figures 1–5 to 1–9 are examples of such artifacts.

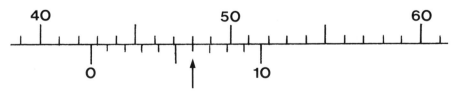

FIG. 1–4. Small and large vernier scales.

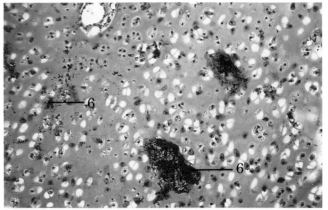

FIG. 1-5 ×62.5

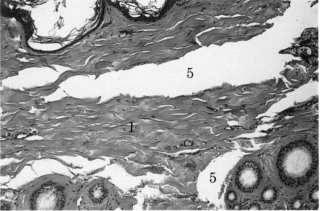

FIG. 1-6 ×62.5

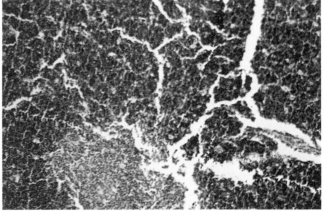

FIG. 1-7 ×62.5

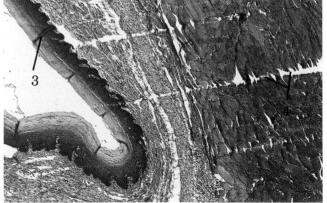

FIG. 1-8 ×25

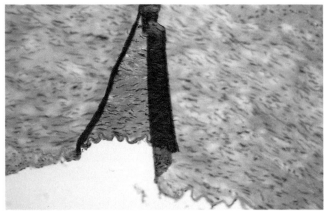

FIG. 1-9 ×62.5

KEY
1. Dermis
2. Epidermis
3. Fold
4. Knife mark
5. Separation artifact
6. Stain precipitate

FIG. 1-5. Stain Precipitate, Cartilage, Dog. Occasionally, solutions accumulate precipitate that may stick to the surface of tissue sections during the staining procedure.

FIG. 1-6. Separation (space) Artifact, Skin, Dog. Tissues may be subjected to excessive pressures, tensions, or shrinkage during processing, resulting in separations within otherwise intact tissue.

FIG. 1-7. Crackling Artifact, Thymus, Horse. Highly cellular tissues, e.g., thymus, liver, pancreas, spleen, often show numerous tiny cracks throughout. Also note that this specimen is not in sharp focus.

FIG. 1-8. Knife Marks and Folds, Esophagus, Horse, Masson's. Knife marks (scratches) in the tissue section may be caused by defects in the microtome knife or by accumulations of debris on the knife edge. Folds occur when the tissue sections fail to spread properly on the surface of the slide.

FIG. 1-9. Fold, Aorta, Pig. In a tissue section, folds are raised areas that frequently overlap. Note that portions of this picture are not in sharp focus.

2

EPITHELIUM

The external and internal surfaces of the body and many of its parts are covered by one or more layers of cells. Collectively, these cellular coverings or linings constitute a tissue called epithelium, whose cells are supported by a basement membrane that separates the epithelium from the underlying connective tissue. Cells are the principal components of the epithelium. Intercellular substance is sparse and is exemplified by the thin layer of material located between cells, which helps to hold them together. The free surface of epithelial cells may have cilia, microvilli, or stereocilia.

Simple epithelia consist of a single layer of cells. The latter may have a **squamous** (flattened), **cuboidal** (more or less square), or **columnar** (tall and rectangular) shape when seen in profile. **Pseudostratified,** a special category, appears in profile to consist of several layers. This, however, is an illusion produced by nuclei located at different levels within cells of different heights. In a simple epithelium, all the cells are in contact with the basement membrane.

Stratified epithelia contain two or more layers of cells. Only the bottom-most layer is in contact with the basement membrane. They are classified as stratified squamous, cuboidal, or columnar, depending on the shape of those cells in their outermost (surface) layer. A category called **transitional** is a special form of stratified epithelium limited to the urinary system. The shape of its cells varies with the amount of tension applied to it.

All glands, endocrine or exocrine, are derived from an epithelium during development. Numerous examples of glands are presented in subsequent chapters.

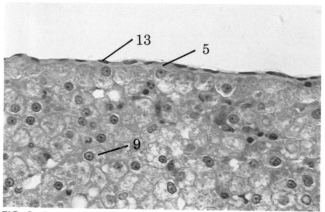

FIG. 2-1 ×250

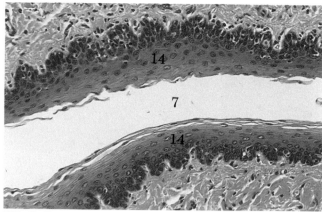

FIG. 2-5 ×125

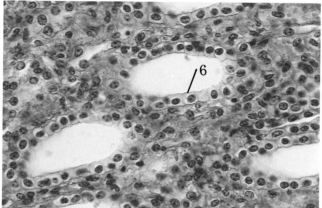

FIG. 2-2 ×250

KEY		
1. Basal cell	**9.** Hepatocyte	
2. Basement membrane	**10.** Lamina propria	
3. Columnar cell	**11.** Lymphocyte	
4. Columnar cell, ciliated	**12.** Smooth muscle cells	
5. Connective tissue	**13.** Squamous cell, nucleus	
6. Cuboidal cell	**14.** Stratified squamous	
7. Esophagus, lumen	epithelium	
8. Goblet cell	**15.** Striated border	

FIG. 2-1. Simple Squamous Epithelium, Mesothelium, Liver, Cat. The surface of the liver is covered by a single layer of squamous cells that lie upon a thin layer of connective tissue. The cytoplasm of the squamous cells is sparse and generally only the nucleus is visible.

FIG. 2-2. Simple Cuboidal Epithelium, Kidney, Cow, Trichrome. The lining of these collecting tubules consists of a layer of cuboidal cells.

FIG. 2-3. Simple Columnar Epithelium, Jejunum, Dog. The jejunum is lined by a simple columnar epithelium. A striated border, consisting of numerous microvilli, is evident. Goblet cells and migrating lymphocytes are present among the columnar cells.

FIG. 2-4. Ciliated Pseudostratified Columnar Epithelium, Trachea, Cow. In this epithelium, the nuclei are at different levels, giving the impression of stratification. All cells, however, contact the basement membrane.

FIG. 2-5. Stratified Squamous Epithelium, Nonkeratinized, Esophagus, Cat. Only cells of the basal layer contact the basement membrane. The name of this epithelium is derived from the squamous cells of its outer layer.

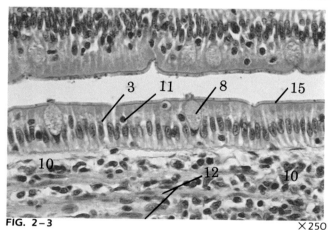

FIG. 2-3 ×250

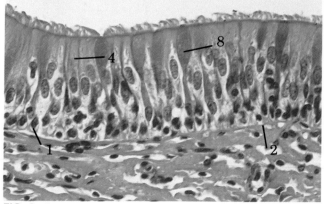

FIG. 2-4 ×250

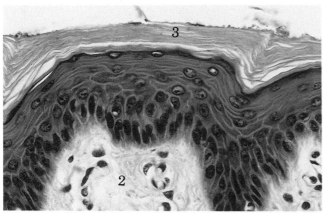

FIG. 2–6   ×250

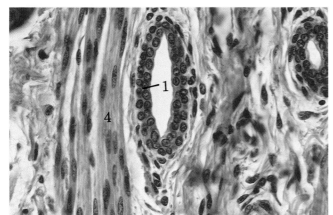

FIG. 2–7   ×250

FIG. 2–8   ×250

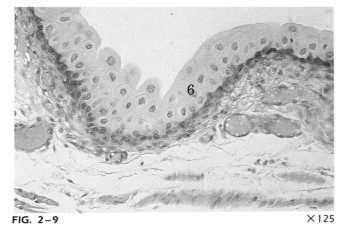

FIG. 2–9   ×125

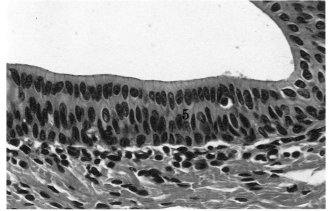

FIG. 2–10   ×125

KEY
1. Bistratified cuboidal epithelium
2. Dermis
3. Keratinized cells
4. Smooth muscle
5. Stratified columnar epithelium
6. Transitional epithelium

FIG. 2–6. Stratified Squamous Epithelium, Keratinized, Wattle, Pig. The wattle is covered by a keratinized stratified squamous epithelium.

FIG. 2–7. Bistratified Cuboidal Epithelium, Esophagus, Dog. Ducts of glands of the esophagus are lined by a bistratified cuboidal epithelium.

FIG. 2–8. Stratified Columnar Epithelium, Urethra, Goat. This portion of the urethra is lined by a stratified columnar epithelium.

FIG. 2–9. Transitional Epithelium, Unstretched, Urinary Bladder, Cat. Surface cells of the transitional epithelial lining are either balloon-shaped or broadly cuboidal when not under tension.

FIG. 2–10. Transitional Epithelium, Stretched, Urinary Bladder, Cat. Surface cells of this epithelium are flattened and elongated when the bladder is full.

CONNECTIVE TISSUE PROPER and EMBRYONAL CONNECTIVE TISSUE

Connective tissue binds together and supports other tissues. It is a composite of various cells and fibers in an amorphous ground substance. The latter two components comprise the extracellular matrix, which typically predominates over the cellular elements.

The **ground substance,** composed largely of glycoproteins and glycosaminoglycans, forms a well hydrated gel that fills the spaces between cells, fibers, and vessels of connective tissue. It acts as a reservoir for interstitial fluid, providing a medium through which oxygen, nutrients, and metabolic by-products diffuse to and from cells of various tissues and the vascular system.

Collagenous, reticular, and elastic fibers occur in connective tissue. **Collagenous fibers,** composed of the fibrous protein collagen, are generally the most abundant. They are strong and flexible, yet able to resist stretch. They may be fine or coarse, and are characteristically unbranched and somewhat wavy. In tissues stained with H&E, they appear pink and refractile. **Reticular fibers** are also formed from the protein collagen. They are delicate, branching fibers that possess a coat of glycoproteins and proteoglycans. They are argyrophilic (silver-loving) and can be stained with silver to distinguish them from other connective tissue fibers. They may also be selectively stained with Schiff's reagent. **Elastic fibers,** formed from the protein elastin, range in diameter from fine to coarse and ordinarily cannot be distinguished from collagenous fibers without the use of special stains such as orcein or Weigert's resorcin fuchsin. In some H&E preparations, however, they become colored more intensely by eosin than the collagenous fibers, from which they can readily be distinguished.

Fibroblasts are generally the most numerous of the cells found in connective tissue. They are responsible for the formation of both fibers and ground substance. **Macrophages** (histiocytes), derivatives of monocytes of the blood, are also common inhabitants of connective tissue. They are phagocytic cells that can often be recognized by the presence of debris in their cytoplasm, which gives them a dirty appearance. Other migrants from the blood that are found in connective tissue are **neutrophils** and **eosinophils. Plasma cells, lymphocytes, adipocytes, mast cells,** and **globular leukocytes** also occur in varying numbers in connective tissue.

All connective tissues are classified on the basis of the arrangement and proportions of their cellular and intercellular components. **Connective tissue proper** includes the general types of connective tissue, loose and dense, as well as the special types, reticular, elastic, and adipose. Mesenchyme and mucous connective tissue are classified as **embryonal connective tissues.**

In **loose** (areolar) **connective tissue,** the ground substance predominates. It contains many scattered cells of various types, vessels, and a loose network of fine collagenous, reticular, and elastic fibers. Loose connective tissue is widespread throughout the body. It surrounds vessels and nerves. It is found in serous membranes such as mesenteries, the lamina propria of mucous membranes, subcutaneous tissue, and the papillary (superficial) layer of the dermis, as well as other places.

In contrast to loose connective tissue, dense connective tissue (often called fibrous tissue) is composed principally of thick collagenous fibers. It contains fewer cells, most of which are fibroblasts. In **dense irregular connective tissue,** the collagenous fibers course in all directions, forming a compact meshwork. **Dense regular connective tissue** is characterized by closely packed, parallel bundles of collagenous fibers. Dense irregular connective tissue occurs in such places as the reticular (deep) layer of the dermis, the submucosa of the diges-tive tract of some species, and the capsules of organs. Tendons, ligaments, and aponeuroses are formed by dense regular connective tissue.

It is helpful to know that there are no sharp lines of distinction between loose and dense irregular connective tissue, or between dense irregular and regular connective tissue. It is not always possible, therefore, to classify these types of connective tissues with great precision.

Reticular tissue is composed of numerous reticular fibers. It forms a supportive network for the parenchyma of structures such as the spleen, lymph node, liver, kidney, and bone marrow.

Elastic tissue is characterized by numerous regularly or irregularly arranged elastic fibers. It is exemplified by the ligamentum nuchae of grazing animals and by the vocal ligaments.

Adipose tissue consists of groups of adipocytes (also called adipose cells or fat cells) within the loose connective tissue of such places as mesenteries, subcutis, and sheaths of vessels and nerves.

Mesenchyme tissue is found in the embryo. It consists of a loose arrangement of pale, star-shaped cells with interconnecting cytoplasmic processes. The mesenchyme cells are embedded in a jelly-like amorphous ground substance that accumulates fine fibers as development progresses.

Mucous connective tissue, another type of embryonal connective tissue, surrounds the vessels of the umbilical cord. It also occurs in limited regions in adult animals, for instance, the dermis of the comb and wattle of the chicken. It is composed of fibroblasts and loosely arranged, fine collagenous fibers in an abundant, amorphous ground substance.

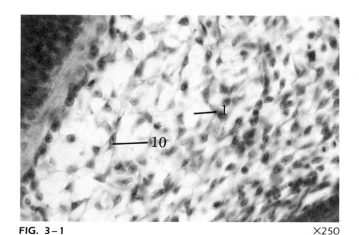

FIG. 3–1   X250

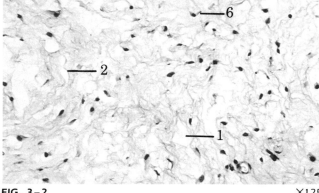
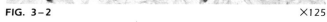

FIG. 3–2   X125

FIG. 3–3   X250

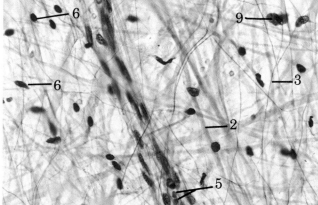

FIG. 3–4   X250

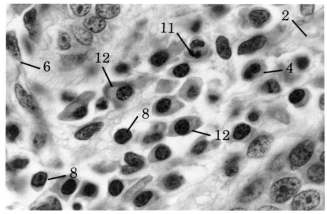

FIG. 3–5   X625

KEY	
1. Amorphous ground substance	**7.** Globular leukocyte
2. Collagenous fiber	**8.** Lymphocyte
3. Elastic fiber	**9.** Mast cell
4. Eosinophil	**10.** Mesenchyme cell
5. Erythrocytes in capillary	**11.** Neutrophil
6. Fibroblast	**12.** Plasma Cell

FIG. 3–1. Mesenchyme, 72 hr. Embryo, Chicken. Mesenchyme consists of stellate cells. Their processes touch, forming a latticework. The cells are surrounded by an amorphous ground substance.

FIG. 3–2. Mucous Connective Tissue, Umbilical Cord, Cow. Mucous connective tissue consists of a loose framework of fibroblasts and collagenous fibers in an amorphous ground substance. Mucous connective tissue of the umbilical cord is often called Wharton's jelly.

FIG. 3–3. Loose Connective Tissue, Mesentery, Cat, LeukoStat and Orcein. The loose arrangement of the connective tissue cells and fibers in this whole mount preparation is evident. Fine, branching elastic fibers appear blue-gray. The thicker, collagenous fibers stain pale pink. Note the mast cell filled with purple granules.

FIG. 3–4. Loose Connective Tissue, Lamina Propria, Duodenum, Cow. A loose meshwork of connective tissue fibers and various cells are contained in an amorphous ground substance.

FIG. 3–5. Plasma Cells, Loose Connective Tissue, Lamina Propria, Jejunum, Dog. Plasma cells are common constituents of the lamina propria of the gastrointestinal tract. They are characterized by a basophilic cytoplasm and large blocks of nuclear heterochromatin. A lightly stained area adjacent to the nucleus, usually eccentric, marks the location of the Golgi apparatus.

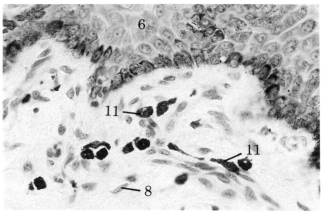

FIG. 3-6   ×250

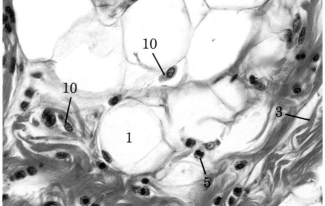

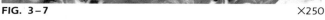

FIG. 3-7   ×250

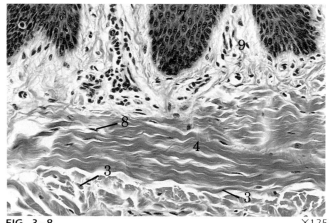

FIG. 3-8   ×125

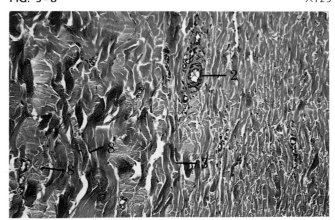

FIG. 3-9   ×62.5

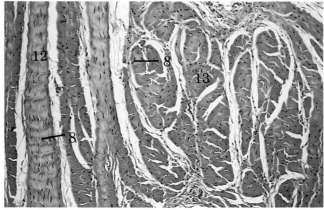

FIG. 3-10   ×62.5

KEY		
1. Adipocyte	**8.** Fibroblast
2. Arteriole	**9.** Loose connective tissue
3. Collagenous fiber	**10.** Macrophage
4. Dense irregular connective tissue	**11.** Mast Cell
5. Eosinophil	**12.** Tendon, l.s.
6. Epithelium, lip	**13.** Tendon, x.s.
7. Epithelium, planum	

FIG. 3-6. Mast Cells, Loose Connective Tissue, Lip, Cat, Toluidine Blue. The granules of mast cells are metachromatic and are colored purple by toluidine blue.

FIG. 3-7. Macrophages, Loose Connective Tissue, Colon, Pig. Wandering macrophages are characterized by their oval shape. The cytoplasm of these cells often contains ingested particles and appears dirty. Eosinophils of the pig contain oval or bilobed nuclei.

FIG. 3-8. Loose and Dense Irregular Connective Tissue, Dermis, Planum Nasolabiale, Cow. Note that the loose connective tissue of the papillary layer of the dermis contains finer fibers and more cells than the dense irregular connective tissue of the reticular layer.

FIG. 3-9. Dense Irregular Connective Tissue, Dermis, Horse. Note the coarse, interwoven collagenous fibers.

FIG. 3-10. Dense Regular Connective Tissue, Tendon, x.s. and l.s., Nose, Pig. In tendons and ligaments, collagenous fibers are arranged in parallel order. Fibroblasts are located between the fibers.

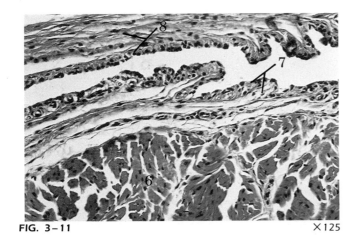

FIG. 3-11   ×125

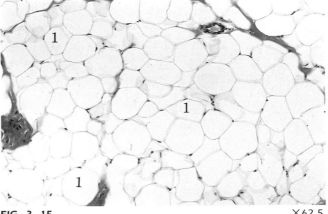

FIG. 3-15   ×62.5

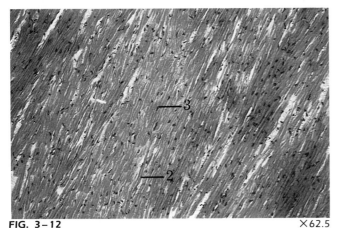

FIG. 3-12   ×62.5

FIG. 3-11. Tendon and Tendon Sheath, x.s., Dog. The tendon sheath is actually made up of two sheaths. The inner sheath attaches to the surface of the tendon. The outer sheath forms a tube around the tendon and attaches to peripheral structures. The space between the two sheaths is filled with synovial fluid in living tissue. The space is not lined by an epithelium, but rather by collagenous fibers and connective tissue cells of the sheaths.

FIG. 3-12. Elastic Tissue, Ligamentum Nuchae, l.s., Sheep. This section shows the parallel arrangement of the elastic fibers within the ligament.

FIG. 3-13. Elastic Tissue, Ligamentum Nuchae, x.s., Sheep, Orcein. Orcein selectively stains elastic fibers red.

FIG. 3-14. Reticular Tissue, Lymph Node, Cow, Silver. Networks of reticular fibers are blackened by silver.

FIG. 3-15. Adipose Tissue, Soft Palate, Cow. Lipid content of each adipocyte (unilocular) was removed during processing, leaving an empty cavity surrounded by a thin rim of cytoplasm. Nuclei occur at the periphery of adipocytes. It is sometimes difficult to distinguish their nuclei from those of other connective tissue cells. See Figure 12-103 for an example of multilocular adipocytes.

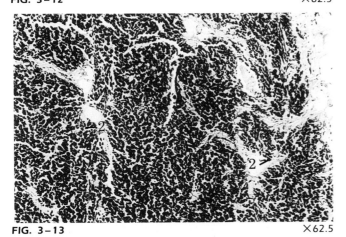

FIG. 3-13   ×62.5

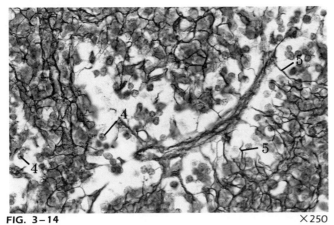

FIG. 3-14   ×250

4

CARTILAGE

Cartilage is a form of connective tissue. There are three basic types of cartilage: **hyaline, elastic,** and **fibrous** (fibrocartilage). Each consists of chondrocytes embedded in an amorphous ground substance (matrix), which is rich in sulfated glycosaminoglycans complexed with protein to form macromolecules called proteoglycans. The latter are bound electrostatically to unit fibrils of collagen. The matrix is firm but flexible.

Hyaline cartilage is the most common type. It forms large parts of the developing vertebrate skeleton, and is also found in epiphyseal discs, articular cartilages, the trachea, bronchi, and elsewhere. Its ground substance is separable into pale and darkly stained areas called **interterritorial** and **territorial matrix,** respectively. The higher concentration of sulfated glycosaminoglycans in the latter is responsible for the darker staining. Chondrocytes are confined to small spaces **(lacunae)** within the matrix. Small clusters of chondrocytes, called **isogenous groups,** are frequently observed. They are the result of cell division of chondrocytes. Each mass of cartilage matrix is invested by a **perichondrium** whose inner layer is chondrogenic, containing cells with the capacity to form chondroblasts. Its outer portion is dense irregular connective tissue.

Elastic cartilage is similar in structure to hyaline cartilage. Its name derives from the presence of large amounts of elastic fibers embedded in the matrix. Among other places, it is found in the epiglottis, parts of the larynx, and the pinna.

Fibrous cartilage is unlike either of the other types. It is dense connective tissue within which are distributed linear groupings of chondrocytes embedded in a small amount of matrix. Fibrous cartilage is found in such places as the intervertebral discs and cardiac skeleton, and within some tendons close to their attachment to bone.

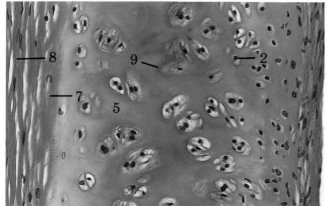

FIG. 4-1   ×125

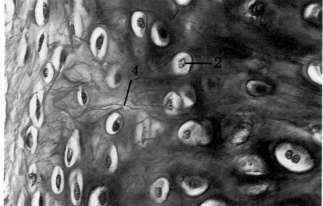

FIG. 4-2   ×250

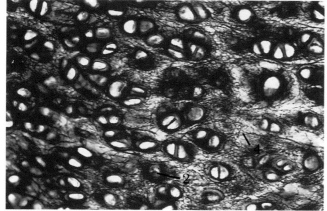

FIG. 4-3   ×125

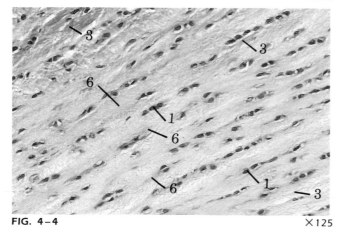

FIG. 4-4   ×125

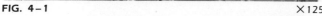

FIG. 4-5   ×125

KEY	
1. Chondrocyte	**6.** Matrix
2. Chondrocyte in lacuna	**7.** Perichondrium,
3. Collagenous fiber	chondrogenic
4. Elastic fiber	**8.** Perichondrium, fibrous
5. Interterritorial matrix	**9.** Territorial matrix

FIG. 4-1. Hyaline Cartilage, Trachea, Cow. The perichondrium consists of an outer fibrous and an inner chondrogenic layer. Isogenous groups and single chondrocytes are scattered throughout the matrix.

FIG. 4-2. Elastic Cartilage, Epiglottis, Dog. Pink elastic fibers can be seen throughout the cartilage matrix.

FIG. 4-3. Elastic Cartilage, Wattle, Pig, Orcein. Elastic fibers are stained red with orcein.

FIG. 4-4. Fibrocartilage, Intervertebral Disc, Horse. Chondrocytes are arranged in rows and framed by a hazy rim of pale blue matrix. Collagenous fibers are visible between rows of chondrocytes.

FIG. 4-5. Fibrocartilage, Claw, Chicken. Rows of chondrocytes are randomly scattered among collagenous fibers. Pale blue matrix is visible around some chondrocytes.

BONE

Bone is a living, dynamic connective tissue. Its hardness and strength are provided by a matrix consisting of hydroxyapatites and collagen, respectively. It is admirably suited to its function as a skeletal substance because of its high tensile strength and relatively light weight.

The structure of bone is unrelated to its mode of development. The **lamellae** of **intramembranous bone** have the same basic structure as those of **endochondral (intracartilaginous) bone. Mature bone,** however, contains fewer osteocytes than the **immature bone** it replaces. The woven form of the latter contains numerous osteocytes and an organic matrix of interlacing collagenous fibers. Its matrix has a bluish cast in preparations stained with hematoxylin and eosin, in contrast to the more uniform acidophilia of the matrix of mature bone.

Deposits of matrix may be dense, with few spaces between matrix elements **(compact bone),** or in the form of delicate three-dimensional latticeworks **(spongy bone).** Compact bone forms the outer shells of the diaphysis and epiphysis, while spongy bone occurs in the interior of the epiphysis or the endosteal surface of portions of the diaphysis. In the compact bone of the diaphysis, matrix appears as **haversian systems, interstitial systems,** and **circumferential lamellae.**

Although **osteocytes** are entrapped within matrix, they are able to communicate, physically, through **canaliculi,** which connect lacunae with each other. **Osteoblasts** and **osteoclasts** lie free on the external surface of the matrix. The former secrete most of the matrix and eventually become surrounded by it. They are then called osteocytes. Osteoclasts, large multinucleate cells derived from monocytes, resorb matrix during bone remodeling or when the need for serum calcium arises.

Bone matrix undergoes remarkable transformations in size and shape during development. These alterations enable the skeleton to accommodate to the growth and the changes in form that occur as an organism matures. This process of bone remodeling is especially well exemplified during the formation of the skull and long bones. In both instances, transformations in shape and increases in size are accomplished by a coupling of the process of bone deposition with that of bone resorption. An important aspect of the growth in length of long bones is the persistence of functional epiphyseal discs. These plates of hyaline cartilage permit the process of intracartilaginous ossification to continue until full growth is achieved, at which time the discs become replaced by bone and no further lengthening is possible.

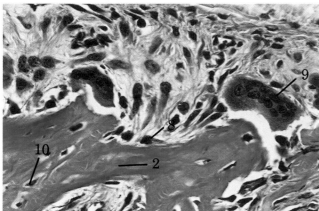

FIG. 5-1 ×62.5

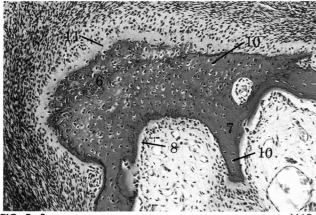

FIG. 5-2 ×250

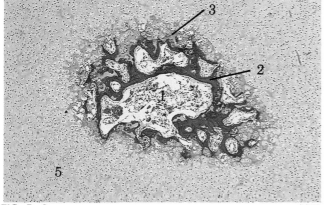

FIG. 5-3 ×62.5

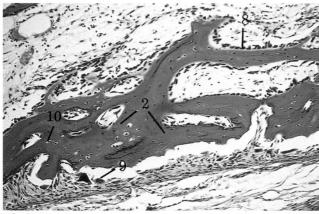

FIG. 5-4 ×25

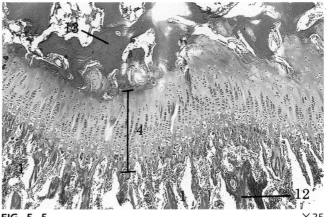

FIG. 5-5 ×25

FIG. 5-1. Membrane Bone, Decalcified, Nose, Dog.
Osteoblasts deposit bone matrix directly within mesenchyme without a preformed cartilage model. Therefore the trabeculae of membrane bone lack calcified cartilage cores.

FIG. 5-2. Membrane Bone, Decalcified, Nose, Dog, Masson's. Osteoclasts are large, multinucleated giant cells.

FIG. 5-3. Immature Bone, Phalanx, Decalcified, Fetus, Horse. Immature bone is characterized by a larger number of osteocytes per unit area than are found in mature bone. Typically, it also shows basophilia. Both characteristics are evident in the micrograph. Note the rather even acidophilia of the matrix of the more mature bone.

FIG. 5-4. Primary Center of Ossification, Phalanx, l.s., Decalcified, Fetus, Horse. Section was taken from the central region of a developing phalanx and shows early endochondral ossification.

FIG. 5-5. Epiphyseal Disc, Humerus, l.s., Decalcified, Cat. The cartilaginous epiphyseal disc (plate) is between the spongy bone of the epiphysis and the diaphysis.

BONE **23**

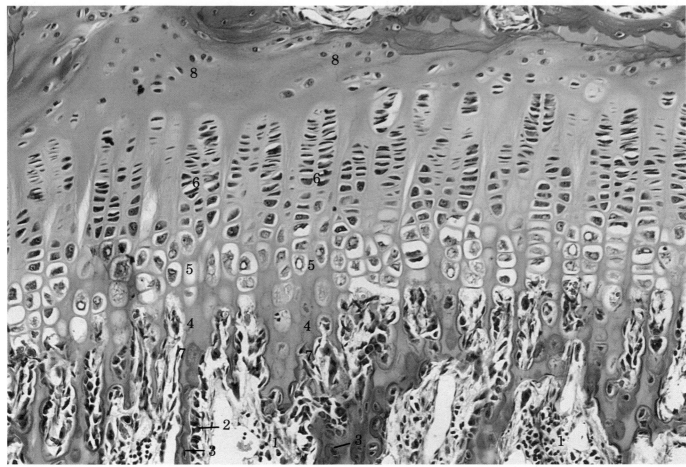

FIG. 5–6   ×130

KEY	
1. Bone marrow	**6.** Zone of multiplication
2. Osteoblast	**7.** Zone of ossification
3. Osteocyte	**8.** Zone of reserve cartilage
4. Zone of calcification	
5. Zone of hypertrophy	

FIG. 5–6. Epiphyseal Disc, Humerus, l.s., Decalcified, Cat.
Various zones of endochondral bone formation. Small,
scattered cartilage cells comprise the zone of reserve
(resting) cartilage. They proliferate and form rows (zone of
multiplication, zone of proliferation). The cells then enlarge
(zone of hypertrophy). The remaining cartilage matrix
between the hypertrophied cells becomes impregnated
with calcium salts (zone of calcification). Osteoblasts
deposit bone matrix (pink) onto the calcified cartilage
matrix (lavender) in the zone of ossification.

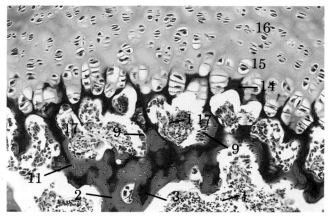

FIG. 5-7   ×62.5

FIG. 5–7. Endochondral Bone, Phalanx, l.s., Decalcified, Dog. The zones of calcification and ossification are distinct in this preparation. Calcified cartilage stains an intense purple, while bone matrix is strongly eosinophilic.

FIG. 5–8. Endochondral Bone, Epiphysis of Radius, Decalcified, Dog. Spicules of bone (pink) with calcified cartilage cores (lavender).

FIG. 5–9. Compact Ground Bone, Femur, x.s., Cat, Unstained. Haversian canals surrounded by concentric bony lamellae constitute a haversian system (osteon). Lacunae with canaliculi (web-like, fine dark lines) are occupied by osteocytes and their processes, respectively, in living tissue. Volkmann's canals, inner circumferential lamellae, and parts of old haversian systems, called interstitial systems, are present.

FIG. 5–10. Compact Bone, Humerus, x.s., Decalcified, Chicken. In decalcified bone, hydroxyapatites have been removed, leaving the collagenous portion of the matrix. Blood vessels, osteocytes, and other tissue elements are also left intact. Compare with Figure 5–9.

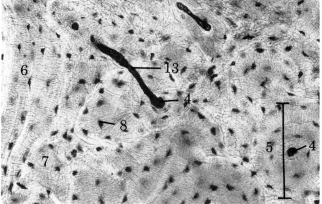

FIG. 5-8   ×62.5

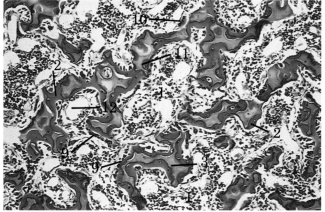

FIG. 5-9   ×125

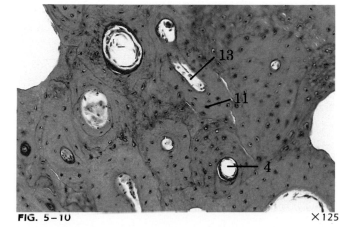

FIG. 5-10   ×125

BONE   **25**

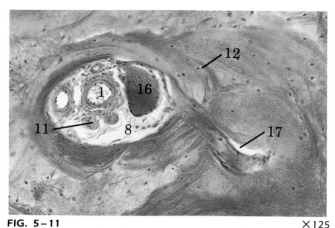

FIG. 5-11   ×125

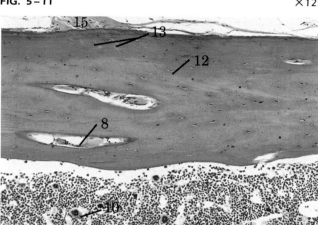

FIG. 5-12   ×62.5

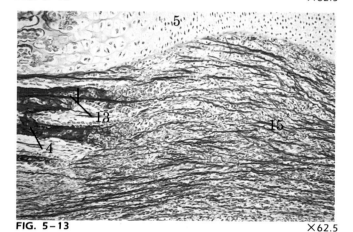

FIG. 5-13   ×62.5

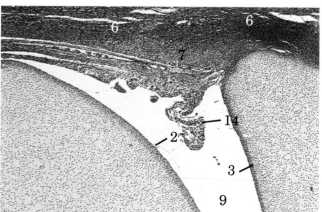

FIG. 5-14   ×25

KEY	
1. Artery	**10.** Megakaryocyte
2. Articulating surface, P_2	**11.** Nerve
3. Articulating surface, P_3	**12.** Osteocyte
4. Bone matrix	**13.** Sharpey's fibers
5. Cartilage	**14.** Synovial fold
6. Extensor tendon	**15.** Tendon
7. Fibrous capsule	**16.** Vein
8. Haversian canal	**17.** Volkmann's canal
9. Joint cavity	

FIG. 5-11. Compact Bone, x.s., Jaw, Decalcified, Dog.
Blood vessels and nerves are evident in this cross section
of a haversian canal.

FIG. 5-12. Compact Bone, Rib, l.s., Decalcified, Cat.
Portions of haversian canals are oriented parallel to the
long axis of the bone. The collagenous fibers of a tendon
extend into the bone as Sharpey's fibers. The large cells in
the bone marrow are megakaryocytes.

**FIG. 5-13. Sharpey's Fibers, Phalanx, l.s., Decalcified,
Fetus, Sheep, Mallory's.** Collagenous fibers of a tendon
become embedded within the bone matrix, where they are
called Sharpey's fibers.

FIG. 5-14. Distal Interphalangeal Joint, l.s., Fetus, Horse.
The mid-dorsal aspect of this developing synovial joint is
shown. The joint capsule is composed of a fibrous portion
and a well vascularized, synovial membrane. The latter
lines the joint cavity, except for the articulating surfaces.
Synovial folds project into the cavity. The outer, more
fibrous portion of the capsule is continuous with the
future periosteum of the phalanges and blends dorsally
with the extensor tendon. The tendon is attached to the
developing extensor process of P_3. Note that the phalanges have not yet begun to ossify. After ossification, a
layer of hyaline cartilage will persist on the articular surfaces.

6

BLOOD

Blood is a special type of connective tissue composed of formed elements in a fluid matrix. **Plasma** is the fluid portion, called **serum** when depleted of fibrinogen. The **formed elements** include erythrocytes (red blood cells), leukocytes (white blood cells), and platelets (thrombocytes in birds).

Blood cells and platelets are usually examined in stained blood smears (blood films). To make such a preparation, a drop of blood is spread thinly on a glass slide, dried, and stained with a Romanovsky-type stain such as Giemsa or Wright's. One end of the film is usually much thinner than the other end. Details of cell morphology are more visible in the thin film, where the cells are more flattened and less crowded. Blood smears should be scanned with the high dry objective. With practice, most cells can be differentiated at this magnification. Oil immersion should be reserved for studying specific cells in more detail.

MAMMALS

Mature **erythrocytes** are small, anucleate cells uniquely adapted to transport oxygen and carbon dioxide to and from tissues. They stain pink because of their high hemoglobin content.

The average diameter of erythrocytes in a dried smear varies with the species. The erythrocytes of the dog are largest (7.0 μm), while those of the goat are the smallest (4.1 μm). Red blood cells from the same animal are all approximately the same size except in the cow, where variation in the size of the erythrocytes (anisocytosis) is not unusual. In most species, the cells are disc-shaped, although in young goats they may also be angulated.

Central pallor, reflecting a biconcave shape, is best defined in the dog, but may be seen in other domestic mammals. Red blood cells sometimes adhere to each other, forming an arrangement resembling a stack of coins, called a rouleau. This occurs readily in the horse and often in the cat, and is rarest in ruminants. Crenated erythrocytes, characterized by pointed cell margins, are observed most often in pigs.

Various factors influence the appearance of red (and white) blood cells. These include the freshness of the blood sample, the use of an anticoagulant, how quickly the smear was dried, and the thickness of the smear. The occurrence of central pallor, rouleaux, and crenation varies not only with the species, but also with each smear and within different regions of the same smear.

Leukocytes are basic cellular components of the immune system. They are nucleated cells that are larger and less numerous than erythrocytes. They are classified, depending on the presence or absence of specific cytoplasmic granules, as either **granulocytes** (neutrophils, eosinophils, and basophils), or **agranulocytes** (lymphocytes and monocytes). Leukocytes tend to accumulate along the edges of a blood smear, so that examples of them, although often distorted, can be found more readily in these regions.

Lymphocytes are the predominant leukocytes in ruminants and pigs. The cells range in size from 6 to 15 μm, and are sometimes classified as small, medium, and large. Most of the lymphocytes in carnivores, horses, and pigs are small. The larger cells occur more often in ruminants.

Small lymphocytes have a relatively large, dense, often eccentric nucleus that is round and may be slightly indented. In the cat, the nucleus is sometimes deeply indented like a kidney. The nucleus tends to be oval in the pig. Some of the lymphocytes of ruminants are binucleate.

Only a thin rim of cytoplasm may be visible in the small lymphocyte. The cytoplasm is basophilic and may show a lighter region near the nucleus, a perinuclear halo. At times, nonspecific azurophilic granules may be seen in the cytoplasm of both small and large lymphocytes.

A large lymphocyte has a less dense nucleus and paler, more abundant cytoplasm than a small lymphocyte. The nucleus may be round, oval, or kidney-shaped.

Monocytes are the largest of the leukocytes (15 to 20 μm in diameter). The nuclear chromatin tends to be diffuse, appearing lacy or sometimes patchy. The shape of the nucleus is highly variable and may be oval, irregular, kidney-shaped, or horseshoe-shaped. In the horse, the nucleus is frequently kidney-shaped. In ruminants it may appear amoeboid, and sometimes has a three-pronged configuration or is shaped like a cloverleaf.

The cytoplasm is generally pale gray-blue and may contain dust-like, azurophilic granules. It often contains vacuoles that give it a foamy appearance. In ruminants, the cytoplasm can be more basophilic and either granular or mottled in appearance.

Neutrophils are the predominant leukocytes in the dog, cat, and horse. The dark-staining nucleus of the mature cell contains very densely packed chromatin. It is long and narrow, and may be monolobed or segmented. The nucleus is sometimes coiled, as it is in the cat and, more often, in the pig. When segmented, the lobes may be separated by slight indentations or thin strands of nucleoplasm. The nuclear membrane may appear irregular or tattered from bulging clumps of chromatin. In the horse, the chromatin is so heavily clumped that the nucleus appears very jagged.

The pale gray cytoplasm of the neutrophil contains pink, dustlike, specific granules that may be difficult to resolve with the light microscope. The granules are smallest in the dog, so that the cytoplasm appears nongranular and very faint. Granulation is most pronounced in the sheep and goat. In these animals, larger, more darkly stained granules occur among the finer pink granules.

Band forms of the neutrophil (and other granulocytes) may be encountered in a smear of peripheral blood. The nucleus of these cells looks like a curved or U-shaped band. It can be distinguished from a mature, monolobed granulocyte by the relatively smooth, rather than ragged, contour of the nucleus. Also, the chromatin is less condensed and the nucleus appears paler and plumper than in the mature cell.

The nucleus of the **eosinophil,** although similar to that of the neutrophil, tends to be less dense and have fewer lobes. In the pig, the nucleus is commonly oval or kidney-shaped rather than segmented. C-shaped, monolobed nuclei are common in ruminants.

The cytoplasm of the eosinophil stains pale blue or gray. Specific granules stain various shades of orange, pink, or red with eosin. The granules of the eosinophil of the dog, unlike those of other domestic mammals, are highly variable in size and do not usually fill the cell. Occasionally, small, clear vacuoles also occur in the cytoplasm. In the cat, the granules are rod-shaped. Large, round to oblong granules are a striking feature of the eosinophil of the horse. They usually fill the cytoplasm and cause the cell membrane to bulge, so that the eosinophil resembles a raspberry. In the pig, sheep, and goat the granules are small, round to oval, and numerous, often distorting the cell membrane. In cows, the granules are round and intensely stained.

Only a small percentage (0.5 to 3%) of the leukocytes of domestic mammals are **basophils.** Hence, they are not often found in blood smears. The basophil nucleus may be irregular, bilobed, or highly segmented. The granules of basophils vary in size, number, and staining intensity. They are often fairly large, round to oval, and stain reddish purple to dark purple. The granules are a dumb-bell or coccoid shape in the pig. The basophil of the cat is much different from that of the other domestic mammals. The granules are small and not deeply stained. They are dull gray to lavender in a lavender cytoplasm.

Because the nuclei of the granulocytes exhibit many forms, the cells are also called **polymorphonuclear leukocytes** (polymorphs, PMNs). These terms, however, are sometimes reserved specifically as synonyms for the neutrophil.

Platelets play an important role in hemostasis. Although also referred to as thrombocytes, they are not cells. They are membrane-bound fragments of cytoplasm from large cells called megakaryocytes, found in the bone marrow and sometimes the lymph nodes and spleen. Platelets are small, stain pale blue, and have purple central granules that may be apparent. They occur singly or in clusters in smears of peripheral blood.

CHICKEN

Mature **erythrocytes** of the chicken are very different from those of domestic mammals. They are large, elongated, flat cells with an oval nucleus. In dried blood smears from White Leghorn chickens, they range from approximately 9 to 12 μm long and 6 to 8 μm wide. Their size varies with the breed and the sex of the bird.

The nucleus contains small, uniformly distributed clumps of chromatin. The cytoplasm stains a pale orange to pink color.

Thrombocytes are nucleated cells, related in function to the platelets of mammals. They are smaller and less elongated than erythrocytes, with a larger, more round nucleus. The pale, dull blue cytoplasm is characterized by a few small magenta granules and vacuoles.

Lymphocytes are the most numerous of the leukocytes in the chicken. Their size varies from small to large, as in mammals. The cytoplasm is slightly basophilic and may appear granular or homogeneous. The nucleus is round, sometimes slightly indented, and usually centrally located. It contains coarse clumps of chromatin that are finer in the larger lymphocytes.

Monocytes are usually larger than lymphocytes. The nuclear chromatin tends to be more diffuse. Vacuoles are often seen in the cytoplasm.

Heterophils are the most abundant of the granulocytes. Both heterophils and eosinophils have acidophilic specific granules. The granules of the heterophil are rod- or spindle-shaped. Their centers sometimes contain a distinctive, ruby red, spheric granule. During staining, there may be partial or complete dissolution of the rods, leaving only the more stable central granule. The granules of the **eosinophil** are round and pink. The cytoplasm stains pale blue, compared to the clear cytoplasm of the heterophil. The nucleus of both of these granulocytes is polymorphic. That of the eosinophil generally has fewer lobes. It also has distinct, dense blocks of chromatin clearly delineated by lighter areas. This contrasts with the less distinctly clumped chromatin of the heterophil.

The **basophils** of the chicken are much more numerous than in mammals. The specific granules are deeply basophilic, and the nucleus is unilobular and pale--staining.

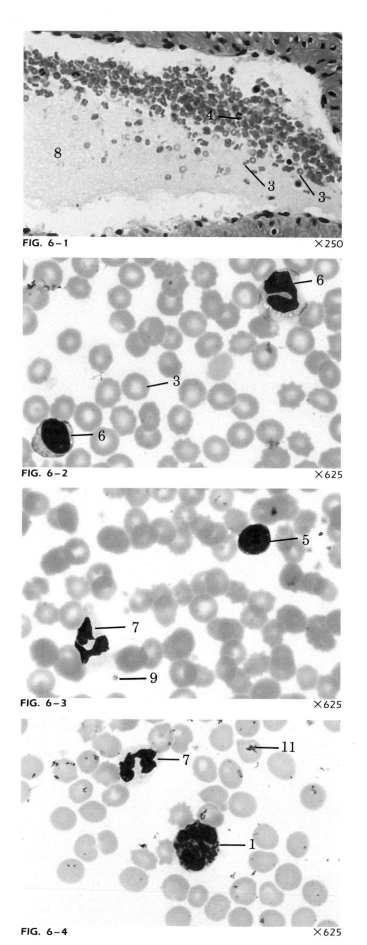

FIG. 6-1　　　　　　　　　　　　　　　×250

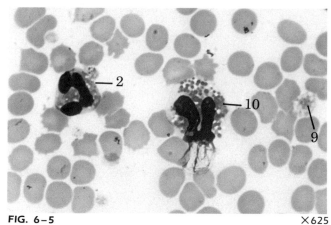

FIG. 6-5　　　　　　　　　　　　　　　×625

FIG. 6-2　　　　　　　　　　　　　　　×625

FIG. 6-3　　　　　　　　　　　　　　　×625

FIG. 6-4　　　　　　　　　　　　　　　×625

KEY		
1. Basophil		**7.** Neutrophil
2. Eosinophil		**8.** Plasma
3. Erythrocyte		**9.** Platelet
4. Leukocyte		**10.** Smudged eosinophil
5. Lymphocyte, small		**11.** Stain precipitate
6. Monocyte		

FIG. 6-1. Blood Cells in Section, Artery, Cat. Biconcave, disc-shaped red blood cells, leukocytes, and plasma (pale pink) are within the lumen of an artery.

FIG. 6-2. Blood, Dog, Giemsa. The cytoplasm of the monocyte is, typically, vacuolated. The nucleus is frequently oval or U-shaped. Central pallor of the erythrocytes in this preparation is evident.

FIG. 6-3. Blood, Dog, Giemsa. The cytoplasm of the small lymphocyte is very sparse and the nuclear chromatin is condensed. The mature neutrophil has a polymorphic nucleus. The pale cytoplasm, barely discernible, is a characteristic of the neutrophil of the dog.

FIG. 6-4. Blood, Dog, Giemsa. The basophil has a polymorphic nucleus and coarse granules of various sizes.

FIG. 6-5. Blood, Dog, Giemsa. In the eosinophil of the dog, the granules vary in size and number. Vacuoles occur in the cytoplasm. The cell on the right is partially smudged.

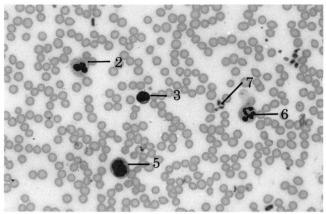

FIG. 6–6 ×250

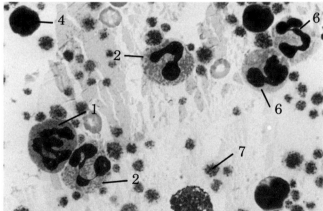

FIG. 6–7 ×625

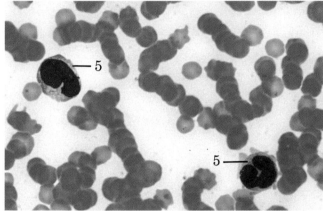

FIG. 6–8 ×625

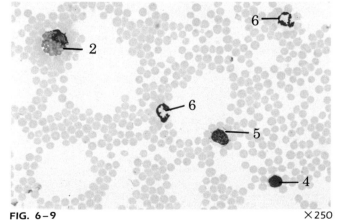

FIG. 6–9 ×250

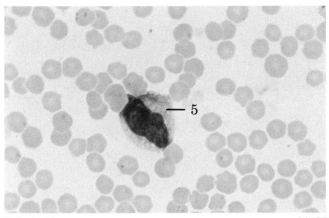

FIG. 6–10 ×625

KEY	
1. Basophil	**5.** Monocyte
2. Eosinophil	**6.** Neutrophil
3. Lymphocyte, medium	**7.** Platelet
4. Lymphocyte, small	

FIG. 6–6. Blood, Cat, Giemsa. Eosinophil, neutrophil, lymphocyte, and monocyte.

FIG. 6–7. Blood, Cat, Giemsa. Two monocytes. Red cells are stacked in rouleaux.

FIG. 6–8. Buffy Coat, Cat, Giemsa. Two eosinophils, two neutrophils, one basophil, three small lymphocytes, and platelets. Eosinophils of the cat have pink, rod-shaped granules. The cytoplasm of the basophil contains numerous small, round, lavender granules that are tightly packed and may be difficult to resolve. Distinct red granules are scattered among the lavender granules. The small lymphocyte of the cat often has a kidney-shaped nucleus.

FIG. 6–9. Blood, Horse, Giemsa. Eosinophil, monocyte, and two neutrophils. In the neutrophil of the horse, the nucleus often appears very jagged.

FIG. 6–10. Blood, Horse, Giemsa. A typical monocyte with pale cytoplasm and linearly arranged chromatin.

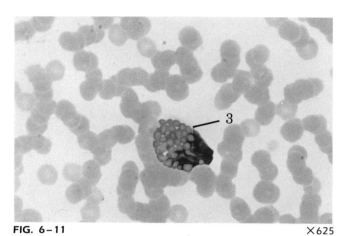

FIG. 6–11   ×625

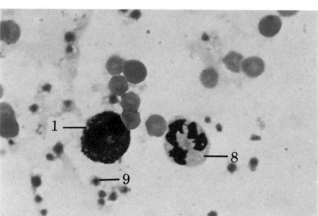

FIG. 6–12   ×625

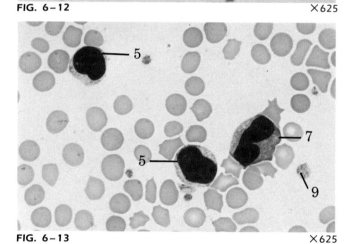

FIG. 6–13   ×625

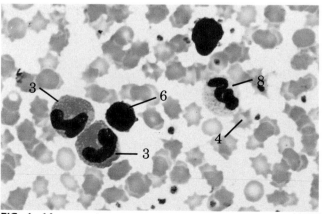

FIG. 6–14   ×625

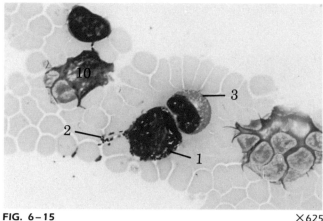

FIG. 6–15   ×625

KEY	
1. Basophil	**7.** Monocyte
2. Basophil granules	**8.** Neutrophil
3. Eosinophil	**9.** Platelet
4. Erythrocyte, crenated	**10.** Smudged cell
5. Lymphocyte, large	
6. Lymphocyte, small	

FIG. 6–11. Blood, Horse, Giemsa. The eosinophil of the horse has characteristic large, round granules. The surface of the cell appears bumpy where granules are pressed against the plasma membrane, giving the cell a raspberry-like appearance. Note the rouleaux, which are common in the horse.

FIG. 6–12. Buffy Coat, Horse, Giemsa. Basophil and neutrophil. Granules of the basophil are purple and vary in size and shape.

FIG. 6–13. Blood, Pig, Giemsa. Two large lymphocytes and a monocyte.

FIG. 6–14. Blood, Pig, Giemsa. Two lymphocytes, one neutrophil, and two eosinophils. The eosinophil of the pig contains numerous pink, round granules that fill the cytoplasm completely. The nucleus of the eosinophil is not highly segmented. It varies from oval to kidney-shaped. Note the coiled appearance of the nucleus of the neutrophil, a common feature in pigs and cats. Crenated red blood cells are commonly seen in blood smears from the pig. Rouleaux are also evident in this field.

FIG. 6–15. Blood, Pig, Giemsa. Eosinophil, basophil, and smudged cell. The granules of the basophil of the pig are dumb-bell or coccoid in shape. Some of the granules have been squeezed from the basophil in this preparation.

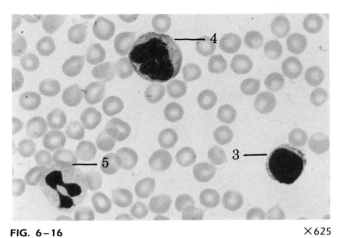

FIG. 6–16   ×625

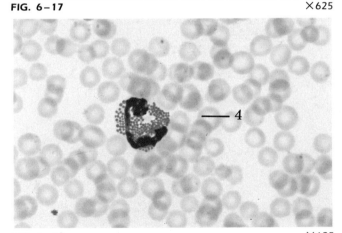

FIG. 6–17   ×625

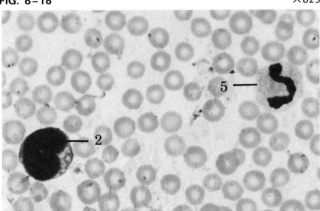

FIG. 6–18   ×625

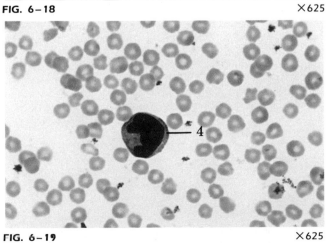

FIG. 6–19   ×625

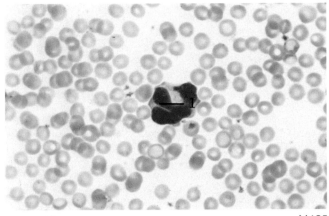

FIG. 6–20   ×625

FIG. 6–16. Blood, Cow, Giemsa. Medium lymphocyte, monocyte, and neutrophil. The cytoplasm of the monocyte is darker and more granular than that of the lymphocyte.

FIG. 6–17. Blood, Cow, Giemsa. Large lymphocyte and neutrophil. Large lymphocytes of the cow often show a deeply indented nucleus. Their cytoplasm is granular and vacuolated.

FIG. 6–18. Blood, Cow, Giemsa. The red granules of the eosinophil are small, round, and intensely stained in the cow. The nucleus may be lobed, but is usually C-shaped.

FIG. 6–19. Blood, Sheep, Giemsa. The nucleus of the monocytes of ruminants may be oval, indented or trilobed. The cytoplasm is gray-blue and vacuolated, and may contain granules.

FIG. 6–20. Blood, Sheep, Giemsa. Monocyte with trilobed nucleus. Compare with Figure 6–19. Our observations have revealed that some monocytes with trilobed nuclei occur in cows and goats also.

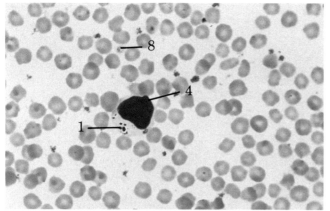

FIG. 6–21　　　　　　　　×625

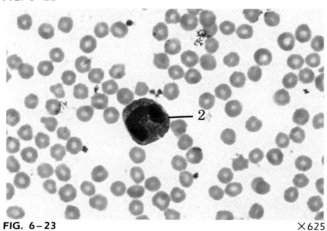

FIG. 6–22

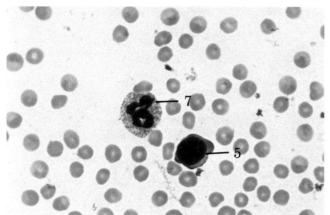

FIG. 6–23　　　　　　　　×625

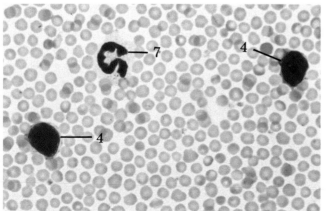

FIG. 6–24　　　　　　　　×625

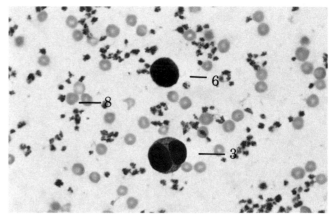

FIG. 6–25　　　　　　　　×625

KEY	
1. Azurophilic granules	**6.** Lymphocyte, small
2. Eosinophil	**7.** Neutrophil
3. Lymphocyte, binucleate	**8.** Platelet
4. Lymphocyte, large	
5. Lymphocyte, medium	

FIG. 6–21. Blood, Sheep, Giemsa. Lymphocyte with azurophilic granules.

FIG. 6–22. Blood, Sheep, Giemsa. Lymphocyte and neutrophil. The cytoplasm of the neutrophil of sheep and goats contains numerous small and a few large pink granules. A perinuclear halo is commonly seen around the periphery of the nucleus of lymphocytes.

FIG. 6–23. Blood, Sheep, Giemsa. The eosinophil of the sheep contains pink, densely packed, oval granules that are uniform in size.

FIG. 6–24. Blood, Goat, Giemsa. Two lymphocytes and a neutrophil. The chromatin of lymphocytes is in the form of closely apposed clumps. Granules are evident in the cytoplasm of the neutrophil.

FIG. 6–25. Buffy Coat, Goat, Giemsa. Some lymphocytes of the cow, sheep, and goat are binucleate.

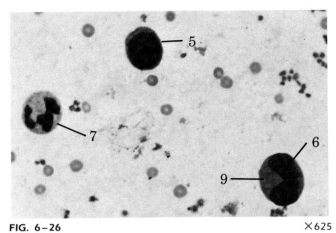

FIG. 6-26   ×625

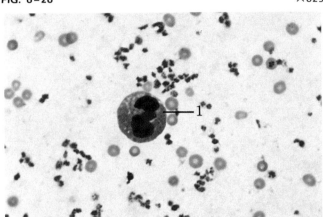

FIG. 6-27   ×625

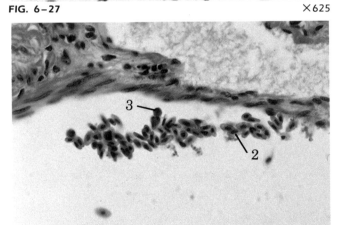

FIG. 6-28   ×250

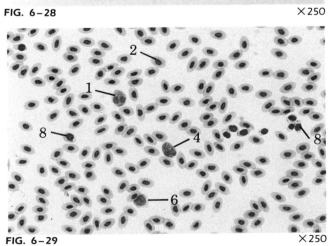

FIG. 6-29   ×250

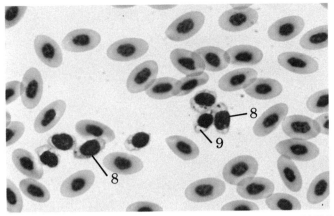

FIG. 6-30   ×625

KEY	
1. Eosinophil	**6.** Monocyte
2. Erythrocyte	**7.** Neutrophil
3. Granulocyte	**8.** Thrombocyte
4. Heterophil	**9.** Vacuole
5. Lymphocyte, large	

FIG. 6-26. Buffy Coat, Goat, Giemsa. Lymphocyte, monocyte, and neutrophil. The cytoplasm of the monocyte is blue and contains vacuoles that are often seen in clusters.

FIG. 6-27. Buffy Coat, Goat, Giemsa. The small, round, acidophilic granules of the eosinophil of the goat almost fill the cytoplasm.

FIG. 6-28. Blood Cells in Section, Chicken. Elongated, nucleated red blood cells and a few granulocytes are shown in the lumen of a blood vessel.

FIG. 6-29. Blood, Chicken, Wright-Giemsa. Erythrocytes, leukocytes, and thrombocytes.

FIG. 6-30. Blood, Chicken, Wright-Giemsa. An oval, coarsely granular nucleus and a vacuolated cytoplasm with one or more magenta granules characterize the thrombocyte.

BLOOD   **35**

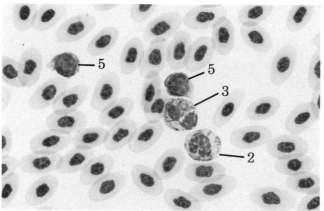

FIG. 6–31 ×625

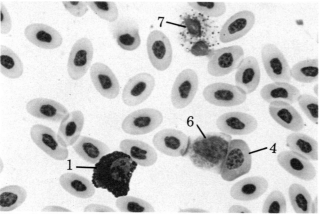

FIG. 6–32 ×625

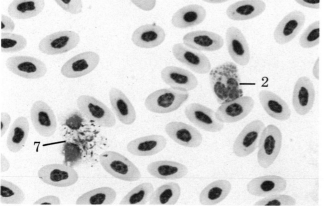

FIG. 6–33 ×625

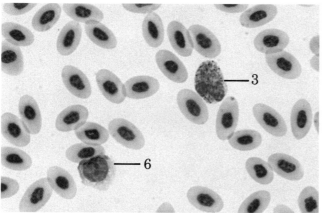

FIG. 6–34 ×625

FIG. 6–31. Blood, Chicken, Wright-Giemsa. Eosinophil, two lymphocytes, and a heterophil. The heterophil has numerous rod-shaped granules. Some of the latter may show a ruby red, spheric center. The nuclear chromatin is coarse and densely packed. In contrast, the eosinophil has fewer, round, pink granules in a pale blue cytoplasm. The nuclear chromatin is block-like, the blocks being distinctly separated from each other.

FIG. 6–32. Blood, Chicken, Wright-Giemsa. Monocyte and heterophil. Many of the rod-shaped granules of the heterophil have a ruby red, spheric granule at their center. This is a common characteristic of the heterophil. The monocyte has a pale, basophilic and vacuolated cytoplasm.

FIG. 6–33. Blood, Chicken, Wright-Giemsa. Basophil, monocyte, smudged heterophil, and immature erythrocyte. The basophil is characterized by large numbers of medium-size basophilic granules. Unlike other granulocytes, the nucleus of this cell is usually unilobed. The cytoplasm of the immature erythrocyte is more basophilic and the nucleus is less condensed than in a mature erythrocyte.

FIG. 6–34. Blood, Chicken, Wright-Giemsa. Eosinophil and smudged heterophil. The rod-shaped granules of the heterophil and the spheric granules of the eosinophil are clearly visible in this preparation.

BONE MARROW

MAMMALS

Red bone marrow is highly cellular and is specialized to produce blood cells and platelets. Along with the spleen and liver, it plays a role in hematopoiesis during prenatal development. At the time of birth, it is the principal source of blood cells and is found throughout the entire skeleton of the animal. In the adult, red marrow is mostly limited to the sternum, ribs, vertebrae, skull, ilia, and the ends of long bones. Yellow marrow, rich in adipose tissue, occupies the remainder of the skeleton of an adult.

Red marrow consists of extravascular hematopoietic tissue and vascular sinusoids. The hematopoietic tissue is rich in blood cells in various stages of formation. It also contains connective tissue cells and is supported by a reticular meshwork. Pluripotent stem cells provide a source of unipotent stem cells committed to the formation of either erythrocytes, granulocytes, agranulocytes, or megakaryocytes. Generally, immature (early) cells of the bone marrow are relatively large, and have a euchromatic nucleus with nucleoli. As they divide and mature, the cells become smaller, the nucleus becomes more heterochromatic, and the nucleoli disappear. Older cells predominate over the immature forms.

The progression of cell stages, from the morphologically indistinct stem cell to a specific mature blood cell, comprises a cell series (cell line). Most of the cells seen in bone marrow preparations belong to either the erythroid or granulocytic (myeloid) series. The cells of these series are presented in this chapter.

The **proerythrocyte** (rubriblast) is a large, round cell with a basophilic cytoplasm. The nucleus is large, with finely granular chromatin and a few nucleoli. This cell undergoes several divisions, giving rise to **basophilic erythroblasts** (prorubricytes). These cells are round with round nuclei. They are the earliest cells of the erythroid series that can be readily identified in smears. The basophilic erythroblast is somewhat smaller than its precursor and has a deeply basophilic cytoplasm. The nuclear chromatin is more coarsely clumped and no nucleoli are visible. Basophilic erythroblasts give rise to **polychromatophilic erythroblasts** (rubricytes), which are smaller cells. The chromatin is more condensed, appearing as blocks separated by light streaks, similar to the chromatin of a plasma cell. The cytoplasm is mottled with pink and blue areas. As hemoglobin synthesis continues and ribosomes diminish, the cytoplasm becomes more pink and less blue. Mitotic division usually ceases in the late polychromatophilic erythroblast stage. **Orthochromatic erythroblasts** (normoblasts, metarubricytes) are characterized by a round, highly condensed, and deeply stained nucleus. Their cytoplasm is distinctly eosinophilic but may show slight tinges of blue. Eventually the nucleus is extruded, leaving an anucleate **reticulocyte** that matures into an erythrocyte.

Myeloblasts are large granuolcytic cells with a grainy, basophilic cytoplasm. The round to oval nucleus contains finely dispersed chromatin. Nucleoli may be present. These cells give rise to the **promyelocyte,** the earliest stage in the development of a granulocyte that can be readily distinguished in smears. This cell contains a relatively large nucleus with nucleoli and chromatin that is beginning to clump. The cytoplasm contains nonspecific azurophilic (magenta) granules. Promyelocytes divide and give rise to **myelocytes.** The myelocyte is smaller and has an oval, often eccentric, nucleus with more condensed chromatin. Specific granules charac-

teristic of neutrophils, eosinophils, or basophils are apparent in the cytoplasm. Late myelocytes lose the capacity to divide. They are known as **metamyelocytes** when the nucleus becomes indented and more condensed. With further modification, the nucleus becomes more elongated in the **band cell** stage before finally assuming a monolobed or segmented shape of the **mature granulocyte.**

Megakaryocytes are situated in the extravascular compartment, close to sinusoids, into which they release platelets. They are very large cells with a polymorphic nucleus and a grainy cytoplasm, and are often seen in bone marrow preparations together with a variety of other cells such as plasma cells, adipocytes, and cells in mitosis. **Osteoblasts** and **osteoclasts,** because of their close relationship with the surface of bone that lines the marrow cavity, may also be encountered in smear preparations of marrow.

CHICKEN

The organization of bone marrow of the chicken is different from that of mammals. Erythropoiesis takes place within the vascular sinusoids, rather than in the extravascular tissue. The immature red blood cells (large cells with a basophilic cytoplasm) are found adjacent to the endothelium of a sinusoid. As division and maturation of these cells progress, the older ones move inward. Thus, mature erythrocytes (with an eosinophilic cytoplasm) accumulate in the center of the vessel. As in mammals, cells of the granulocytic series (heterophils, eosinophils, and basophils) develop in the extravascular spaces of the marrow.

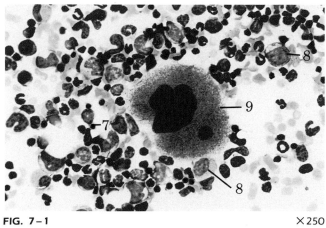

FIG. 7-1 ×250

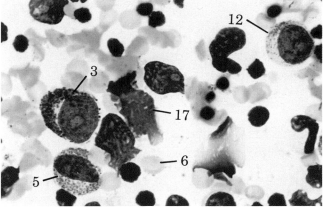

FIG. 7-5 ×625

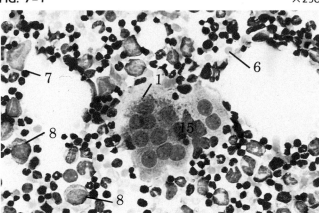

FIG. 7-2 ×250

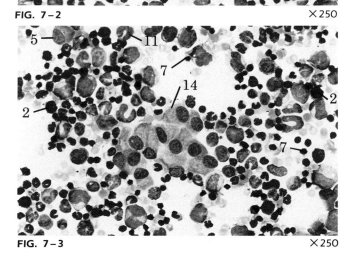

FIG. 7-3 ×250

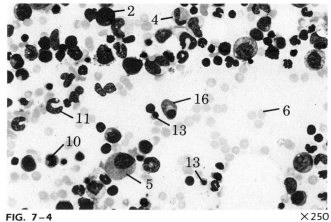

FIG. 7-4 ×250

KEY	
1. Azurophilic debris	**10.** Mitotic figure
2. Basophilic erythroblast	**11.** Neutrophilic band cell
3. Basophilic myelocyte	**12.** Neutrophilic myelocyte
4. Eosinophilic band cell	**13.** Orthochromatic
5. Eosinophilic myelocyte	erythroblast
6. Erythrocyte	**14.** Osteoblast
7. Erythroid cell, late	**15.** Osteoclast
8. Granulocytic cell, early	**16.** Plasma cell
9. Megakaryocyte	**17.** Smudged cell, nucleus

FIG. 7-1. Megakaryocyte, Bone Marrow, Cat, Giemsa. The megakaryocyte is a large cell with a polymorphic nucleus and grainy cytoplasm. Blood platelets are derived from fragments of the cytoplasm. Forces generated during the formation of the smear appear to have separated a segment of the nucleus.

FIG. 7-2. Osteoclast, Bone Marrow, Cat, Giemsa. The osteoclast is a large multinucleate cell formed from fused macrophages. Azurophilic bone debris can be seen in the cytoplasm of this specimen.

FIG. 7-3. Osteoblasts, Bone Marrow, Cat, Giemsa. Osteoblasts are characterized by the presence of an eccentric nucleus and basophilic cytoplasm. A perinuclear clear zone, representing the site of the Golgi apparatus, may be visible. In smears, these cells often occur in clusters.

FIG. 7-4. Bone Marrow, Cat, Giemsa. A variety of different cells of the bone marrow can be identified at this magnification.

FIG. 7-5. Bone Marrow, Cat, Giemsa. Basophilic, neutrophilic, and eosinophilic myelocytes are represented in this field.

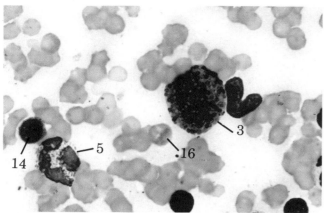

FIG. 7-6 ×625

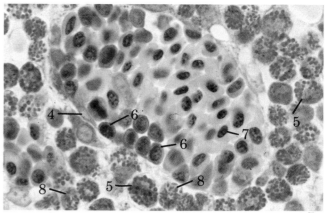

FIG. 7-10 ×625

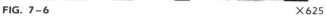

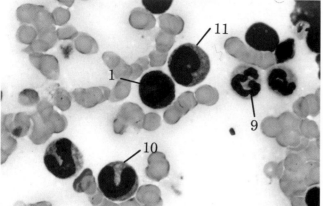

FIG. 7-7 ×625

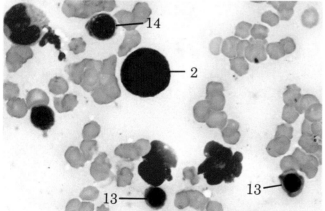

FIG. 7-8 ×625

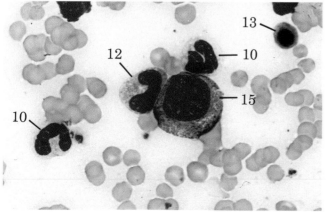

FIG. 7-9 ×625

KEY	
1. Basophilic band cell	**11.** Neutrophilic
2. Basophilic erythroblast	metamyelocyte
3. Basophilic myelocyte	**12.** Neutrophilic
4. Endothelial cell, nucleus	metamyelocyte, late
5. Eosinophil	**13.** Orthochromatophilic
6. Erythrocyte, early	erythroblast
7. Erythrocyte, mature	**14.** Polychromatophilic
8. Heterophil	erythroblast
9. Neutrophil	**15.** Promyelocyte
10. Neutrophilic band cell	**16.** Reticulocyte

FIG. 7-6. Bone Marrow, Cat, Wright-Giemsa. A basophilic myelocyte, segmented eosinophil, and polychromatophilic erythroblast are evident.

FIG. 7-7. Bone Marrow, Cat, Wright-Giemsa. Various myeloid developmental stages are shown in this field.

FIG. 7-8. Bone Marrow, Cat, Wright-Giemsa. Various erythroid developmental stages are shown in this field.

FIG. 7-9. Bone Marrow, Cat, Wright-Giemsa. The largest cell seen in this field is a promyelocyte. Note the presence of numerous magenta, azurophilic granules in its cytoplasm.

FIG. 7-10. Bone Marrow, Plastic Section, Chicken, Giemsa. Intravascular developmental stages of erythrocytes are shown. In the extravascular compartment, heterophils and eosinophils can be distinguished.

CHAPTER

8

MUSCLE

A unique characteristic of muscle cells is the presence of a substructure of myofilaments that provides them with the ability to contract. Although the arrangement of the myofilaments in smooth muscle cells differs from that of skeletal and cardiac muscle cells, the contraction process is the same, and occurs when the filaments slide past one another.

Smooth muscle is involuntary. Its cells are long and tapered, with an elongated nucleus located about midway between the ends of each cell. Smooth muscle tissue consists of groups of these cells bound together by connective tissue fibers. Students often encounter difficulty in distinguishing smooth muscle from the surrounding connective tissue. It is helpful to know, therefore, that smooth muscle presents an overall dull appearance in hematoxylin and eosin preparations, while connective tissue fibers are considerably more refractile and appear bright and shiny by comparison. Smooth muscle is found in a variety of places, for example, the digestive tract, blood vessels, urinary bladder, capsules of some organs, and bronchi.

Skeletal muscle is striated and voluntary. Cells are multinucleated and may be 3 or 4 cm long. Cross-striations result from the precise registration of the A, I, H, and M bands of the sarcomeres of their myofibrils. Nuclei are located peripherally, immediately below the sarcolemma. Individual cells are arranged into fascicles. Each fascicle, in turn, is surrounded by a **perimysium** of loose connective tissue, and each cell within a fascicle is closely invested by delicate reticular fibers, the **endomysium.** Bundles of fascicles are bound together by a superficial layer of dense connective tissue called the **epimysium.** Collagenous fibers of tendons insert into invaginations at the ends of the muscle cell and anchor the tendon to the external lamina, which is adherent to the sarcolemma.

Cardiac muscle is striated and involuntary. It forms the myocardium of the heart and occurs in the walls of the major vessels immediately adjacent to the heart, including the aorta, pulmonary artery, pulmonary vein, and vena cava. Each cell has one nucleus (centrally located), and may branch and anastomose with adjacent cells. As in skeletal muscle, cross-striations are present and are formed from the alignment of sarcomeric bands. Special cell surface modifications, called **intercalated discs,** join cardiac muscle cells together end to end. Some cardiac muscle cells are modified to form a conducting system (sinoatrial node, atrioventricular node, Purkinje fibers), which helps to coordinate the heartbeat.

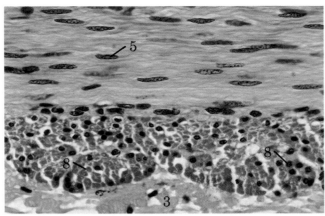

FIG. 8–1 ×250

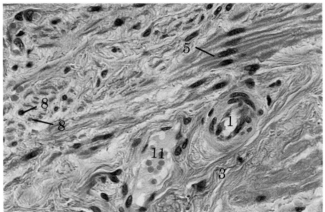

FIG. 8–2 ×250

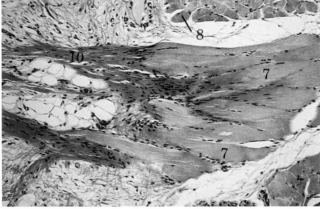

FIG. 8–3 ×62.5

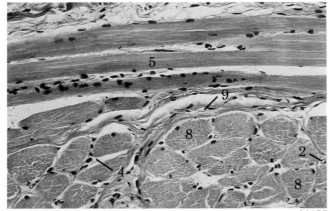

FIG. 8–4 ×125

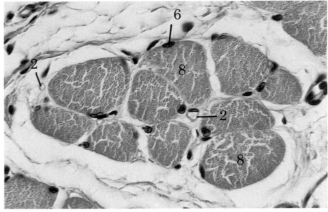

FIG. 8–5 ×250

KEY	
1. Arteriole	**7.** Muscle cell, oblique cut
2. Capillary, x.s.	**8.** Muscle cell, x.s.
3. Connective tissue	**9.** Perimysium
4. Endomysium	**10.** Tendon
5. Muscle cell, l.s.	**11.** Venule
6. Muscle cell, nucleus	

FIG. 8–1. Smooth Muscle, x.s. and l.s., Muscularis Externa, Jejunum, x.s., Sheep. Smooth muscle cells have a single, elongated nucleus. This is apparent in cells that have been sectioned longitudinally. Cross sections of smooth muscle cells vary in diameter, depending on where they were transected along their length. If the cell was transected through its middle region, the nucleus is seen and appears round. If the cut was closer to the tapered extremity of the cell, no nucleus is evident and the cell has a smaller diameter.

FIG. 8–2. Smooth Muscle, x.s. and l.s., Urinary Bladder, Pig. The tapered form of the smooth muscle cell is evident.

FIG. 8–3. Skeletal Muscle and Tendon, oblique cut, Tongue, Horse. The collagenous fibers of a tendon can be seen blending with skeletal muscle cells.

FIG. 8–4. Skeletal Muscle, x.s. and l.s., Tongue, Horse. Skeletal muscle cells are large and possess numerous, peripheral nuclei. Cross-striations are evident in cells cut longitudinally.

FIG. 8–5. Skeletal Muscle, x.s., Tongue, Horse. Transected myofibrils can be clearly seen within each cell.

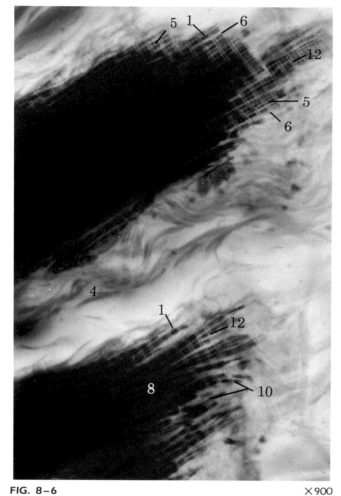

FIG. 8–6 ×900

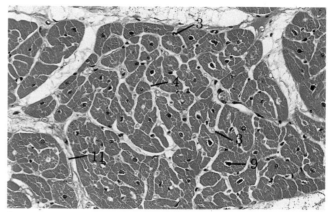

FIG. 8–9 ×125

FIG. 8–6. Skeletal Muscle, l.s., Lip, Dog, Masson's. Portions of two skeletal muscle cells showing individual myofibrils and cross-striations.

FIG. 8–7. Cardiac Muscle, l.s., Heart, Cat. Bifurcated muscle cells and intercalated discs are visible.

FIG. 8–8. Cardiac Muscle, l.s., Cat. Cross-striations and intercalated discs are apparent in this preparation.

FIG. 8–9. Cardiac Muscle, x.s., Pig. Note the centrally located nuclei of the muscle cells.

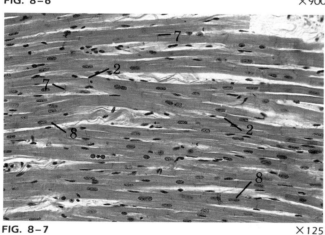

FIG. 8–7 ×125

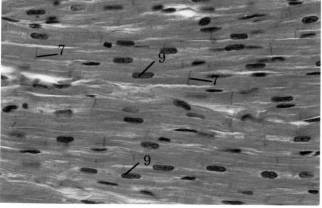

FIG. 8–8 ×250

9

NERVOUS SYSTEM

One can hardly examine a histologic preparation of any sort without finding some evidence of nervous tissue, for example, sections through myelinated or unmyelinated nerves, isolated neurons, encapsulated nerve endings, or perhaps a nerve plexus.

The nervous system consists of neurons of various sizes and kinds, including their supporting elements, and is basically similar in all domestic animals. In the central nervous system is a structural framework provided by neuroglia cells and their processes. In contrast, the peripheral nervous system is held together by various types of connective tissue proper. For example, axons and bundles of axons of peripheral nerves are fastened together by both loose and dense irregular connective tissue. Connective tissue meninges surround the brain and spinal cord, providing support and protection.

Selected examples of nervous system elements as they appear, typically, in histologic preparations of various kinds are presented. Additionally, sections through portions of the brain, brain stem, and spinal cord have been included. The organs of special sense, the eye and ear, are treated in separate chapters.

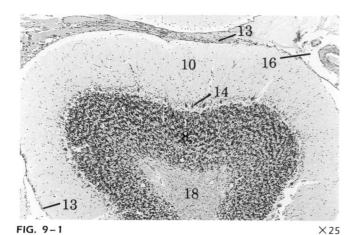

FIG. 9–1 ×25

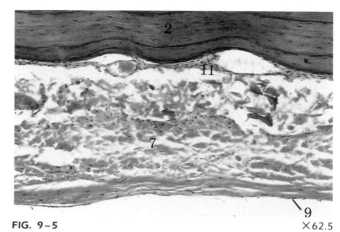

FIG. 9–5 ×62.5

KEY	
1. Arachnoid layer	**10.** Molecular layer
2. Bone, skull	**11.** Periosteum
3. Capillary	**12.** Perivascular space
4. Cerebrospinal fluid	**13.** Pia mater
5. Connective tissue wisp	**14.** Purkinje cell
6. Dendrite	**15.** Small artery
7. Dura mater	**16.** Subarachnoid space
8. Granular layer	**17.** Venule
9. Mesothelium	**18.** White matter

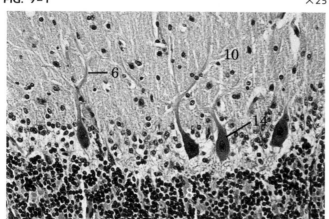

FIG. 9–2 ×125

FIG. 9–1. Cerebellum, Sheep. The molecular and granular layers of the gray matter and Purkinje cells are shown. The white matter lies deep to the gray matter.

FIG. 9–2. Cerebellum, Sheep. Portions of the dendritic tree of the multipolar Purkinje cells are visible.

FIG. 9–3. Meninges, Cerebellum, Sheep, Mallory's. The arachnoid layer, subarachnoid space, and pia mater are shown. The subarachnoid space is filled with cerebrospinal fluid, which is stained purple. Wisps of connective tissue (blue) can be seen within the subarachnoid space. These connect the arachnoid layer with the pia.

FIG. 9–4. Cerebellum, Dog. Portion of a sulcus containing a venule. The perivascular space surrounding the vessel is continuous with the subarachnoid space and separates the vessel from the pia mater on either side.

FIG. 9–5. Dura Mater, Goat. The dura remains attached to the skull when the latter is separated from the brain. It is a dense fibroelastic layer lined by a mesothelium. The dura merges with the periosteum of the skull.

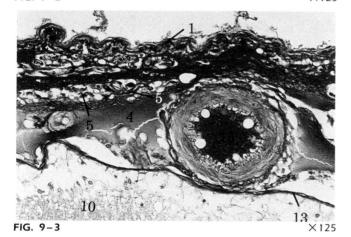

FIG. 9–3 ×125

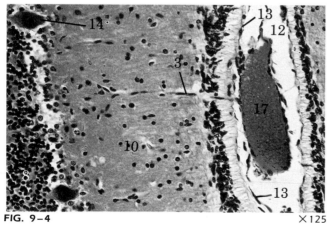

FIG. 9–4 ×125

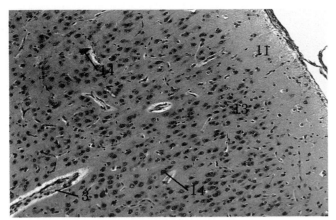

FIG. 9–6 ×62.5

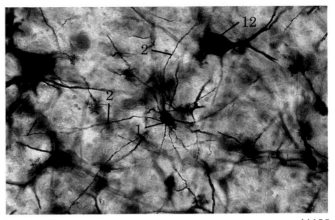

FIG. 9–10 ×125

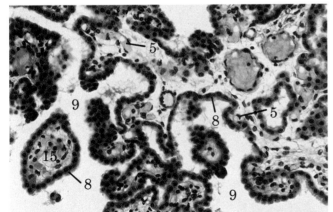

FIG. 9–7 ×12.5

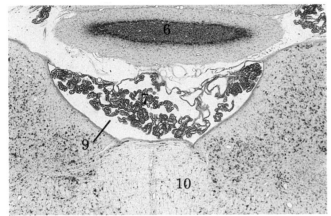

FIG. 9–8 ×125

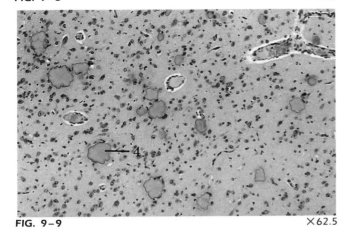

FIG. 9–9 ×62.5

KEY	
1. Astrocyte, cell body	**9.** Fourth ventricle
2. Astrocyte, process	**10.** Medulla
3. Blood vessel	**11.** Molecular layer
4. Brain sand	**12.** Neuron
5. Capillary	**13.** Outer granular layer
6. Cerebellum, vermis	**14.** Pyramidal cell
7. Choroid plexus	**15.** Villus, x.s
8. Epithelium	

FIG. 9–6. Cerebral Cortex, Dog. Outer portion of cerebral cortex with numerous blood vessels.

FIG. 9–7. Choroid Plexus, Cat, Cresyl Violet. Portion of the fourth ventricle with choroid plexus in the roof of the medulla.

FIG. 9–8. Choroid Plexus, Dog. The simple cuboidal epithelium and large, thin-walled capillaries are major constituents of the villi of the choroid plexus.

FIG. 9–9. Brain Sand, Hypothalamus, Dog. Calcified, granular material called brain sand can be found dispersed through various parts of the brain, including the hypothalamus, cerebellum, and pineal gland.

FIG. 9–10. Fibrous Astrocyte, Medulla, Cat, Golgi. These neuroglia cells have long processes that show little or no branching.

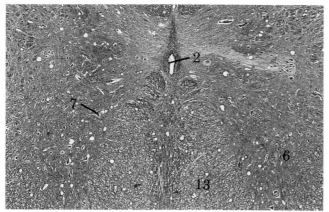

FIG. 9-11 ×12.5

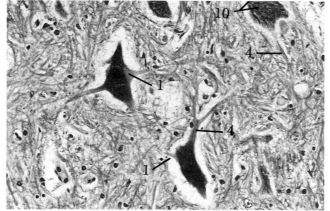

FIG. 9-12 ×125

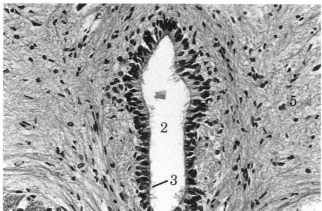

FIG. 9-13 ×125

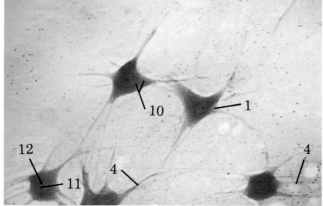

FIG. 9-14 ×62.5

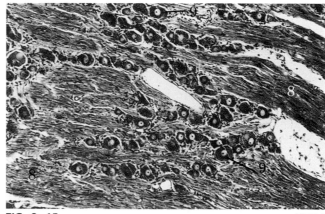

FIG. 9-15 ×62.5

KEY	
1. Axon hillock	**8.** Nerve fibers
2. Central canal	**9.** Neuron cell body
3. Cilia	**10.** Nissl granules
4. Dendrite	**11.** Nucleolus
5. Gray matter	**12.** Nucleus
6. Gray matter, ventral horn	**13.** White matter
7. Multipolar neuron	

FIG. 9-11. Spinal Cord, Cervical, x.s., Sheep, Masson's. The central canal, gray matter, and white matter are shown.

FIG. 9-12. Central Canal, Spinal Cord, x.s., Sheep. Tall ependymal cells, some of which are ciliated, line the central canal.

FIG. 9-13. Multipolar Neurons, Spinal Cord, Sheep. The axon hillock of two neurons can be seen. Nissl granules are absent from the hillock region, but extend into the dendrites.

FIG. 9-14. Multipolar Neurons, Spinal Cord, Cow. Several multipolar neurons are shown in this smear preparation. Note prominent nucleoli and Nissl granules.

FIG. 9-15. Dorsal Root Ganglion, Dog, Luxol Fast Blue/Cresylecht Violet. Portion of a dorsal root ganglion showing neurons and nerve fibers. *(Photomicrograph of a histologic section borrowed from the College of Veterinary Medicine, Iowa State University.)*

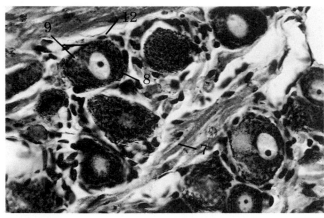

FIG. 9–16 ×250

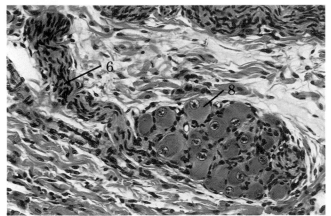

FIG. 9–17 ×125

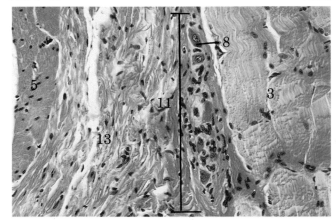

FIG. 9–18 ×125

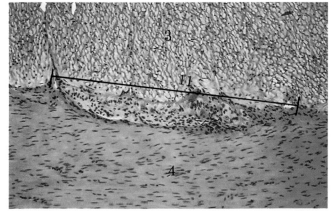

FIG. 9–19 ×62.5

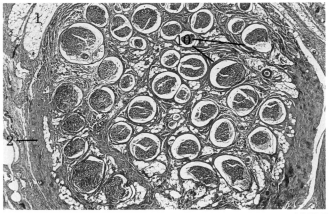

FIG. 9–20 ×12.5

KEY	
1. Adipose tissue	**8.** Neuron cell body
2. Epineurium	**9.** Nissl granules
3. Muscularis externa, inner circular	**10.** Perineurium
4. Muscularis externa, outer longitudinal	**11.** Plexus
5. Muscularis mucosae	**12.** Satellite cell
6. Nerve	**13.** Submucosa
7. Nerve fiber	

FIG. 9–16. Dorsal Root Ganglion, Dog, Luxol Fast Blue/Cresylecht Violet. Flattened satellite cells envelop the round neuron cell bodies of the unipolar neurons. *(Photograph of a histologic section borrowed from the College of Veterinary Medicine, Iowa State University.)*

FIG. 9–17. Parasympathetic Ganglion, Pulmonary Artery, Dog. A ganglion and associated nerve located in the adventitia of the artery.

FIG. 9–18. Meissner's Plexus, Esophagus, x.s., Pig. These parasympathetic plexuses are located in the submucosa of the digestive tract. Note the characteristic large "owl's eye" nucleus of the neurons.

FIG. 9–19. Auerbach's Plexus, Jejunum, l.s., Dog. These parasympathetic plexuses are located between the inner circular and outer longitudinal layers of the muscularis externa of the digestive tract.

FIG. 9–20. Nerve, Myelinated, x.s., Pig, Masson's. The nerve shown is composed of many fascicles bounded by a connective tissue sheath, the epineurium. Each fascicle is surrounded by a perineurium and contains numerous axons.

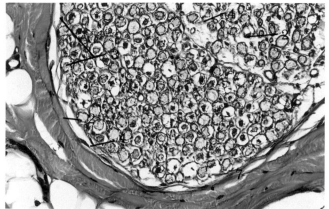

FIG. 9–21 ×125

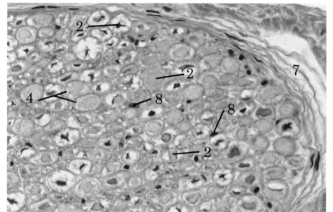

FIG. 9–22 ×250

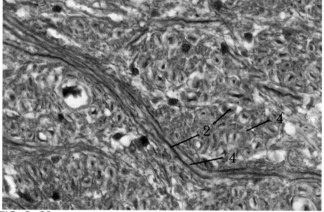

FIG. 9–23 ×250

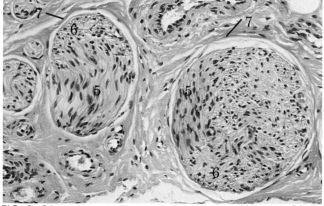

FIG. 9–24 ×125

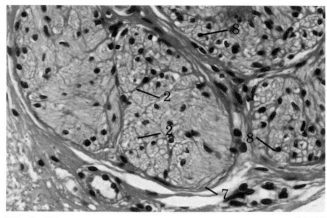

FIG. 9–25 ×250

KEY	
1. Adipose tissue	**5.** Nerve fibers, l.s.
2. Axon	**6.** Nerve fibers, x.s.
3. Endoneurium	**7.** Perineurium
4. Myelin sheath	**8.** Schwann cell, nucleus

FIG. 9–21. Nerve Fascicle, Myelinated, x.s., Pig, Masson's. Delicate connective tissue fibers of the endoneurium are visible around individual myelinated axons.

FIG. 9–22. Nerve, Myelinated, Thoracic Wall, Cat. Myelin sheaths (pink) often present a scalloped or vacuolated appearance, an artifact of processing. Axons in this preparation are blue-gray and round, oval, or shriveled.

FIG. 9–23. Axons, Myelinated, Medulla, Horse, Hagguist. Axons (blue) with myelin sheaths (pink) are seen in longitudinal and cross sections.

FIG. 9–24. Nerve Fascicles, Unmyelinated, Ureter, Pig. Note the wavy appearance of the fibers that have been cut longitudinally. See Figure 9–25 for comment on relationship of axons to Schwann cells.

FIG. 9–25. Nerve Fascicles, Unmyelinated, Left Ventricle, Pig. Each Schwann cell enwraps several unmyelinated axons within grooves of its plasma membrane. The grooves appear as vesicles in this preparation. Axons may be seen within some of these vesicles and appear as small pink dots.

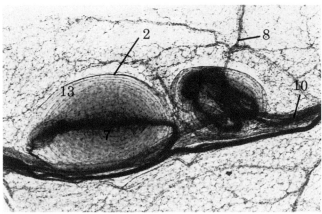

FIG. 9-26   ×25

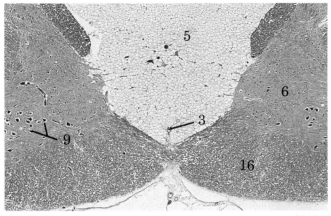

FIG. 9-30   ×12.5

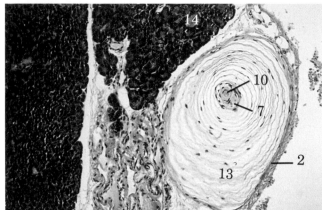

FIG. 9-27   ×62.5

KEY	
1. Arteriovenous shunt	**9.** Multipolar neurons
2. Capsule	**10.** Nerve
3. Central canal	**11.** Nuclear bag fiber
4. Fluid-filled space	**12.** Nuclear chain fiber
5. Glycogen body	**13.** Outer core
6. Gray matter	**14.** Pancreas
7. Inner core	**15.** Skeletal muscle, x.s.
8. Mesenteric blood vessel	**16.** White matter

FIG. 9-26. Pacinian Corpuscle, whole mount, Mesentery, Cat, Carmine. Two corpuscles (one somewhat distorted) are shown. Each is surrounded by a connective tissue capsule, within which are located concentric laminae of flattened cells that form the core. A nerve ending courses through the center of the corpuscle. The closely packed inner core cells surround the nerve. The peripheral laminae form a looser, outer core.

FIG. 9-27. Pacinian Corpuscle, x.s., Pancreas, Cat. This corpuscle is frequently seen in the pancreas of carnivores. See Figure 9-26 for description.

FIG. 9-28. Small Encapsulated Nerve Endings, Dermis, Planum, Cow. Numerous encapsulated sensory nerve endings occur in the dermis of the planum near the epithelium.

FIG. 9-29. Neuromuscular Spindle, x.s., Thoracic Muscle, Cat. A neuromuscular spindle is a proprioceptor located within a muscle. It consists of sensory and motor nerve endings and intrafusal fibers, which are narrow, modified skeletal muscle cells. Nuclear chain fibers are intrafusal fibers with a single row of nuclei, while nuclear bag fibers are intrafusal fibers that contain many closely packed nuclei. A capsule encloses the fluid-filled space that surrounds the intrafusal fibers.

FIG. 9-30. Glycogen Body, Lumbosacral Enlargement, Spinal Cord, x.s., Chicken. The glycogen body is found only in birds. It consists of polyhedral, vesicular cells, each containing a central mass of glycogen and a peripherally displaced nucleus.

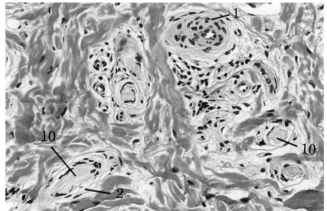

FIG. 9-28   ×125

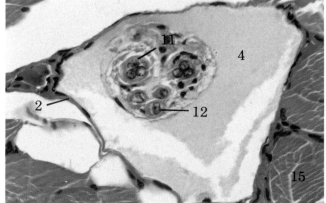

FIG. 9-29   ×250

NERVOUS SYSTEM   **51**

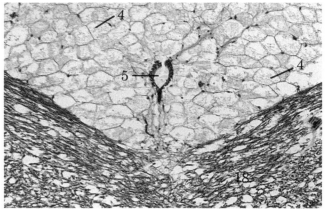

FIG. 9–31 ×62.5

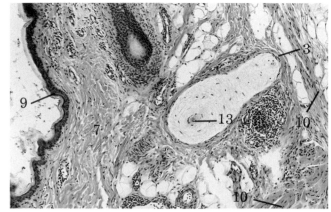

FIG. 9–35 ×62.5

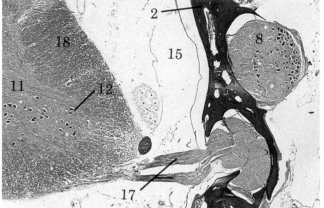

FIG. 9–32 ×12.5

KEY	
1. Axon	**10.** Feather muscle
2. Bone	**11.** Gray matter
3. Capsule	**12.** Multipolar neuron
4. Cell of glycogen body	**13.** Nerve
5. Central canal	**14.** Sharpey's fibers
6. Core	**15.** Space artifact
7. Dermis	**16.** Unipolar neuron
8. Dorsal root ganglion	**17.** Ventral root
9. Epidermis	**18.** White matter

FIG. 9–31. Glycogen Body, Lumbosacral Enlargement, Spinal Cord, x.s., Chicken. Cells of the glycogen body in detail. See Figure 9–30 for description.

FIG. 9–32. Dorsal Root Ganglion, Lumbosacral Enlargement, Spinal Cord, x.s., Chicken. Portions of the spinal cord, ventral root of a spinal nerve, dorsal root ganglion, and vertebra.

FIG. 9–33. Dorsal Root Ganglion, Lumbosacral Enlargement, Spinal Cord, x.s., Chicken. Neuron cell bodies of unipolar neurons and myelinated axons are shown.

FIG. 9–34. Herbst Corpuscle, Upper Beak, x.s., Chicken. These encapsulated nerve endings occur frequently in the skin of the bird. They are similar to Pacinian corpuscles of mammals and consist of an outer connective tissue capsule, a laminated core, and an axial sensory nerve ending.

FIG. 9–35. Herbst Corpuscle, Skin, Neck, Chicken. The Herbst corpuscles associated with follicles of feathered skin are sausage-shaped.

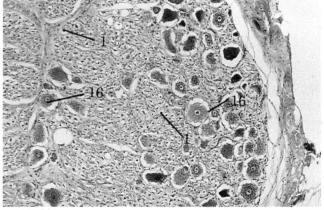

FIG. 9–33 ×62.5

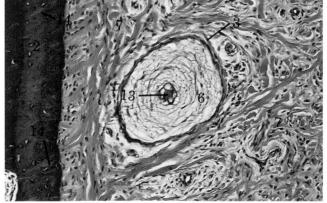

FIG. 9–34 ×125

10

CARDIOVASCULAR SYSTEM

The heart pumps blood and conveys it to the tissues and organs through blood vessels. Fluid that escapes from the blood is returned to the venous system by lymphatic vessels.

Vessels of the cardiovascular system are lined by an **endothelium,** which is, typically, a single layer of squamous cells. The smallest of the blood vessels, **capillaries,** are tiny endothelial tubes. They are easily overlooked in histologic sections, especially if they are compressed or collapsed.

The walls of arteries and veins are arranged into concentric layers: the inner **tunica intima,** middle **tunica media,** and outer **tunica adventitia.** The composition and thickness of these layers vary with the size and type of vessel. The tunica media is not always present.

Small arteries can be defined, arbitrarily, as possessing up to eight or nine layers of smooth muscle cells in the tunica media. The smallest of these vessels is usually termed an **arteriole.** Its wall is composed of an endothelium (tunica intima), one or two layers of circularly arranged smooth muscle cells (tunica media), and a bit of surrounding loose connective tissue (tunica adventitia). Some of the larger small arteries have an **internal elastic membrane.** Small arteries are accompanied by **small veins.** The smallest of these are called **venules.** These are similar to arterioles, but have relatively thin walls and lack a tunica media of smooth muscle. An internal elastic membrane is not found in small veins.

As the diameter of a vessel increases, the tunics become larger and more elaborate. For example, the tunica intima of a **medium artery** contains connective tissue interspersed between the endothelium and internal elastic membrane. The thick tunica media, with varying proportions of smooth muscle and elastic fibers, comprises the bulk of the wall. The connective tissue of the tunica adventitia contains collagenous and elastic fibers, small blood vessels **(vasa vasorum),** and nerves. A **medium vein,** in contrast, has less smooth muscle and fewer elastic fibers in the tunica media and a thicker tunica adventitia.

Arteries appear round in cross section and have an obvious rippled internal elastic membrane. Conversely, accompanying veins are larger in diameter, with an irregular or collapsed lumen, thinner walls and, except for some of the largest, have no internal elastic membrane. The lumens of blood vessels in tissue sections often contain blood cells, plasma, or both. Although it can be difficult to distinguish between veins and **lymphatic vessels,** the latter have thinner walls than veins of similar size and normally do not contain erythrocytes. **Valves** may occur in both veins and lymphatic vessels.

There are several variations from the "typical" blood vessels: The tunica adventitia of large veins adjacent to the heart contains cardiac, rather than smooth, muscle. Some arteries have smooth muscle in the tunica intima as well as the tunica media. Smooth muscle may be oriented either longitudinally or circularly. The tunica adventitia of some vessels may be abundant or scant.

The arteries of **arteriovenous anastomoses** lack an internal elastic membrane, but possess epithelioid-like, longitudinally arranged smooth muscle cells. Special structures, the aortic and carotid bodies, are closely associated with the tunica adventitia of their respective arteries.

Many special vessels unique to certain organs, such as the sinusoids of the liver, postcapillary venules of lymph nodes, and helicine arteries of the penis, are presented elsewhere with their appropriate organ systems.

The **heart** is a muscular organ whose wall is composed of an **endocardium, myocardium,** and **epicardium.** The thickness and composition of the wall vary, being thickest in the ventricles and thinnest in the atria. The middle layer of cardiac muscle, the myocardium, predominates. Connective tissue valves, covered by an endothelium, are extensions of the endocardium. Regions of the heart, including the base of the aorta and pulmonary trunk, as well as the atrioventricular orifices and septum, are supported by the **cardiac skeleton.** This may be in the form of dense irregular connective tissue, fibrocartilage, hyaline cartilage, or bone, and varies with age and among individuals.

A small amount of fluid occurs in the pericardial cavity between the epicardium (visceral pericardium) and the parietal pericardium.

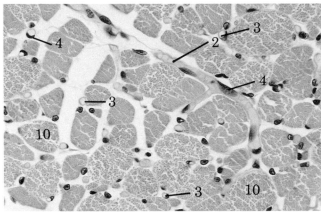

FIG. 10–1 ×250

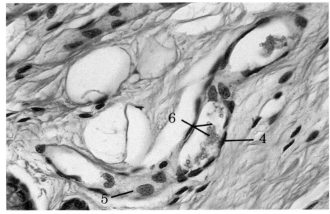

FIG. 10–5 ×250

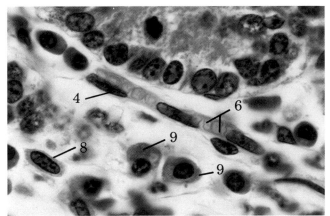

FIG. 10–2 ×625

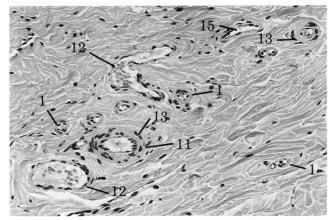

FIG. 10–3 ×125

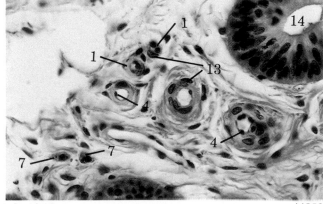

FIG. 10–4 ×250

KEY	
1. Arteriole, x.s.	**9.** Plasma cell
2. Capillary, l.s.	**10.** Skeletal muscle cell, x.s.
3. Capillary, x.s.	**11.** Small artery, x.s.
4. Endothelial cell, nucleus	**12.** Small vein
5. Endothelial cell, surface cut	**13.** Smooth muscle cell, nucleus
6. Erythrocytes	**14.** Uterine gland
7. Macrophage	**15.** Venule
8. Mast cell	

FIG. 10–1. Capillaries, x.s. and l.s., Diaphragm, Dog.
Extensive capillary networks occur around muscle cells.

FIG. 10–2. Capillary, l.s., Lamina Propria, Duodenum, Sheep. Erythrocytes fill the lumen of this capillary.

FIG. 10–3. Arterioles and Venules, Eyelid, Pig. Small blood vessels of various sizes are present in the dermis.

FIG. 10–4. Arterioles, x.s., Endometrium, Uterus, Dog. The smallest of the arterioles shown have only one layer of smooth muscle in their walls.

FIG. 10–5. Venule, l.s., Connective Tissue, Epiglottis, Goat. The wall of the venule consists of an endothelium and a small amount of connective tissue.

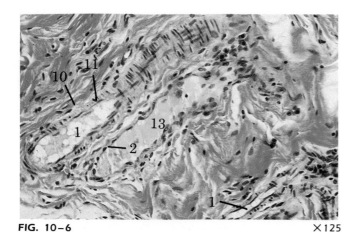

FIG. 10–6 ×125

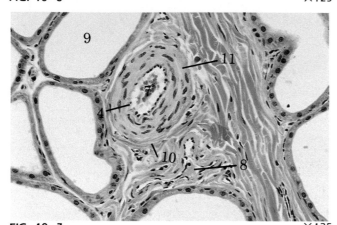

FIG. 10–7 ×125

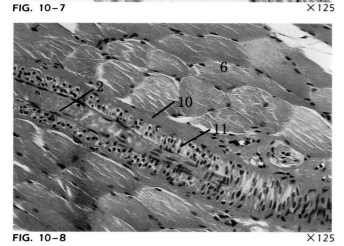

FIG. 10–8 ×125

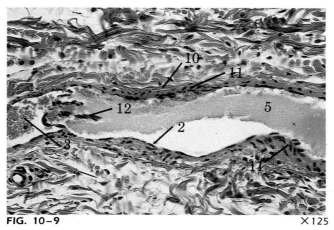

FIG. 10–9 ×125

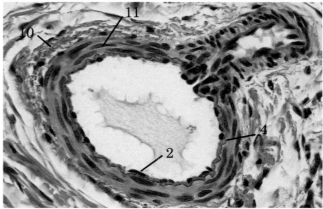

FIG. 10–10 ×250

KEY	
1. Arteriole	**8.** Small vein, x.s.
2. Endothelial cell, nucleus	**9.** Sweat gland
3. Erythrocytes	**10.** Tunica adventitia
4. Internal elastic membrane	**11.** Tunica media
5. Plasma	**12.** Valve
6. Skeletal muscle	**13.** Venule
7. Small artery, x.s.	

FIG. 10–6. Arterioles and Venule, l.s., Submucosa, Esophagus, Cat. In the region where the arterioles have been cut tangentially, the circular arrangement of the smooth muscle of the tunica media can be seen.

FIG. 10–7. Small Artery and Vein, x.s., Eyelid, Pig. These vessels are surrounded by portions of sweat glands in the dermis. Veins, such as the one shown, often have an irregular or collapsed lumen.

FIG. 10–8. Small Artery, l.s., Esophagus, Pig.

FIG. 10–9. Small Vein with Valve, l.s., Nose, Sheep. Valves are thin flaps of connective tissue covered on both sides by an endothelium.

FIG. 10–10. Small Artery, x.s., with Branch, Subcutis, Dog.

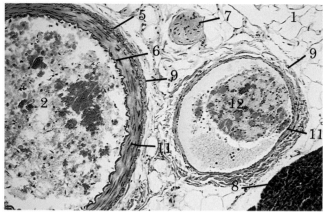

FIG. 10–11 ×62.5

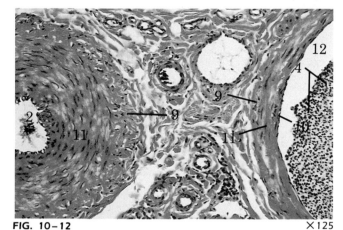

FIG. 10–12 ×125

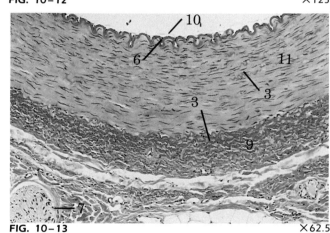

FIG. 10–13 ×62.5

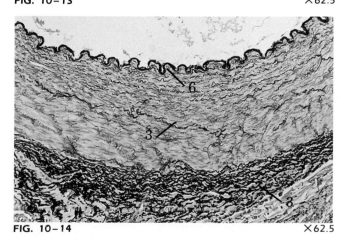

FIG. 10–14 ×62.5

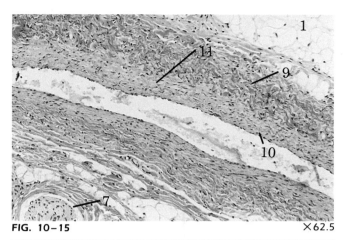

FIG. 10–15 ×62.5

KEY	
1. Adipose tissue	**8.** Pancreas
2. Artery	**9.** Tunica adventitia
3. Elastic fiber	**10.** Tunica intima, endothelium
4. Erythrocytes	**11.** Tunica media
5. External elastic membrane	**12.** Vein
6. Internal elastic membrane	
7. Nerve	

FIG. 10–11. Small Artery, Vein, and Nerve, x.s., Pancreas, Cat. Note that both of the vessels have a sparse adventitia.

FIG. 10–12. Artery and Vein, x.s., Wattle, Rooster. Note the especially thick tunica media of the artery.

FIG. 10–13. Medium Artery, x.s., Lymph Node, Pig. The rich pink color of the elastic fibers contrasts with the paler pink color of the collagenous fibers and smooth muscle.

FIG. 10–14. Medium Artery, x.s., Lymph Node, Pig, Orcein. Elastic fibers are stained reddish-brown with orcein.

FIG. 10–15. Medium Vein, l.s., Lymph Node, Pig. This vein accompanied the artery in Figures 10–13 and 10–14.

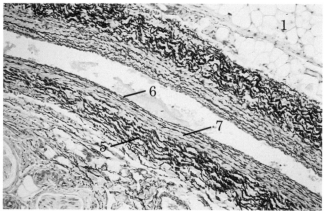

FIG. 10–16   ×62.5

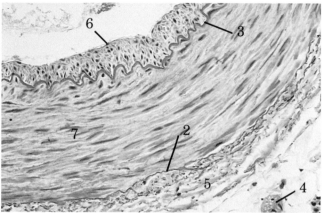

FIG. 10–17   ×125

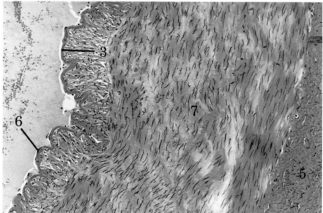

FIG. 10–18   ×62.5

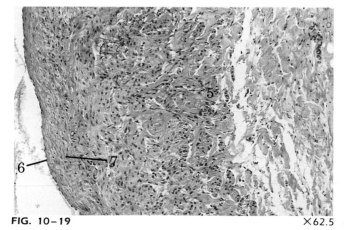

FIG. 10–19   ×62.5

FIG. 10–20   ×25

KEY	
1. Adipose tissue	**6.** Tunica intima, endothelium
2. External elastic membrane	**7.** Tunica media
3. Internal elastic membrane	**8.** Valve
4. Nerve	
5. Tunica adventitia	

FIG. 10–16. Medium Vein, l.s., Lymph Node, Pig, Orcein. Elastic fibers are stained red-brown with orcein.

FIG. 10–17. Medium Artery, x.s., Lymph Node, Cat. Longitudinally oriented smooth muscle is present in the tunica intima between the endothelium and internal elastic membrane.

FIG. 10–18. Renal Artery, Near Aorta, x.s., Pig. Note both an inner and outer layer of smooth muscle in the tunica media. The inner layer is arranged longitudinally.

FIG. 10–19. Portal Vein, x.s., Dog. Note the bundles of longitudinally arranged smooth muscle in the tunica adventitia, a characteristic of large veins.

FIG. 10–20. Vein with Valves, x.s., Lip, Pig.

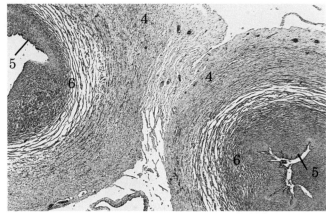

FIG. 10–21   ×12.5

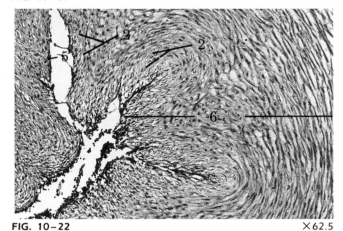

FIG. 10–22   ×62.5

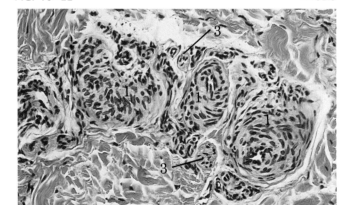

FIG. 10–23   ×125

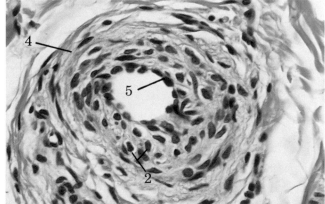

FIG. 10–24   ×250

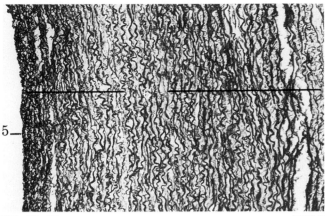

FIG. 10–25   ×62.5

KEY
1. Anastomotic artery
2. Epithelioid cells
3. Nerve
4. Tunica adventitia
5. Tunica intima, endothelium
6. Tunica media

FIG. 10–21. Umbilical Artery (Right) and Vein (Left), x.s., Horse, Masson's. The tunica media of the umbilical artery is thicker than that of the umbilical vein.

FIG. 10–22. Umbilical Artery, x.s., Horse, Masson's. The umbilical artery lacks an internal elastic membrane. The innermost smooth muscle cells of the tunica media are epithelioid (epithelial-like) and oriented longitudinally.

FIG. 10–23. Glomus, Nose, Pig. The highly convoluted anastomotic artery, surrounding connective tissue, and nerves forming this organized arteriovenous anastomosis can be seen.

FIG. 10–24. Arteriovenous Anastomosis, x.s., Lip, Pig. Longitudinally directed smooth muscle cells of the tunica media are characteristically epithelioid (epithelial-like) in an anastomotic artery. These arteries lack an internal elastic membrane and have a small lumen.

FIG. 10–25. Aorta, x.s., Dog, Orcein. This specimen was stained with orcein to emphasize elastic tissue (red-brown).

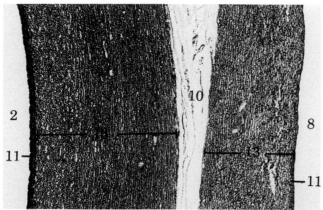

FIG. 10–26   ×12.5

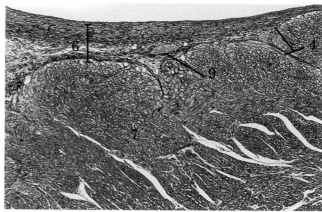

FIG. 10–30   ×25

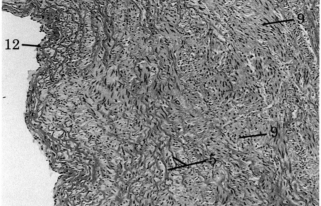

FIG. 10–27   ×62.5

KEY	
1. Adipose tissue	**9.** Smooth muscle
2. Aorta, lumen	**10.** Tunica adventitia
3. Cardiac muscle	**11.** Tunica intima
4. Collagenous fibers	**12.** Tunica intima, endothelium
5. Elastic fibers	**13.** Tunica media
6. Endocardium	**14.** Vasa vasorum
7. Myocardium	
8. Pulmonary artery, lumen	

FIG. 10–26. Aorta (Left) and Pulmonary Artery (Right), x.s., Pig, Orcein. This preparation was stained with orcein to highlight elastic tissue (red-brown).

FIG. 10–27. Pulmonary Artery, x.s., Sheep. Portion of the tunica intima and tunica media. Smooth muscle of the tunica media is oriented in various directions. Wavy, pink elastic fibers occur among the smooth muscle.

FIG. 10–28. Vena Cava, x.s., Dog. This section was taken from a region near the heart. The tunica adventitia consists largely of cardiac muscle and adipose tissue.

FIG. 10–29. Right Auricle, Pig, Orcein. The section was stained with orcein to show the distribution of elastic fibers (red-brown).

FIG. 10–30. Right Auricle, Pig, Mallory's. This preparation shows the distribution of smooth muscle in the endocardium.

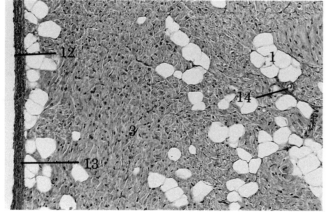

FIG. 10–28   ×62.5

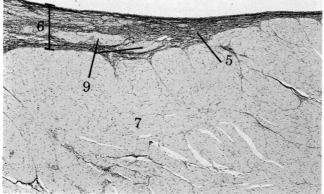

FIG. 10–29   ×25

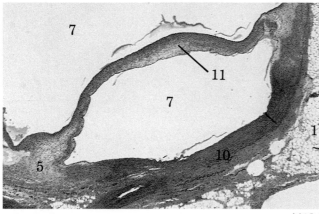

FIG. 10-31 ×12.5

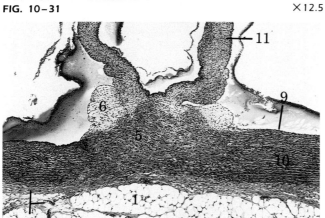

FIG. 10-32 ×25

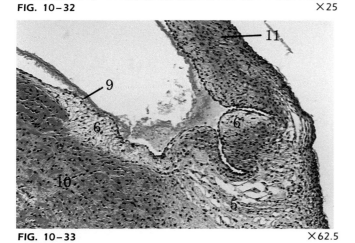

FIG. 10-33 ×62.5

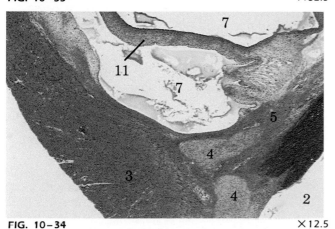

FIG. 10-34 ×12.5

KEY	
1. Adipose tissue	**7.** Pulmonary artery, lumen
2. Aorta, lumen	**8.** Tunica adventitia
3. Atrium, myocardium	**9.** Tunica intima, endothelium
4. Cardiac skeleton, cartilaginous	**10.** Tunica media
5. Cardiac skeleton, fibrous	**11.** Valve
6. Mesenchyme-like tissue	

FIG. 10-31. Pulmonic (Semilunar) Valve, x.s., Dog.
Pulmonic valves are located in the pulmonary artery near the heart. The section shows a portion of the fibrous cardiac skeleton.

FIG. 10-32. Pulmonic (Semilunar) Valve, x.s., Dog, Masson's. Portions of two adjacent pulmonic valves are visible. The connective tissue of the valves and the tunica media of the pulmonary artery blend with the fibrous cardiac skeleton. A cushion of mesenchyme-like connective tissue lies adjacent to the cardiac skeleton.

FIG. 10-33. Pulmonic (Semilunar) Valve, x.s., Dog. The valve consists of a core of dense irregular connective tissue sandwiched between two layers of endothelium.

FIG. 10-34. Pulmonic (Semilunar) Valve, x.s., Dog. A portion of the atrial wall, pulmonary artery, aorta, and cardiac skeleton (cartilaginous and fibrous) are visible.

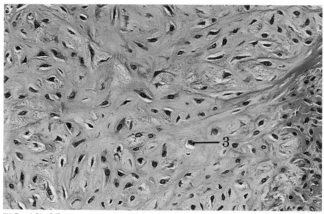

FIG. 10-35   ×125

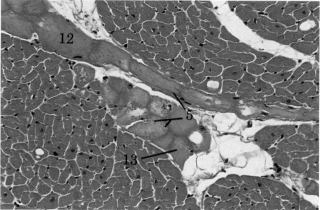

FIG. 10-36   ×125

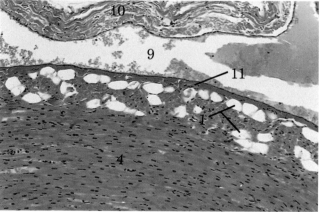

FIG. 10-37   ×62.5

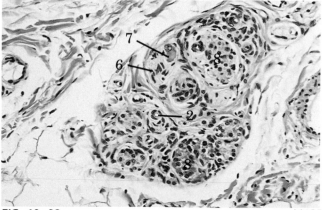

FIG. 10-38   ×125

KEY	
1. Adipose tissue	**8.** Parenchyma cells
2. Arteriole	**9.** Pericardial cavity
3. Chondrocyte	**10.** Pericardium, parietal
4. Myocardium, right ventricle	**11.** Pericardium, visceral
5. Myofibrils	**12.** Purkinje cell, l.s.
6. Nerve	**13.** Purkinje cell, x.s.
7. Neuron cell body	

FIG. 10-35. Cardiac Skeleton, Dog. The cartilaginous portion of the cardiac skeleton of the dog is formed from fibrocartilage containing numerous scattered chondrocytes.

FIG. 10-36. Purkinje Cells, x.s. and l.s., Left Ventricle, Goat. Myofibrils are limited to the periphery of these large, modified cardiac muscle cells.

FIG. 10-37. Visceral and Parietal Pericardium, Cat. The pericardium consists of a mesothelium (simple squamous epithelium) and underlying connective tissue. The mesothelium of the visceral pericardium (epicardium) covers the surface of the heart. The remainder of the pericardial cavity is lined by the mesothelium of the parietal pericardium.

FIG. 10-38. Aortic Body, Pig. The aortic body is located between the pulmonary artery and aorta. It is a small, encapsulated structure containing blood vessels, nerves, and two types of parenchyma cells (see Fig. 10-39).

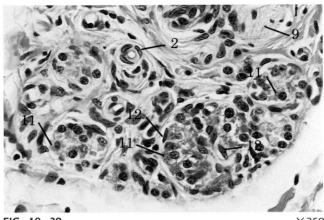

FIG. 10–39   ×250

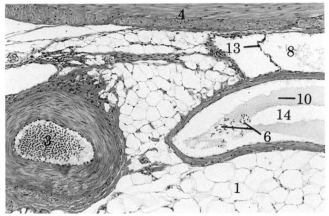

FIG. 10–40   ×62.5

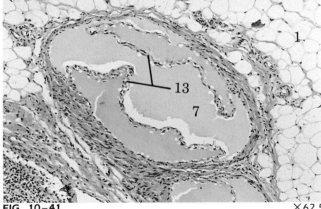

FIG. 10–41   ×62.5

FIG. 10–42   ×62.5

KEY	
1. Adipose tissue	**9.** Nerve
2. Arteriole	**10.** Plasma
3. Artery	**11.** Type I cell
4. Cecum, wall	**12.** Type II cell
5. Endothelium	**13.** Valve
6. Erythrocytes	**14.** Vein
7. Lymph	**15.** Venule
8. Lymphatic vessel	

FIG. 10–39. Aortic Body, Pig. Two types of parenchyma cells can be distinguished in the aortic body. The type I (glomus) cell has a round nucleus and a granular cytoplasm. The type II (sustentacular) cell has few or no cytoplasmic granules and an oval nucleus. Type I cells usually occur in clusters surrounded by Type II cells and connective tissue.

FIG. 10–40. Lymphatic Vessel with Valve, Artery, and Vein, Cecal Tonsil, Chicken. Lymphatic vessels have a large lumen and a relatively thin wall. Valves may be present.

FIG. 10–41. Lymphatic Vessel with Valve, Lymph Node, Pig. The valves of lymphatic vessels consist of a connective tissue core surrounded on each side by an endothelium.

FIG. 10–42. Large Lymphatic Vessel, Submucosa, Cecum, Horse. The wall of the lymphatic vessel consists of an endothelium surrounded by a small amount of connective tissue. The latter blends with the connective tissue of the submucosa.

CARDIOVASCULAR SYSTEM   **63**

LYMPHATIC SYSTEM

Lymphatic tissue consists predominantly of lymphocytes. These and a variable number of plasma cells, macrophages, and other cells occur among a framework of reticular cells and fibers. In H&E preparations, lymphatic tissue appears purple because of numerous small lymphocytes, each with a basophilic nucleus and little cytoplasm.

MAMMALS

Diffuse lymphatic tissue is characterized by a moderate concentration of scattered lymphocytes. A round, oval, or irregularly circumscribed aggregation of mostly small, densely packed lymphocytes is called a **lymphatic nodule.** A nodule may contain a central pale area, the **germinal center.** Because the majority of cells of the germinal center are larger lymphocytes with more cytoplasm and lightly-staining nuclei, this region appears pale in contrast with the dense **corona** (marginal zone, peripheral zone) of small lymphocytes. Diffuse lymphatic tissue and lymphatic nodules are components of most lymphatic organs. They also appear in the connective tissue of the digestive, respiratory, urinary, and reproductive organs, among other locations.

Aggregations of lymphatic nodules form **Peyer's patches** in the lamina propria and submucosa of the small intestine, particularly the ileum.

Tonsils are collections of lymphatic nodules and diffuse lymphatic tissue. They occur in the connective tissue below the epithelium in specific regions of the tongue, pharynx, and larynx. **Tonsils with crypts** (follicular tonsils) are characterized by deep invaginations of the surface epithelium called crypts. A crypt with its associated lymphatic tissue constitutes a **tonsillar follicle,** and several follicles form the tonsil. Examples of tonsils with crypts include the following: **lingual tonsils** of the horse, pig, and cow; **tubal tonsils** of the pig; **paraepiglottic tonsils** of the pig, sheep, and goat; **palatine tonsils** of the horse, pig, and ruminant. In the palatine tonsils of ruminants, the crypts lead into a common sinus, which then opens onto the surface. **Tonsils without crypts** have a smooth, somewhat folded, or bulging surface but lack deep invaginations of the epithelium. **Tubal tonsils** of ruminants, the **paraepiglottic tonsil** of the cat, and **palatine tonsils** of carnivores are examples. Salivary glands associated with tonsils are typically mucous, except in carnivores, where they are mixed (mucous and serous combined).

A **lymph node** contains diffuse and nodular lymphatic tissue and lymphatic sinuses that are organized into a cortical and medullary region. Lymphatic nodules occupy the **cortex** and may be particularly large in cows. Diffuse lymphatic tissue occurs between the nodules and in the **deep cortex** (paracortex), and continues inward as **medullary cords** containing lymphocytes, other leukocytes, macrophages, and plasma cells.

A **capsule** of connective tissue, with some smooth muscle and elastic fibers, covers the lymph node. Parts of the capsule extend inward as **trabeculae.** Lymph flows through communicating channels, from afferent lymphatic vessels that enter the capsule, through the **subcapsular and cortical sinuses** of the cortex, to **medullary sinuses** that lead to efferent lymphatic vessels at the hilus. The sinuses are less cellular than the parenchyma and appear as light areas. They are lined by a discontinuous endothelium, spanned by a webwork of cytoplasmic processes of reticular cells, and contain some free cells such as lymphocytes and macrophages.

Most blood vessels enter and leave the node from the hilus. Unique vessels of the deep cortex, **postcapillary venules,** are lined by elongated cells that appear cuboidal in cross section. Lymphocytes are frequently seen migrating between these cells.

Not all lymph nodes have a typical appearance. The amount or arrangement of cortical and medullary tissue can vary. The lymph node of the pig is characteristically atypical, with the location of the cortical and medullary tissue, as well as the flow of lymph, being reversed.

Hemal nodes occur along blood vessels of ruminants. They are characterized by blood-filled sinuses between cellular cords. Connective tissue and some smooth mus-cle form the capsule and trabeculae (which are sparse). Hemal nodes lack lymphatic vessels. **Hemolymph nodes,** in contrast, have lymphatic vessels and their sinuses receive a mixture of blood and lymph.

The **capsule** of the **spleen** is rich in smooth muscle and elastic fibers. In horses and cows, two or three layers of muscle are oriented perpendicular to each other, while in carnivores, pigs, sheep, and goats, the muscle fibers are interwoven. The capsule is thickest in the horse and cow, and thinnest in carnivores. **Trabeculae,** which continue inward from the capsule, tend to be especially large in cows and sheep.

The parenchyma of the spleen is divisible into the white and red pulp. Dense accumulations of lymphocytes, arranged around central arteries, form the **periarterial lymphatic sheaths** (PALS). These, along with lymphatic nodules, comprise the **white pulp.** White pulp appears purple in H&E preparations because of the density of numerous small lymphocytes. **Red pulp,** because of the large numbers of erythrocytes it contains in its reticular meshwork and vessels, appears red overall.

The **splenic artery** enters the hilus of the spleen and branches into **trabecular arteries.** As these enter the parenchyma of the spleen and become surrounded by white pulp, they are called **central arteries** (not necessarily located in the center of the PALS). On leaving the white pulp, the central artery branches into a group of **pulp arteries.** These, in turn, branch into two or three **arterioles,** which terminate in two or more **capillaries.** Commonly, the pulp arteries and their branches are called a **penicillus** because, collectively, they resemble the bristles of an artist's brush. A portion of the capillaries of the penicillus becomes surrounded by concentric layers of macrophages contained in a reticular framework. These cellular and fibrous thickenings are called **ellipsoids** (pericapillary macrophage sheaths). The term **sheathed capillary** is used by some authors for the combined unit consisting of the capillary and the ellipsoid. Ellipsoids are especially abundant in the **marginal zone,** the region between the red and white pulp. They are very large and numerous in pigs. The capillaries of the ellipsoids continue as terminal arterial capillaries. Arterial capillaries may join venous sinuses or pulp veins (closed circulation), or they may empty first into the spaces of the reticular meshwork of the red pulp (open circulation).

The spleen of the dog is a **sinusal** spleen. The red pulp contains typical **venous** (splenic, vascular) **sinuses.** These are wide channels lined by elongated, longitudinally oriented endothelial cells. The spleens of the cat, horse, pig, and ruminant are classified as **nonsinusal,** having poorly developed or no sinuses. Wisps of smooth muscle in the red pulp are most numerous in pigs and ruminants.

The **thymus** is covered by a thin connective tissue capsule that projects inward as **septa,** partially dividing the organ into **lobules.** The parenchyma of each lobule is organized into a **cortex** of mostly small, densely packed lymphocytes and a **medulla** with fewer and larger lymphocytes. The medulla is continuous between lobules. The thymus lacks lymphatic nodules and is supported by a unique cytoreticulum of stellate, epithelial reticular cells and only a few reticular fibers. **Hassall's** (thymic) **corpuscles** are a special feature of the thymus and occur in the medulla. They are acidophilic, concentric whorls of flattened reticular cells that may become swollen, keratinized, and calcified centrally. With age, much of the thymus becomes replaced by adipose tissue.

CHICKEN

Lymph nodes are absent in the chicken, although diffuse lymphatic tissue and lymphatic nodules are widespread.

The **spleen** is covered by a muscular capsule as in mammals, but lacks trabeculae. Areas of red and white pulp are less distinct than those of the mammalian spleen. **White pulp** is diffusely scattered throughout the spleen and is composed primarily of small lymphocytes. It contains **sheathed arteries** and, occasionally, lymphatic nodules. **Red pulp** is formed from venous sinuses and anastomosing cords of reticular cells, macrophages, lymphocytes, and blood cells.

As in mammals, the **thymus** is arranged into incompletely separated lobules of cortical and medullary tissue. Typical Hassall's corpuscles, similar to those found in mammals, are seen infrequently. Instead, diffuse forms of Hassall's corpuscles, called **reticular structures**, are abundant in the medulla. These are pale, irregular masses of reticular cells with vesicles that contain acidophilic material and degenerating cells. **Myoid cells,** characterized by a fibrous cytoplasm, also lie in the medulla.

The **bursa of Fabricius** is a sac-like dorsal diverticulum of the proctodeum that is unique to birds. It is characterized by tall, thick mucosal **folds** (plicae) filled with numerous polyhedral **follicles.** Each follicle, composed of lymphatic tissue, is divided into a **cortex** and **medulla.** A layer of **undifferentiated epithelial cells** occupies the periphery of the medulla, which is separated from the cortex by a **capillary layer.** The bursa is lined by a pseudostratified columnar epithelium, except at the apex of each follicle, which is covered by a simple columnar **epithelial tuft.**

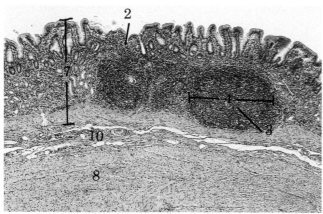

FIG. 11–1 ×25

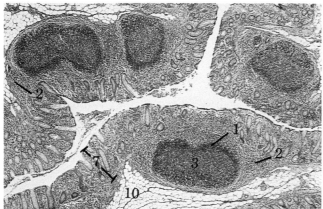

FIG. 11–2 ×12.5

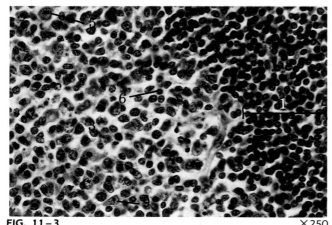

FIG. 11–3 ×250

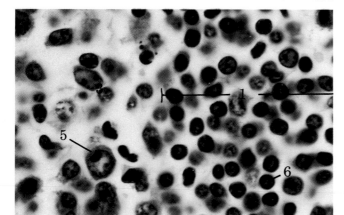

FIG. 11–4 ×250

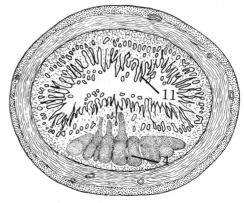

FIG. 11–5

KEY		
1. Corona		**7.** Mucosa
2. Diffuse lymphatic tissue		**8.** Muscularis externa
3. Germinal center		**9.** Reticular cell
4. Lymphatic nodule		**10.** Submucosa
5. Lymphocyte, large		**11.** Villus
6. Lymphocyte, small		

FIG. 11–1. Lymphatic Nodules and Diffuse Lymphatic Tissue, Pyloric Stomach, Cat. Dense aggregations of lymphocytes form lymphatic nodules in the lamina propria.

FIG. 11–2. Lymphatic Nodules and Diffuse Lymphatic Tissue, Colon, x.s., Pig. The mucosa and submucosa contain diffuse lymphatic tissue and large lymphatic nodules with germinal centers. Lymphatic nodules are especially numerous in the digestive tract of the pig.

FIG. 11–3. Lymphatic Nodule, Colon, Pig. Cells of the germinal center and corona. Many small lymphocytes occur in the peripheral corona; fewer and larger cells are seen in the germinal center.

FIG. 11–4. Lymphatic Nodule, Colon, Pig. Detail of cells of the germinal center and corona. Small lymphocytes are characterized by a heterochromatic nucleus and scant cytoplasm.

FIG. 11–5. Peyer's Patch, Ileum, x.s., Cat. A Peyer's patch is an aggregation of lymphatic nodules in the lamina propria and submucosa of the small intestine.

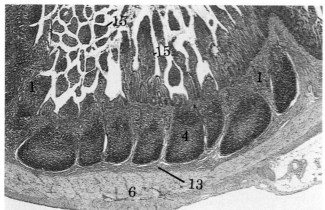

FIG. 11–6 ×12.5

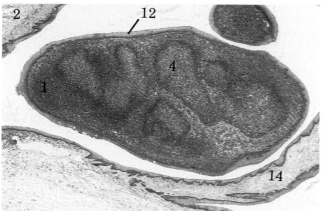

FIG. 11–7 ×12.5

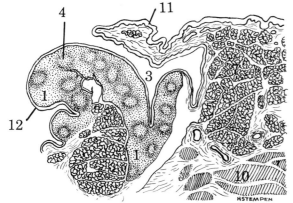

FIG. 11–8

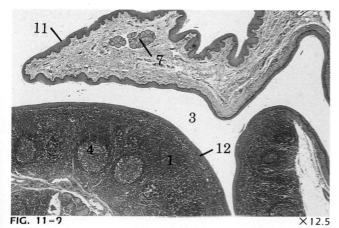

FIG. 11–9 ×12.5

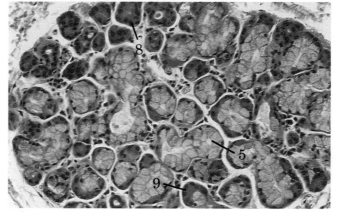

FIG. 11–10 ×125

KEY	
1. Diffuse lymphatic tissue	**10.** Skeletal muscle
2. Epiglottis	**11.** Stratified squamous
3. Fossa	epithelium, semilunar fold
4. Lymphatic nodule	**12.** Stratified squamous
5. Mucous acinus	epithelium, tonsil
6. Muscularis externa	**13.** Submucosa
7. Salivary glands	**14.** Vestibular fold
8. Serous acinus	**15.** Villus
9. Serous demilune	

FIG. 11–6. Peyer's Patch, Ileum, x.s., Dog. Eight lymphatic nodules of a portion of a Peyer's patch are visible in this section.

FIG. 11–7. Paraepiglottic Tonsil, Larynx, l.s., Cat. In the cat, an accumulation of lymphatic tissue in the lateral wall of the larynx, between the epiglottis and the vestibular fold, forms a tonsil without crypts.

FIG. 11–8. Palatine Tonsil, Dog. In the dog, the entire tonsil lies within a fossa (a small hollow), and is covered in part by a semilunar fold. The palatine tonsils of carnivores lack crypts.

FIG. 11–9. Palatine Tonsil, Dog. A portion of a tonsil and semilunar fold.

FIG. 11–10. Palatine Tonsil, Dog. Mixed salivary glands are associated with the wall of the tonsils in carnivores. In other species, only mucous glands are present.

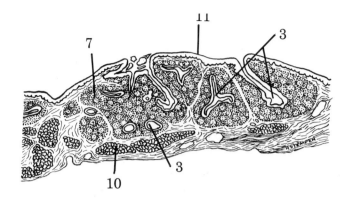

FIG. 11–11

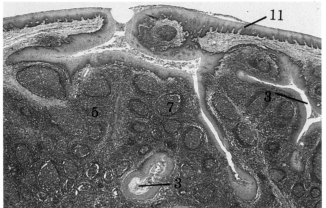

FIG. 11–12   ×12.5

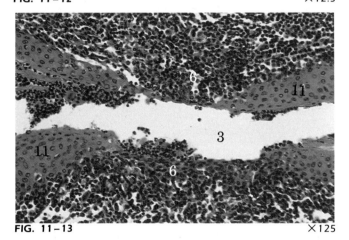

FIG. 11–13   ×125

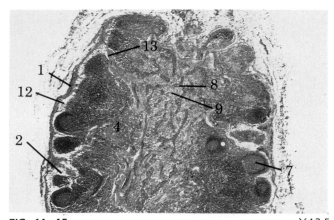

FIG. 11–15   ×12.5

KEY	
1. Capsule	**8.** Medullary cord
2. Cortical sinus	**9.** Medullary sinus
3. Crypt	**10.** Salivary glands, mucous
4. Deep cortex	**11.** Stratified squamous
5. Diffuse lymphatic tissue	epithelium
6. Leukocyte infiltration	**12.** Subcapsular sinus
7. Lymphatic nodule	**13.** Trabecula

FIG. 11–11. Palatine Tonsil, Horse. The palatine tonsils of noncarnivores have crypts (surface invaginations lined by stratified squamous epithelium).

FIG. 11–12. Palatine Tonsil, Horse. Note that the continuity of each crypt with the surface is not always evident.

FIG. 11–13. Palatine Tonsil, Horse. Lymphocytes and other leukocytes have infiltrated and partly obliterated the epithelial lining of this crypt.

FIG. 11–14. Lymph Node, Cow. The lymph node is surrounded by a capsule. Trabeculae project inward from the capsule. The cortex contains sinuses, diffuse lymphatic tissue, and lymphatic nodules. The medulla is composed of medullary cords and sinuses.

FIG. 11–15. Lymph Node, Dog.

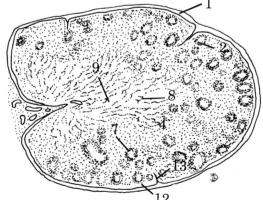

FIG. 11–14

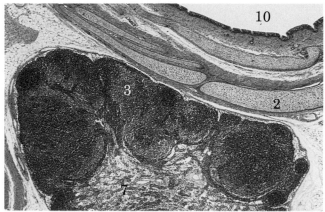

FIG. 11-16 ×12.5

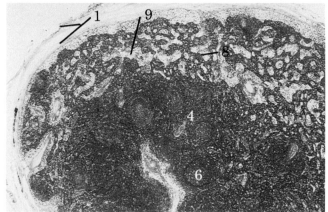

FIG. 11-17 ×12.5

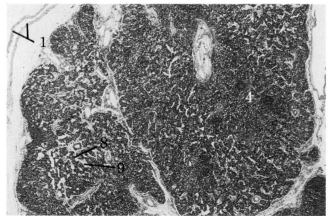

FIG. 11-18 ×12.5

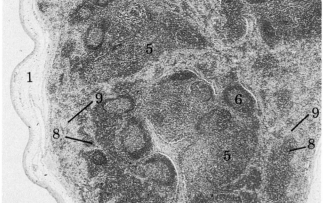

FIG. 11-19 ×12.5

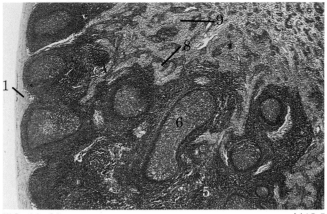

FIG. 11-20 ×12.5

KEY	
1. Capsule	**6.** Lymphatic nodule
2. Cartilage plate, bronchus	**7.** Medulla, lymph node
3. Cortex, lymph node	**8.** Medullary cord
4. Cortical tissue	**9.** Medullary sinus
5. Diffuse lymphatic tissue	**10.** Primary bronchus, lumen

FIG. 11-16. Tracheobronchial Lymph Node, Dog. This lymph node is adjacent to the wall of a primary bronchus near the tracheal bifurcation.

FIG. 11-17. Lymph Node, Horse. The arrangement of cortical and medullary tissues may be atypical in some of the lymph nodes of mammals. In the example shown, the distribution of cortical and medullary components is the reverse of that commonly expected.

FIG. 11-18. Lymph Node, Horse. Not only is the arrangement of cortical and medullary components reversed in this section, but the proportion of the medullary tissue is much greater than usual.

FIG. 11-19. Lymph Node, Pig. The lymph nodes of pigs consistently show an atypical pattern. In this section, cortical tissue is predominantly central, while medullary tissue occurs both superficially and internally.

FIG. 11-20. Lymph Node, Cow. The lymph node of the cow is often characterized by the presence of large lymphatic nodules.

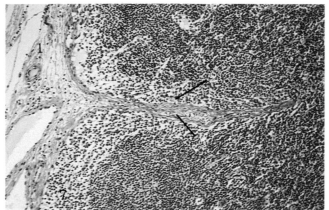

FIG. 11-21   ×62.5

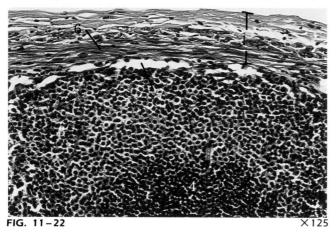

FIG. 11-22   ×125

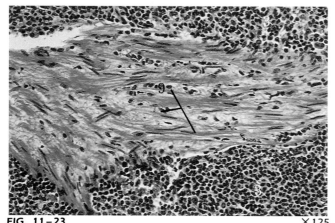

FIG. 11-23   ×125

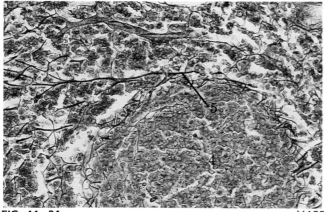

FIG. 11-24   ×125

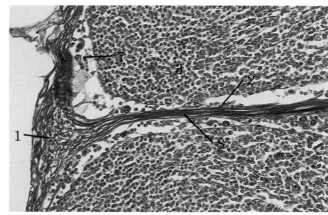

FIG. 11-25   ×125

KEY	
1. Capsule	**5.** Reticular fiber
2. Cortical sinus	**6.** Smooth muscle
3. Diffuse lymphatic tissue	**7.** Subcapsular sinus
4. Lymphatic nodule	**8.** Trabecula

FIG. 11-21. Cortex, Lymph Node, Horse. The subcapsular sinus below the capsule continues as cortical sinuses that parallel the trabeculae through the cortex.

FIG. 11-22. Cortex, Lymph Node, Cow, Masson's. The inner portion of the capsule contains smooth muscle (pink).

FIG. 11-23. Cortex, Lymph Node, Cow. The trabecula contains smooth muscle.

FIG. 11-24. Cortex, Lymph Node, Cow, Silver. A network of fine, branching reticular fibers provides a supportive framework for the diffuse and nodular lymphatic tissue.

FIG. 11-25. Cortex, Lymph Node, Sheep, Mallory's. Continuity of the subcapsular sinus with the cortical sinus is evident.

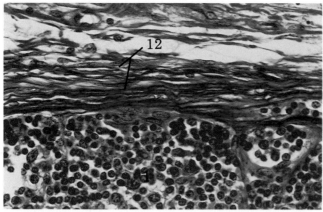

FIG. 11–26 ×250

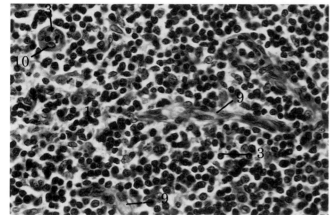

FIG. 11–27 ×250

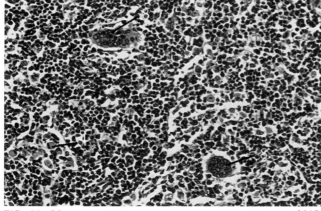

FIG. 11–28 ×125

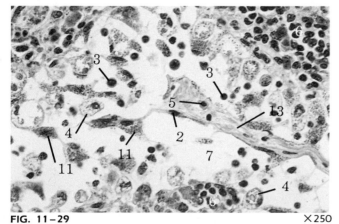

FIG. 11–29 ×250

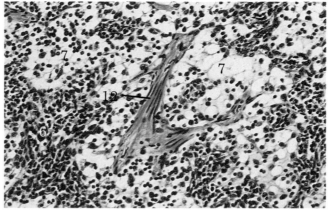

FIG. 11–30 ×125

KEY		
1. Diffuse lymphatic tissue	**8.** Multinucleate giant cell
2. Endothelial cell, nucleus	**9.** Postcapillary venule, l.s.
3. Lymphocyte	**10.** Postcapillary venule, x.s.
4. Macrophage	**11.** Reticular cell
5. Mast cell	**12.** Smooth muscle
6. Medullary cord	**13.** Trabecula
7. Medullary sinus	

FIG. 11–26. Cortex, Lymph Node, Sheep, Mallory's. Smooth muscle cells (pink) among collagenous fibers (blue) of the capsule.

FIG. 11–27. Deep Cortex, Lymph Node, Dog. Postcapillary venules, l.s. and x.s. These vessels are lined by elongated cells that appear cuboidal in cross section. Lymphocytes migrate between the endothelial cells of the postcapillary venules.

FIG. 11–28. Cortex, Lymph Node, Horse. Multinucleate giant cells, derived from macrophages, are sometimes found in lymph nodes.

FIG. 11–29. Medulla, Lymph Node, Cow. In this preparation, reticular cells, endothelial cells, and macrophages contain numerous pigment granules.

FIG. 11–30. Medulla, Lymph Node, Sheep. Smooth muscle is distributed throughout the medullary sinuses.

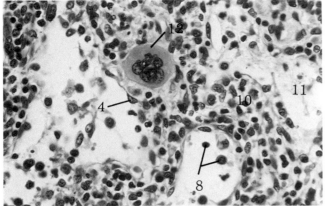

FIG. 11–31   ×250

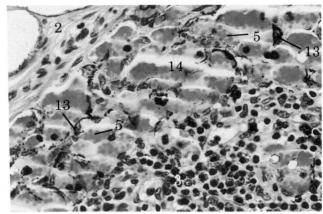

FIG. 11–34   ×250

KEY	
1. Adipose tissue	**9.** Macrophage with
2. Capsule	erythrocytes
3. Diffuse lymphatic tissue	**10.** Medullary cord
4. Endothelial cell, nucleus	**11.** Medullary sinus
5. Erythrocytes	**12.** Megakaryocyte
6. Granulocyte	**13.** Reticular cell
7. Lymphatic nodule	**14.** Subcapsular sinus
8. Lymphocyte	

FIG. 11–31. Medulla, Lymph Node, Dog. Cellular medullary cords surround medullary sinuses that are lined incompletely by endothelial cells. A megakaryocyte is present in a medullary cord.

FIG. 11–32. Medulla, Lymph Node, Dog. Macrophages containing phagocytized erythrocytes are evident in the medullary sinuses.

FIG. 11–33. Hemal Node, Sheep. The general organization is much like that of a lymph node, but the sinuses are filled with blood. Lymphatic nodules are scarce, and connective tissue trabeculae are not apparent.

FIG. 11–34. Hemal Node, Sheep. The subcapsular (marginal) sinus is filled with blood. Reticular cells of the sinus contain phagocytized material.

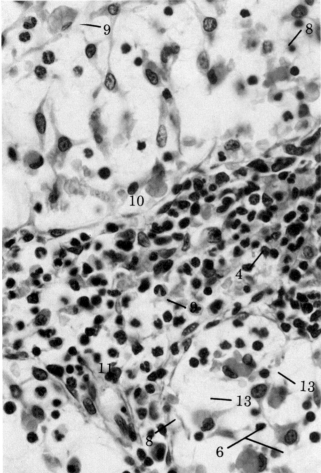

FIG. 11–32   ×360

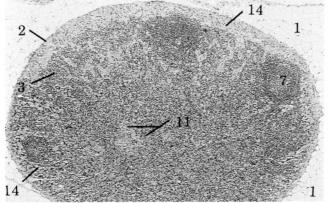

FIG. 11–33   ×25

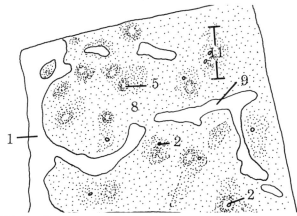

FIG. 11−35

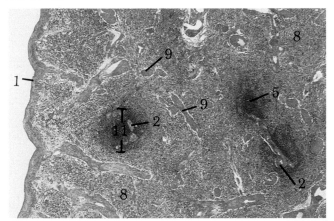

FIG. 11−36　　　　　　　　　　×12.5

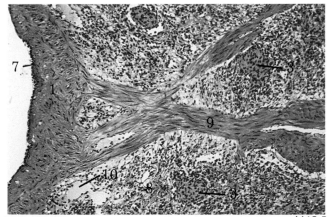

FIG. 11−37　　　　　　　　　　×62.5

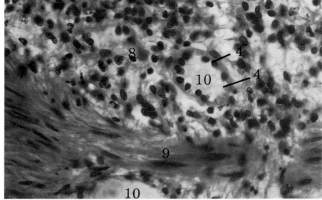

FIG. 11−38　　　　　　　　　　×250

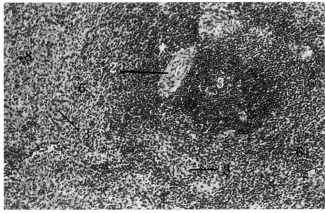

FIG. 11−39　　　　　　　　　　×62.5

KEY	
1. Capsule	**7.** Mesothelium
2. Central artery	**8.** Red pulp
3. Ellipsoid	**9.** Trabecula
4. Endothelial cell	**10.** Venous sinus
5. Lymphatic nodule	**11.** White pulp
6. Marginal zone	

FIG. 11−35. Spleen, Dog. This drawing is of a small portion of the spleen.

FIG. 11−36. Spleen, Dog. The parenchyma of the spleen is organized into red pulp and white pulp (periarterial lymphatic sheaths and lymphatic nodules). Trabeculae extend inward from the capsule and are seen throughout the red pulp.

FIG. 11−37. Spleen, Dog. Note the smooth muscle in the capsule and trabeculae. The spleen of the dog is a sinusal spleen, containing venous sinuses (see Fig. 11−38).

FIG. 11−38. Spleen, Dog. Venous sinuses are lined by longitudinally oriented, elongated endothelial cells. The nuclei may or may not be apparent in cross sections of such lining cells. Erythrocytes fill the sinuses and the spaces of the red pulp.

FIG. 11−39. Spleen, Dog. Ellipsoids can be seen in the marginal zone between the periarterial lymphatic sheath (white pulp) and the red pulp. They are also present in the red pulp.

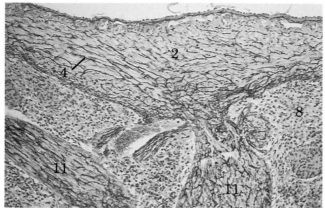

FIG. 11–40 ×125

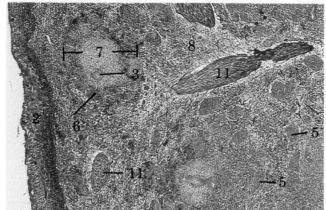

FIG. 11–41 ×25

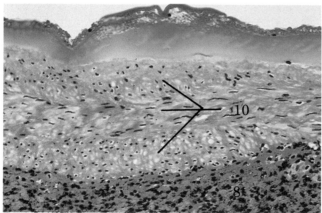

FIG. 11–42 ×62.5

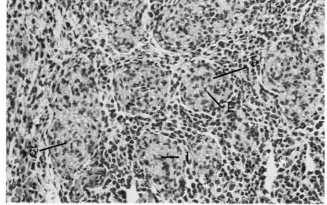

FIG. 11–43 ×125

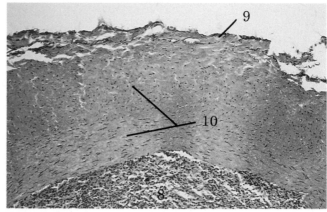

FIG. 11–44 ×62.5

KEY	
1. Capillary lumen	**7.** Periarterial lymphatic
2. Capsule	sheath
3. Central artery	**8.** Red pulp
4. Elastic fiber	**9.** Serosa
5. Ellipsoid	**10.** Smooth muscle
6. Marginal zone	**11.** Trabecula

FIG. 11–40. Capsule, Spleen, Horse. The capsule of the spleen of the horse and cow contains smooth muscle arranged in perpendicular layers oriented at right angles to each other, rather than interwoven as in carnivores, pigs, sheep, and goats. In this preparation, there are three distinct layers of muscle. Compare with Figures 11–37, 11–44, and 11–45.

FIG. 11–41. Spleen, Pig, Mallory's. Ellipsoids are abundant in the pig. These are especially numerous in the vicinity of the marginal zone of a periarterial lymphatic sheath.

FIG. 11–42. Spleen, Pig, Orcein. The capsule and trabeculae are rich in elastic fibers (red-brown).

FIG. 11–43. Spleen, Pig. Ellipsoids are especially abundant in the spleen of the pig. Each consists of macrophages and reticular fibers that surround a capillary.

FIG. 11–44. Capsule, Spleen, Cow. The capsule contains two thick layers of smooth muscle arranged perpendicular to each other.

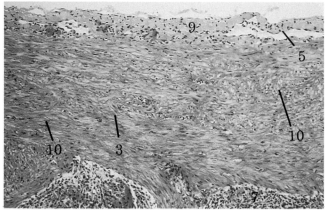

FIG. 11–45 ×62.5

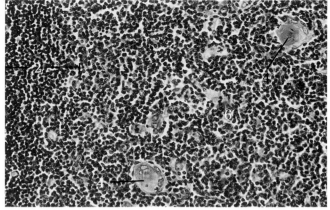

FIG. 11–49 ×125

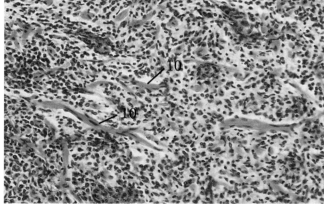

FIG. 11–46 ×25

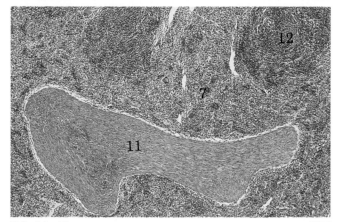

FIG. 11–47 ×125

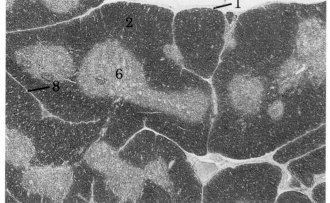

FIG. 11–40 ×12.5

KEY	
1. Capsule	**7.** Red pulp
2. Cortex	**8.** Septum
3. Elastic fiber	**9.** Serosa
4. Hassall's corpuscle	**10.** Smooth muscle
5. Lymphatic vessel	**11.** Trabecula
6. Medulla	**12.** White pulp

FIG. 11–45. Capsule, Spleen, Sheep. In sheep, the bulk of the capsule contains many interwoven smooth muscle cells. The smooth muscle in the capsule of the spleen of carnivores (Fig. 11–37), pigs, and goats has a similar arrangement (compare with Figs. 11–40 and 11–44). Elastic fibers can be observed as faint pink spirals.

FIG. 11–46. Spleen, Sheep. Note the thick trabecula. Characteristically, the spleens of cows and sheep have thick trabeculae (compare with Fig. 11–41).

FIG. 11–47. Red Pulp, Spleen, Sheep. Wisps of smooth muscle are scattered throughout the red pulp.

FIG. 11–48. Thymus, Puppy. A thin connective tissue capsule covers the thymus. Lobules, incompletely divided by connective tissue septa, consist of an outer, dark cortex and an inner, pale medulla. The medulla is continuous between adjacent lobules.

FIG. 11–49. Thymus, Puppy. Portion of the medulla and cortex. The cortex consists predominantly of small lymphocytes. The lymphocytes of the medulla are larger and less abundant. The medulla contains concentrically arranged, swollen and keratinized reticular cells that form Hassall's corpuscles, which are characteristic of the thymus.

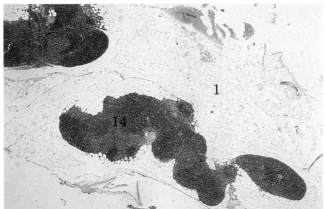

FIG. 11–50 ×12.5

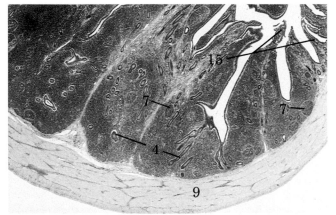

FIG. 11–51 ×12.5

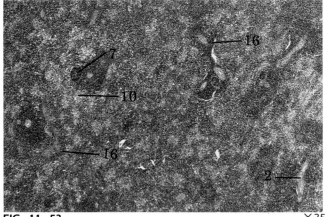

FIG. 11–52 ×25

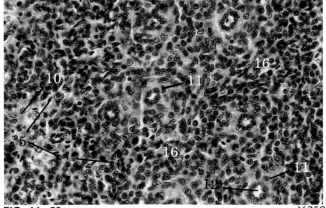

FIG. 11–53 ×250

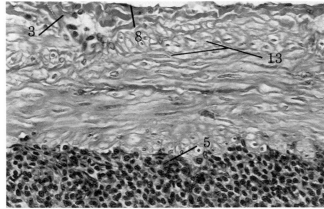

FIG. 11–54 ×250

KEY	
1. Adipose tissue	**9.** Muscularis externa
2. Blood vessel	**10.** Red pulp
3. Connective tissue	**11.** Reticular cell
4. Crypt of Lieberkühn	**12.** Sheathed artery, lumen
5. Erythrocyte	**13.** Smooth muscle
6. Granulocyte	**14.** Thymic tissue
7. Lymphatic nodule	**15.** Villus
8. Mesothelium	**16.** White pulp

FIG. 11–50. Thymus, Cat (old). In older animals, functional thymic tissue is largely supplanted by adipose tissue.

FIG. 11–51. Cecal Tonsil, x.s., Chicken. The accumulation of diffuse and nodular lymphatic tissue in the lamina propria and submucosa near the opening of each cecum is called the cecal tonsil.

FIG. 11–52. Spleen, Chicken. Red pulp (pink) intermingles with white pulp (purple). The white pulp contains a few lymphatic nodules. Connective tissue trabeculae are absent.

FIG. 11–53. Spleen, Chicken. Sheathed arteries, x.s., in white pulp. These vessels are lined by plump endothelial cells surrounded by reticular cells.

FIG. 11–54. Capsule, Spleen, Chicken. Layers of smooth muscle make up a substantial part of the capsule.

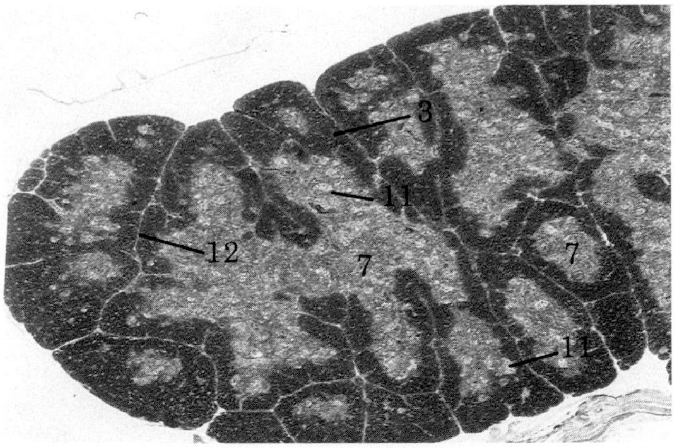

FIG. 11–55 ×12.5

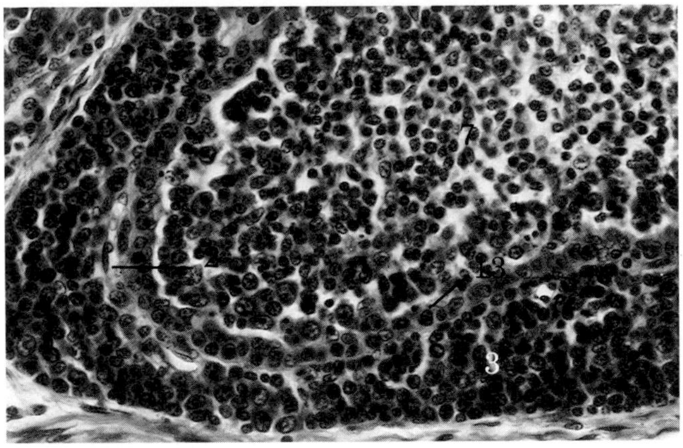

FIG. 11–59 ×250

KEY

1. Bursa, lumen	**9.** Myoid cell
2. Capillary layer	**10.** Pseudostratified epithelium
3. Cortex	**11.** Reticular structure
4. Epithelial tuft	**12.** Septum
5. Follicle	**13.** Undifferentiated epithelial cell
6. Lamina propria	**14.** Vesicle
7. Medulla	
8. Muscularis	

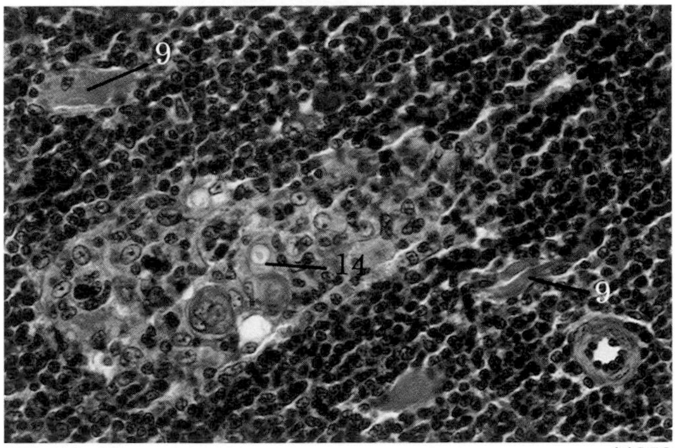

FIG. 11–56 ×250

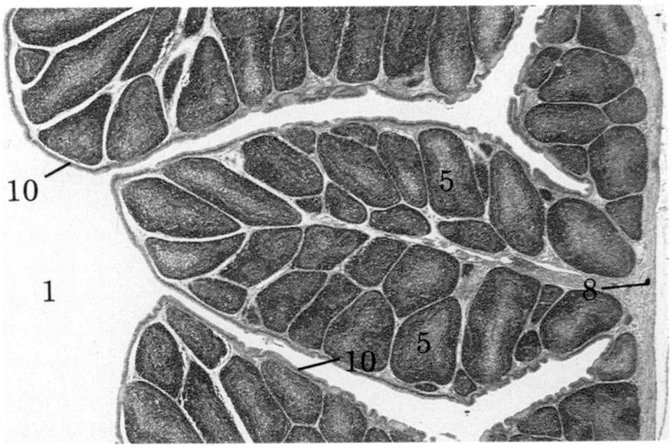

FIG. 11–57 ×12.5

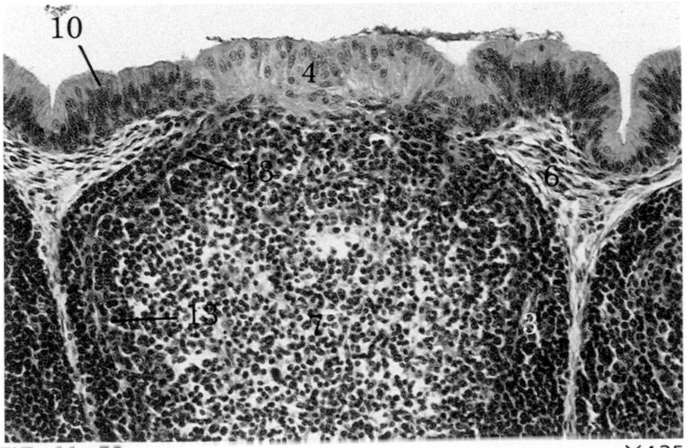

FIG. 11–58 ×125

FIG. 11–55. Thymus, Chicken. The thymus is similar to that of mammals. The pale areas throughout the medullary regions of the lobules are called reticular structures. See Figure 11–56.

FIG. 11–56. Medulla, Thymus, Chicken. Myoid cells, cut obliquely, are characterized by a fibrous cytoplasm and peripheral nuclei. The pale-staining reticular structure in this section is considered a diffuse form of a Hassall's corpuscle. It consists of diffuse groups of reticular cells and scattered vesicles. The vesicles may contain eosinophilic material or degenerating cells.

FIG. 11–57. Bursa, Chicken. Portions of the long mucosal folds (plicae) project into the lumen of the bursa. Numerous follicles, each composed of a cortex and medulla, fill the lamina propria of each fold.

FIG. 11–58. Bursa, Chicken. Where the apex of a follicle contacts the epithelium, tall, pale columnar cells with apical nuclei form an epithelial tuft. Elsewhere, mucosal folds are lined by a pseudostratified columnar epithelium.

FIG. 11–59. Bursa, Chicken. A portion of a follicle. The darkly stained cortex is composed mostly of many small lymphocytes. The paler medulla contains fewer cells of various sizes. A layer of undifferentiated epithelial cells, which are cuboidal with an acidophilic cytoplasm, occupies the periphery of the medulla. A capillary network separates the cortex and the medulla.

INTEGUMENT

The integument includes the skin and its derivatives. Skin consists of an epidermis and dermis joined to underlying structures, such as muscle and bone, by the subcutis (subcutaneous tissue). Sweat, sebaceous, and mammary glands, as well as hair and feather follicles, are epidermal structures that are located in the dermis and subcutis. The highly keratinized claws and hooves of mammals and the beak, claws, and scales of fowl are also skin derivatives.

MAMMALS

The **epidermis** of **thick skin** is a keratinized stratified squamous epithelium. The **stratum basale** is a single layer of cuboidal to columnar cells that lies on a basement membrane adjacent to the dermis. These cells give rise to the **stratum spinosum,** a layer of variable thickness, whose polygonal cells become squamous toward the surface. Cells of the **stratum granulosum** contain basophilic keratohyalin granules in their cytoplasm. The **stratum lucidum** is a thin, pale eosinophilic, translucent layer. It is limited to regions where the epidermis is very thick, such as the digital pads of carnivores. In structures composed of hard keratin (rather than soft keratin), such as hooves and claws, both the stratum granulosum and stratum lucidum are absent. The most superficial layer of skin, the **stratum corneum,** is composed of dead, keratinized squamous cells that slough from the surface. Cytokinesis of cells of the stratum basale and stratum spinosum allows continued growth of the epidermis.

The epidermis of **thin skin** is composed of relatively few cells, but the number varies with the location. Thin skin lacks a stratum lucidum. The stratum granulosum is not always evident.

The **dermis** consists of loose and dense irregular connective tissue containing blood vessels, lymphatic vessels, and nerves. In thick skin, the superficial, loose connective tissue of the dermis, the **papillary layer,** forms projections called **dermal papillae** that interdigitate with the epidermis and serve to anchor the two layers. The deep layer of dense irregular connective tissue is called the **reticular layer.** Dermal papillae are reduced or absent in thin skin. For this reason, when both loose and dense irregular connective tissue layers can be distinguished in the dermis of thin skin, they are best referred to as the superficial and deep layers, respectively.

Hairs are associated with regions of the body covered by thin skin. They arise from **germinal (matrix) cells of the hair bulb** at the base of the follicle. A hair near its origin consists of a central **medulla** of cuboidal cells, a **cortex** of flattened cells oriented parallel to the long axis of the hair, and an outer **cuticle.** As the cells of the hair are pushed toward the surface, they become keratinized. The cuticle consists of scale-like cells that partially overlap so that their free edges are directed upward. Within the hair, the medulla may become reduced distally, and is absent entirely in wool hairs.

Hair follicles are set obliquely in the dermis or subcutis, although in sheep they tend to be vertical. A vascular **dermal papilla** projects into the hair bulb. **Melanocytes,** located close to the dermal papilla among matrix cells, have cytoplasmic processes that provide pigment to the hair cells. The germinal cells of the matrix, in addition to forming hair, give rise to the **inner root sheath** of the follicle. The **cuticle of the inner root sheath** is composed of overlapping, scale-like cells similar to those of the cuticle of the hair, but their free edges are directed downward, so that the hair and inner root sheath interlock. The inner root sheath becomes keratinized and tapers distally, ending near where sebaceous glands open into the follicle. The peripheral **external root sheath** represents a downward continuation of the epidermis. A **connective tissue** (dermal) **sheath** abuts the **basement** (glassy) **membrane** of the external root sheath, surrounds the follicle, and blends with the rest of the dermal connective tissue. The **arrector pili muscle** (smooth muscle) attaches to the connective tissue sheath of the follicle and the superficial layer of the dermis.

Single (simple) **hair follicles** are evenly distributed in the skin of horses and ruminants and occur in groups of three in pigs. In carnivores, most of the follicles are **compound follicles.** Each compound follicle is formed from a single primary follicle and several secondary follicles. The follicles unite at the level of the openings of the sebaceous glands, forming a common follicle, which extends from the point of union to the skin surface. The hairs that are produced exit as a group to the surface through the common follicular opening. **Sinus** (tactile) **hairs** are limited to the face region. They are produced by large follicles that are well innervated and that contain blood-filled sinuses within their connective tissue sheaths. In horses, pigs, and ruminants, the sinus is trabeculated throughout its length. In carnivores, the upper region is nontrabeculated, forming an annular sinus.

The short ducts of **sebaceous glands** usually empty into hair follicles, although they may also empty directly onto the skin surface. Basal (stem) cells of sebaceous glands divide and give rise to vacuolated secretory cells that synthesize lipid. The innermost, mature secretory cells degenerate, forming sebum. This is a form of holocrine secretion.

Sweat glands may be winding (serpentine) or highly coiled, and either tubular or sac-like. They empty their secretion through a duct, either into a hair follicle or onto the skin surface. The epithelium of the secretory portion varies from flattened to columnar. Contractile **myoepithelial cells** surround the secretory cells and the initial portion of their ducts.

In merocrine secretion, secretory vesicles release their contents directly to the exterior after fusing with the cell membrane (exocytosis). In apocrine secretion, small blebs of cytoplasm containing the secretion are pinched off from the secretory cell. Traditionally, sweat glands have been classified as either merocrine or apocrine. Recent evidence, however, has suggested that this may not be true and that all sweat glands may release their products using the merocrine mode. We have chosen to use the traditional nomenclature until the matter is resolved.

Special regions in the skin of various species have numerous, well developed glands. The carpal glands of pigs consist of masses of merocrine sweat glands. Numerous apocrine sweat glands characterize the mental organ of pigs and the interdigital and inguinal pouches of sheep. The submental organ of cats, the supracaudal gland of carnivores, the infraorbital pouch of sheep, and the scent (horn) glands of goats contain many large sebaceous glands.

The skin of the **nose** of horses is thin with fine hairs, sebaceous and sweat glands, and occasional sinus hairs. The planum of the nose of the other domestic mammals is covered by a thick, highly keratinized epidermis. The planum nasale of carnivores is devoid of glands and hairs. In cats, the epidermis forms numerous small bumps, while that of the dog is rather flat with surface grooves. The planum rostrale of the pig contains numerous merocrine sweat glands and sparse hairs. The planum nasolabiale of the cow and the planum nasale of sheep and goats are hairless and contain compound acinar glands that produce a serous secretion.

Digital pads of cats and dogs are covered by a very thick epidermis which is smooth in the dog and roughened by conical papillae in the cat. Coiled merocrine sweat glands occur in the dermis and the digital cushion of the pads.

Lobules of **mammary glands** are situated in the subcutis and consist of tubuloacinar glands and intralobular ducts. When the gland is active, secretory tissue is prominent, and intralobular and interlobular connective tissue is reduced. When the gland is inactive, only the duct system is evident. Cellular thickenings at the termination of intralobular ducts represent gland remnants or precursors in the inactive gland. Interlobular ducts, with a bistratified cuboidal to columnar lining, drain the lobules and lead to the lactiferous ducts and lactiferous sinuses at the base of the teat. The teat sinus, with a bistratified columnar to cuboidal lining, leads to the teat canal that opens onto the tip of the teat. The teat canal is lined by a stratified squamous epithelium that is continuous with the skin. Single ducts pass through the teats of ruminants, while the teats of carnivores, horses, and pigs contain multiple ducts, each opening onto the surface. The skin surface of the teat of cows and pigs lacks sebaceous glands, sweat glands, and hairs.

Chestnuts and **ergots** are epidermal thickenings characteristic of the horse. The **claws** of carnivores, **hooves** of ungulates, and **horns** of ruminants are highly specialized derivatives of the skin composed of hard keratin.

CHICKEN

The **epidermis** of the chicken is generally thinner than that of mammals. It is composed of an inner **stratum germinativum** and an outer **stratum corneum.** The stratum germinativum includes a **basal layer, an intermediate layer** of one to several layers of polygonal cells, and a thin **transitional layer** of flat vacuolated cells just below the stratum corneum.

The **dermis** of feathered skin lacks papillae and is nonglandular. Mutlilocular as well as unilocular adipocytes occur in the **subcutis.**

The epidermally derived **feathers** may be classified into three main types in the adult chicken: contour, down, and filoplume. A **contour feather** has a central shaft which is divisible into a hollow **calamus** (quill) and a **rachis.** A **vein** extends laterally from each side of the rachis and is composed of **barbs** and **barbules** with interlocking **hooklets.** Down feathers are soft and fluffy. Their barbules lack hooklets. **Filoplumes** are small, hair-like feathers.

Feathers are situated in tube-like **follicles** oriented obliquely in the dermis or subcutis. The follicle wall of a developing feather is lined by a stratum corneum and underlying stratum germinativum surrounded by a layer of connective tissue. The **epidermal collar,** a thick ring of epidermal cells at the base of the follicle, gives rise to the feather. It surrounds the **dermal** (feather) **papilla,** which gives rise to a well vascularized, mesenchyme-like **feather pulp** that is present during growth of the feather. A network of **feather muscles,** each composed of one to several bundles of smooth muscle, attaches the follicles to each other. No muscles are associated with the follicles of filoplumes.

Wattles and **combs** are appendages of the skin whose dermis contains an extensive, superficial network of sinus capillaries and abundant mucous connective tissue. The sinus capillaries are responsible for the striking red color of the appendages.

Digital pads are covered by a thick stratum corneum and contain a cushion of adipose tissue in their subcutis. **Scales, claws,** and **beaks** are keratinized derivatives of the skin.

The **uropygial** (preen) **gland** is a bilobed holocrine gland located in the dorsal base of the tail. It produces an oily secretion. Simple tubular glands radiate outward from the lumen of each lobe like the bristles of a bottle brush. Each tubule is divided into a **sebaceous zone** and a **glycogen zone,** named according to their histochemical staining properties. The glycogen zone is continuous with the lumen of the lobe. Each lobe is drained by a **primary duct** that passes through the **isthmus** to the **papilla** (nipple) to open onto the surface.

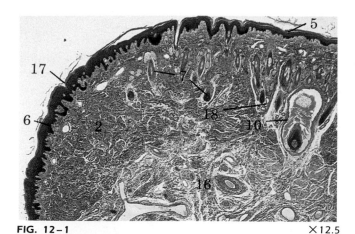

FIG. 12–1   ×12.5

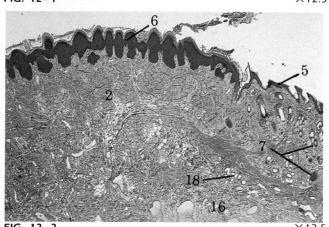

FIG. 12–2   ×12.5

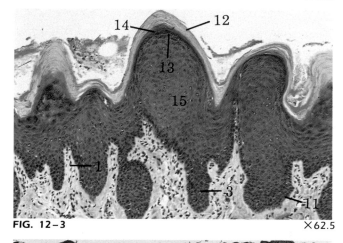

FIG. 12–3   ×62.5

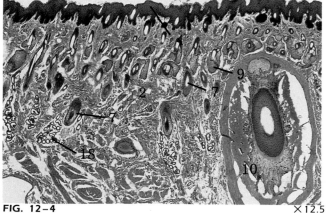

FIG. 12–4   ×12.5

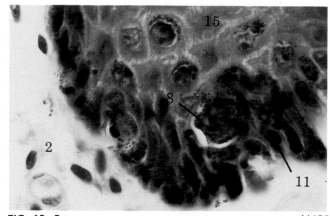

FIG. 12–5   ×625

KEY		
1. Dermal papilla	**11.** Stratum basale	
2. Dermis	**12.** Stratum corneum	
3. Epidermal peg	**13.** Stratum granulosum	
4. Epidermis	**14.** Stratum lucidum	
5. Epithelium, hairy skin	**15.** Stratum spinosum	
6. Epithelium, planum	**16.** Subcutis	
7. Hair follicle	**17.** Surface groove	
8. Melanocyte	**18.** Sweat gland	
9. Sebaceous gland		
10. Sinus hair follicle		

FIG. 12–1. Planum Nasale and Hairy Skin, Nose, Dog. Junction of the hairless planum nasale (thick skin) and the hairy portion (thin skin) of the nose. No glands are associated with the planum of carnivores. There are surface grooves in the planum of the dog.

FIG. 12–2. Planum Nasale and Hairy Skin, Nose, Cat. No hairs or glands are associated with the planum of carnivores. The surface of the planum bears numerous small raised tubercles that are characteristic of the cat.

FIG. 12–3. Epithelium, Planum Nasale, Cat. Portions of the small tubercles typical of the cat's planum. All layers of the epidermis are evident. Note how the papillae of the dermis interdigitate with the epidermal pegs.

FIG. 12–4. Nose, Horse. Numerous small sebaceous glands, sweat glands, fine hairs, and the follicle of a sinus hair are evident. The epidermis is heavily pigmented.

FIG. 12–5. Nose, Horse. A melanocyte with numerous pigment granules is located in the deep portion of the epidermis. Surrounding cells have phagocytized melanin granules produced by melanocytes. The granules are aggregated like a cap just above the nucleus of some of the cells of the stratum spinosum.

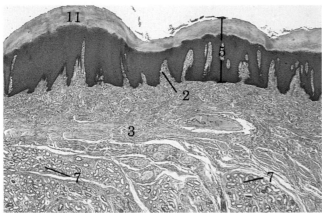

FIG. 12–6   ×12.5

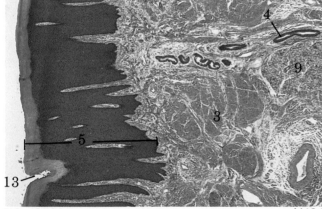

FIG. 12–7   ×250

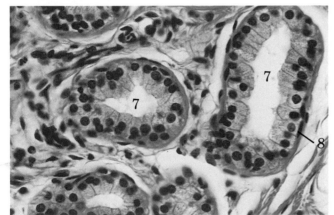

FIG. 12–8   ×12.5

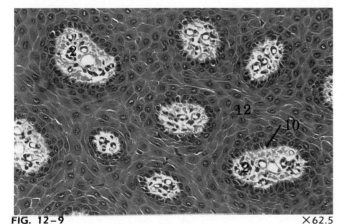

FIG. 12–9   ×62.5

FIG. 12–10   ×250

KEY	
1. Cytoplasmic bridges	**8.** Myoepithelial cell, nucleus
2. Dermal papilla	**9.** Nasolabial glands
3. Dermis	**10.** Stratum basale
4. Duct	**11.** Stratum corneum
5. Epidermis	**12.** Stratum spinosum
6. Keratinocyte, nucleus	**13.** Surface groove
7. Merocrine sweat gland	

FIG. 12–6. Planum Rostrale, Pig. The very thick epidermis of the snout of the pig has low, wide elevations and an especially thick stratum corneum. Long dermal papillae project into the epidermis. Numerous merocrine sweat glands occur in the subcutis. Hairs, which are sparse on the planum of the pig, are not shown.

FIG. 12–7. Planum Rostrale, Pig. Detail of the merocrine sweat glands. Secretory cells are either columnar or cuboidal and are surrounded by myoepithelial cells.

FIG. 12–8. Planum Nasolabiale, Cow. The surface of the planum of the cow is hairless and marked by grooves. Long dermal papillae project into the thick epidermis. Glands are abundant in the subcutis of the planum of ruminants.

FIG. 12–9. Planum Nasolabiale, Cow. The tissue was cut parallel to the surface of the planum, so that cross sections of dermal papillae appear in the stratum spinosum. Each papilla is surrounded by cells of the stratum basale and contains several vessels.

FIG. 12–10. Planum Nasolabiale, Cow. During tissue processing, the keratinocytes of the stratum spinosum shrink away from each other, but remain attached at multiple sites where desmosomes are located. This gives the appearance of cytoplasmic (intercellular) bridges or spines between the cells.

INTEGUMENT   **85**

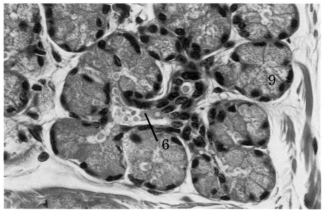

FIG. 12-11 ×250

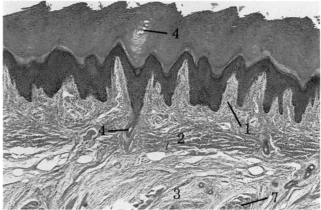

FIG. 12-12 ×25

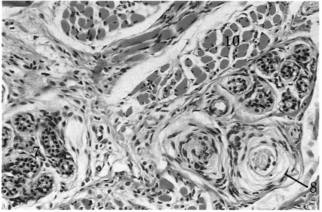

FIG. 12-13 ×125

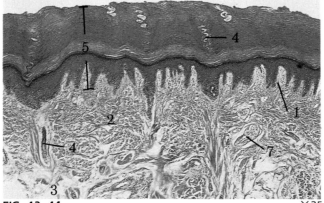

FIG. 12-14 ×25

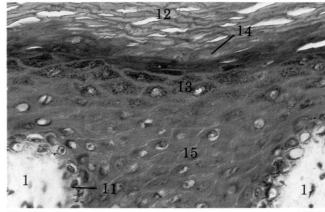

FIG. 12-15 ×250

KEY	
1. Dermis, papillary layer	9. Secretory acinus
2. Dermis, reticular layer	10. Skeletal muscle
3. Digital cushion	11. Stratum basale
4. Duct of sweat gland	12. Stratum corneum
5. Epidermis	13. Stratum granulosum
6. Intralobular duct	14. Stratum lucidum
7. Merocrine sweat gland	15. Stratum spinosum
8. Pacinian corpuscle	

FIG. 12-11. Planum Nasolabiale, Cow. The planum of the cow, sheep, and goat contains many tubuloacinar serous glands. Branches of an intralobular duct can be seen entering portions of the secretory acini.

FIG. 12-12. Digital Pad, Dog. The digital pad is hairless and covered by a very thick epidermis that is roughened by small conical projections in the dog (compare with Fig. 12-14). Portions of merocrine sweat glands lie in the dermis and digital cushion (subcutis).

FIG. 12-13. Digital Pad, Dog. Coiled merocrine sweat glands and Pacinian corpuscles among skeletal muscle and loose connective tissue of the footpad.

FIG. 12-14. Digital Pad, Cat. The surface of the digital pad of the cat is smooth, lacking the conical papillae that are typical of the dog. Portions of the excretory ducts of sweat glands spiral through the stratified squamous epithelium.

FIG. 12-15. Digital Pad, Cat. Detail of the epidermis and dermis shown in Figure 12-14. All five layers of the epidermis are evident.

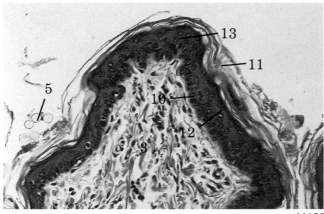

FIG. 12-16 ×125

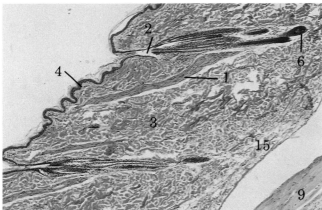

FIG. 12-17 ×25

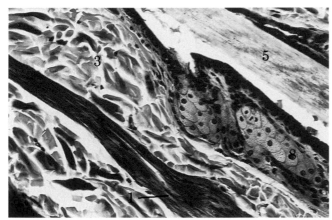

FIG. 12-18 ×125

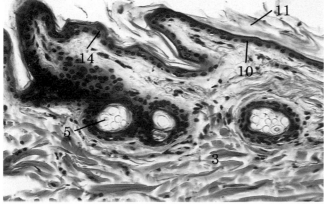

FIG. 12-19 ×125

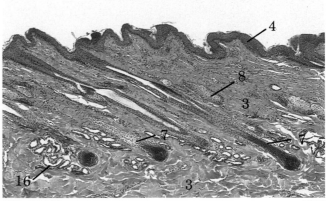

FIG. 12-20 ×25

KEY	
1. Arrector pili muscle	**10.** Stratum basale
2. Common follicular opening	**11.** Stratum corneum
3. Dermis	**12.** Stratum granulosum
4. Epidermis	**13.** Stratum spinosum
5. Hair	**14.** Stratum spinosum cell,
6. Hair bulb	nucleus
7. Hair follicle	**15.** Subcutis
8. Sebaceous gland	**16.** Sweat gland
9. Skeletal muscle	

FIG. 12-16. Skin, Mid-Ventral Abdomen, Dog. The epidermis is thin and consists of four layers. Note that only a few layers of cells comprise the stratum spinosum. The stratum corneum is also relatively thin, and the keratinized cells have loosened and separated from the surface.

FIG. 12-17. Skin, Back, Cat. Two compound follicles in the dermis. In carnivores, the hairs of compound follicles merge at the level of the sebaceous glands and share a common follicular opening to the surface. Bits of hairs are evident in the follicles as shiny, yellow-brown structures. The arrector pili muscles of the skin of the back are especially well developed in cats and dogs. A space artifact separates the subcutis from the underlying skeletal muscle.

FIG. 12-18. Skin, Back, Cat, Masson's. Portions of an arrector pili muscle, sebaceous gland, and a hair within a follicle.

FIG. 12-19. Skin, Caudal Abdomen, Cat. The epidermis is extremely thin. Cells of the stratum spinosum are sparse, and those of the stratum granulosum are visible only as occasional dark granular areas just beneath the stratum corneum. Hairs are visible within the compound follicles.

FIG. 12-20. Skin, Neck, Horse. Simple hair follicles occur in the skin of noncarnivores.

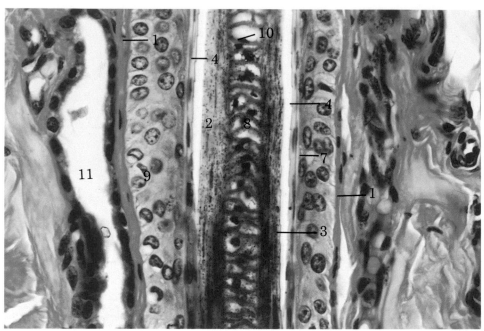

FIG. 12-21   ×360

KEY	
1. Connective tissue sheath	**7.** Inner root sheath
2. Cortex, hair	**8.** Medulla, hair
3. Cuticle, hair	**9.** Outer root sheath
4. Cuticle, inner root sheath	**10.** Pyknotic nucleus
5. Dermal papilla	**11.** Sweat gland
6. Dermis	

FIG. 12-21. Skin, Neck, Horse. Mid-region of a longitudinal section of a hair follicle. Large, clear cells of the medulla of the hair have round nuclei that become pyknotic as they progress distally from the hair bulb. The pigment-laden cortex of the hair is formed from closely packed elongated cells that have become keratinized. Scale-like, keratinized cells of the cuticle of the hair partially overlap so that their free edges point upward. They interlock with cells of the cuticle of the inner root sheath, whose free edges are directed downward.

FIG. 12-22. Skin, Neck, Horse. A dermal papilla projects into the hair bulb at the base of the follicle. Cells of the cortex of the hair are nearly obscured by pigment granules provided by melanocytes of the bulb.

FIG. 12-22   ×125

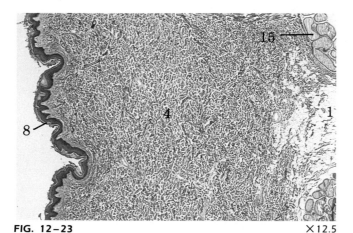

FIG. 12-23 ×12.5

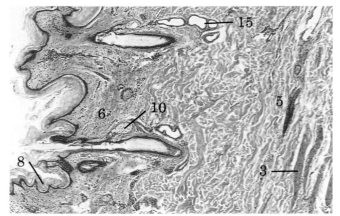

FIG. 12-27 ×25

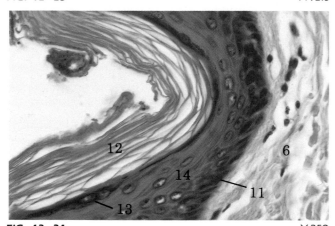

FIG. 12-24 ×250

KEY	
1. Adipose tissue	**9.** Hair bulb
2. Collagenous fiber	**10.** Sebaceous gland
3. Dartos muscle	**11.** Stratum basale
4. Dermis	**12.** Stratum corneum
5. Dermis, deep layer	**13.** Stratum granulosum
6. Dermis, superficial layer	**14.** Stratum spinosum
7. Elastic fiber	**15.** Sweat gland
8. Epidermis	

FIG. 12-23. Skin, Dorsal Neck, Pig. Note the extremely thick dermis. Sweat glands and adipose tissue are seen in the subcutis.

FIG. 12-24. Skin, Dorsal Neck, Pig. The epidermis and part of the dermis are shown in detail.

FIG. 12-25. Skin, Dorsal Neck, Pig, Orcein. The dermis of the skin contains numerous branching elastic fibers. The fibers of the superficial layer are fine, while those of the deep layer are coarse.

FIG. 12-26. Skin, Back, Sheep. Various portions of numerous hair follicles are embedded in the thick superficial layer of the dermis. The hair follicles of sheep tend to be arranged vertically, rather than diagonally, in the dermis (compare with Figs. 12-17 and 12-20).

FIG. 12-27. Scrotum, Goat. The epidermis of the scrotum is remarkably thin. Portions of two simple hair follicles are located in the dermis. Smooth muscle bundles among fibroelastic tissue in the dermis comprise the tunica dartos.

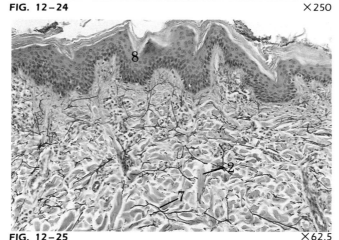

FIG. 12-25 ×62.5

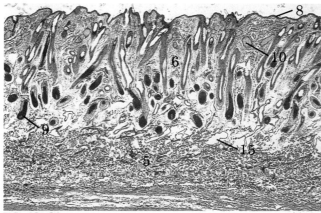

FIG. 12-26 ×12.5

89

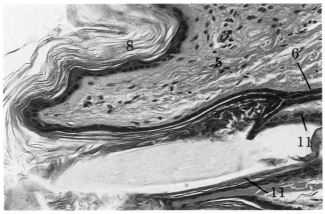

FIG. 12-28 ×125

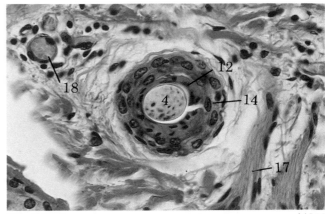

FIG. 12-32 ×250

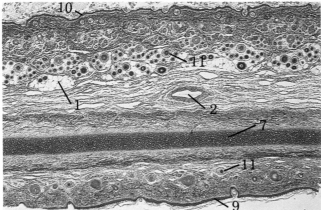

FIG. 12-29 ×12.5

FIG. 12-28. Scrotum, Goat. The thin epidermis and a portion of a hair follicle are shown in detail.

FIG. 12-29. Pinna (Auricle), External Ear, Dog. A plate of elastic cartilage is covered by the skin of the outer (convex) and inner (concave) surfaces of the pinna. Hair follicles are more numerous in the skin of the outer surface.

FIG. 12-30. Pinna, External Ear, Dog. Clusters of compound hair follicles cut in cross section vary in appearance at different levels of the dermis. The cells of the cortex and medulla of the hairs are evident in the deepest portions of the follicles. More superficially, the cells become keratinized and appear shiny pink (medulla) and yellow (cortex). Several hairs have merged to share a common follicle wall near the epidermis.

FIG. 12-31. Pinna, External Ear, Dog. Detail of follicles, in cross section, from the deep region of the dermis, similar to those in Figure 12-30.

FIG. 12-32. Skin, Back, Sheep. A wool hair, shown in cross section, lacks a medulla.

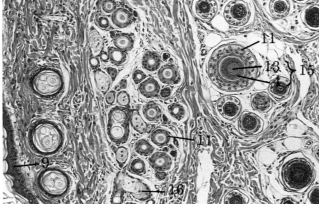

FIG. 12-30 ×62.5

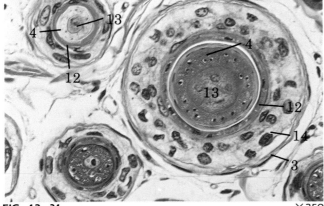

FIG. 12-31 ×250

90 COLOR ATLAS OF VETERINARY HISTOLOGY

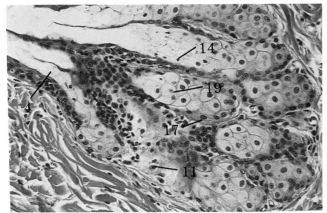

FIG. 12–36 ×125

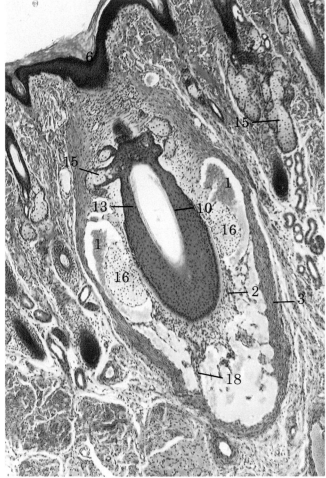

FIG. 12–33 ×360

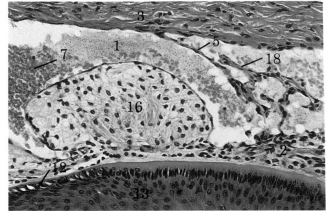

FIG. 12–34 ×125

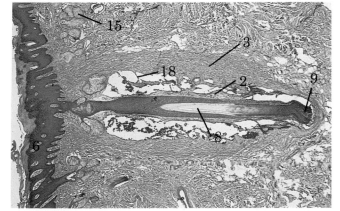

FIG. 12–35 ×12.5

KEY	
1. Annular sinus	**10.** Inner root sheath
2. Connective tissue sheath, inner	**11.** Mast cell
	12. Merkel's cell
3. Connective tissue sheath, outer	**13.** Outer root sheath
	14. Pyknotic nucleus
4. Duct	**15.** Sebaceous gland
5. Endothelial cell, nucleus	**16.** Sinus pad
6. Epidermis	**17.** Stem cell
7. Erythrocytes	**18.** Trabecula
8. Hair	**19.** Vacuolated cell
9. Hair bulb	

FIG. 12–33. Sinus Hair Follicle, oblique section, Nose, Dog. The large sinus hair follicle contains a blood-filled sinus, lined by an endothelium, between the inner and outer layers of the connective tissue sheath. In carnivores, only the lower region of the sinus is spanned by a network of connective tissue trabeculae. The upper region contains an annular sinus, free of trabeculae, into which protrudes a thickening of the inner connective tissue sheath called the sinus pad.

FIG. 12–34. Sinus Hair Follicle, Nose, Dog. Detail of Figure 12–33. Portion of the sinus pad, annular sinus, and trabeculated sinus. Note the Merkel's cells, associated with tactile stimulation, in the external root sheath.

FIG. 12–35. Sinus Hair Follicle, l.s., Nose, Cow. In sinus hair follicles of ruminants, horses, and pigs, the entire length of the blood-filled sinus is crossed by numerous trabeculae.

FIG. 12–36. Sebaceous Gland, Lip, Cat. The cell types comprising this holocrine gland are evident: small, flat peripheral stem cells; maturing, round cells with pale, vacuolated cytoplasm; inner, degenerating cells with pyknotic nuclei. The vacuolated cells arise from the stem cells, accumulate lipid (lost during tissue processing), and then break down, forming sebum.

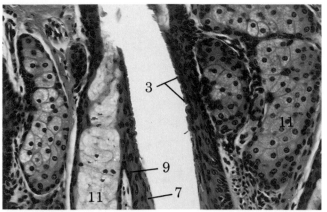

FIG. 12–37   ×125

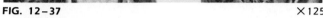

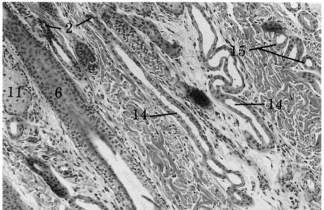

FIG. 12–38   ×62.5

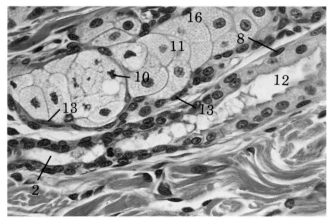

FIG. 12–39   ×250

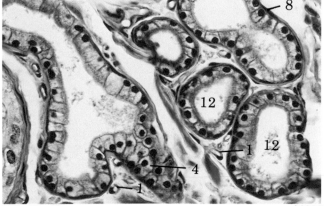

FIG. 12–40   ×250

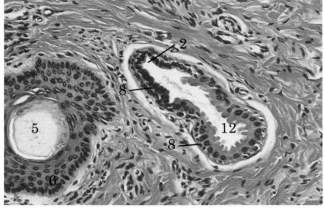

FIG. 12–41   ×125

KEY		
1. Capillary	**10.** Pyknotic nucleus	
2. Duct	**11.** Sebaceous gland	
3. Follicular folds	**12.** Secretory portion, sweat	
4. Gland cells, surface cut	gland	
5. Hair	**13.** Stem cell	
6. Hair follicle	**14.** Sweat gland, l.s.	
7. Inner root sheath	**15.** Sweat gland, x.s.	
8. Myoepithelial cell, nucleus	**16.** Vacuolated cell	
9. Outer root sheath		

FIG. 12–37. Sebaceous Gland and Hair Follicle, l.s., Lip, Sheep. The inner root sheath forms follicular (circular) folds below the entrance of sebaceous glands into the follicle.

FIG. 12–38. Nose, Dog. Longitudinal sections of two serpentine sweat glands. Their tubular structure is evident.

FIG. 12–39. Sebaceous Gland and Sweat Gland, Nose, Dog. The secretory portion of a sweat gland, lined by cuboidal to columnar cells, is continuous with the bistratified, flattened cells of its duct.

FIG. 12–40. Sweat Gland, Skin, Horse, Trichrome. Cross and oblique sections of a coiled sweat gland in the dermis are lined by cuboidal to columnar cells and surrounded by myoepithelial cells. The solid sheet of several cells represents a surface cut through the wall of the gland.

FIG. 12–41. Sweat Gland and Duct, Teat, Sheep. Low columnar secretory cells with apical blebs end abruptly where the duct epithelium begins. Both the secretory cells and the initial segment of the duct are surrounded by myoepithelial cells. The cytoplasm of the myoepithelial cells appears as a pink, sometimes rippled band.

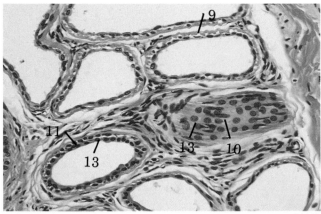

FIG. 12–42 ×125

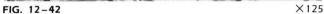

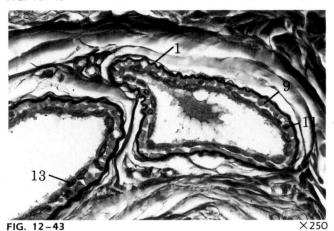

FIG. 12–43 ×250

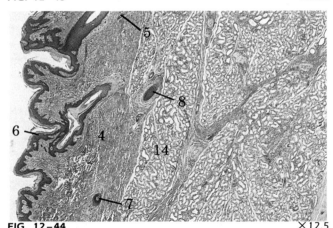

FIG. 12–44 ×12.5

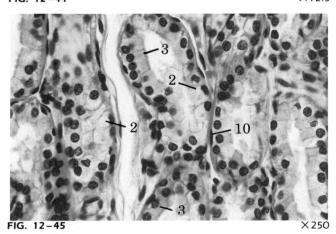

FIG. 12–45 ×250

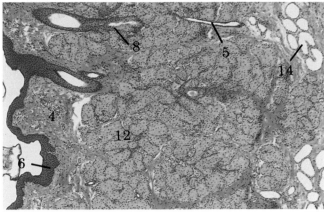

FIG. 12–46 ×25

KEY	
1. Basement membrane	**10.** Myoepithelial cell, nucleus, l.s.
2. Clear cell	**11.** Myoepithelial cell, nucleus, x.s.
3. Dark cell	
4. Dermis	**12.** Sebaceous gland
5. Duct of sweat gland	**13.** Secretory cell, nucleus
6. Epidermis	**14.** Sweat gland
7. Hair bulb	
8. Hair follicle	
9. Myoepithelial cell, cytoplasm	

FIG. 12–42. Sweat Gland, Teat, Sheep. The secretory cells of sweat glands vary from squamous to tall columnar. They are squamous in this preparation, but are columnar in Figure 12–41. Note that one of the secretory portions is cut tangentially, revealing the elongated shape of the myoepithelial cells.

FIG. 12–43. Sweat Gland, Teat, Sheep, Silver and Eosin. The basement membrane of a sweat gland is blackened with silver. Myoepithelial cells occur between the flattened secretory cells and the basement membrane.

FIG. 12–44. Carpal Gland, Pig. Lobules of merocrine sweat glands occur in the subcutaneous tissue on the medial side of the carpus of the pig.

FIG. 12–45. Carpal Gland, Pig. Dark and clear cells of the secretory units of these merocrine sweat glands are surrounded by myoepithelial cells.

FIG. 12–46. Infraorbital Pouch (Sinus), Sheep. Many large sebaceous glands occupy the wall of the infraorbital pouch of sheep. Some apocrine sweat glands lie deep to the sebaceous glands.

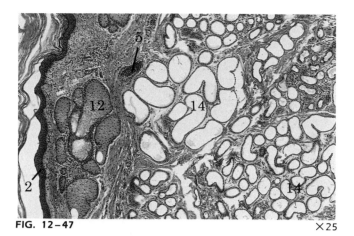

FIG. 12–47 ×25

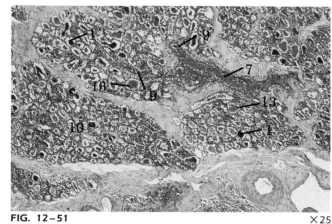

FIG. 12–51 ×25

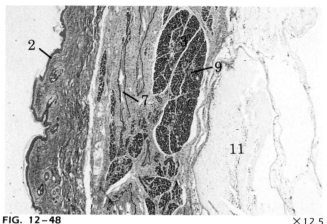

FIG. 12–48 ×12.5

FIG. 12–47. Inguinal Pouch, Sheep. The skin of the inguinal pouch of sheep contains a few hairs, sebaceous glands, and an abundance of apocrine sweat glands.

FIG. 12–48. Mammary Gland, Inactive, Cat. Lobules of glandular tissue and ducts are surrounded by fibroelastic subcutaneous tissue. The overlying skin contains a few hairs. Large lymphatic vessels lie deep to the parenchyma.

FIG. 12–49. Mammary Gland, Inactive, Cow. Abundant interlobular connective tissue and components of the duct system are evident in an inactive gland. Interlobular ducts branch into the lobules as intralobular ducts.

FIG. 12–50. Mammary Gland, Inactive, Cow. Lobules are composed of intralobular ducts and intralobular connective tissue, which is moderately rich in cells. Thickenings at the terminations of intralobular ducts represent remnants or precursors of glandular epithelium. When these are cut in cross section, they cannot always be distinguished from ducts.

FIG. 12–51. Mammary Gland, Active, Cow. In the active gland, secretory parenchyma is well developed and connective tissue is reduced (compare with Fig. 12–49). The lumens of the secretory glands and ducts are filled with secretion (deep pink).

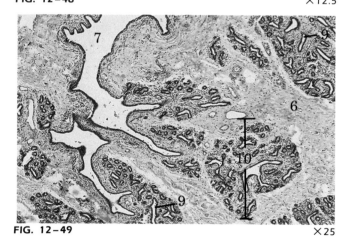

FIG. 12–49 ×25

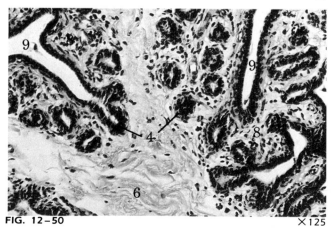

FIG. 12–50 ×125

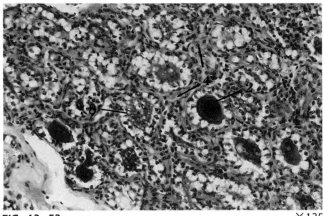

FIG. 12-52 ×125

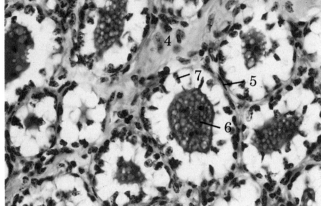

FIG. 12-53 ×250

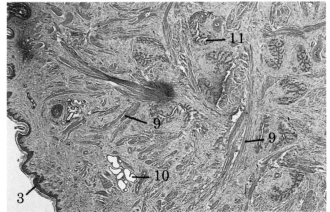

FIG. 12-54 ×12.5

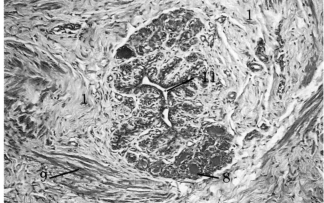

FIG. 12-55 ×62.5

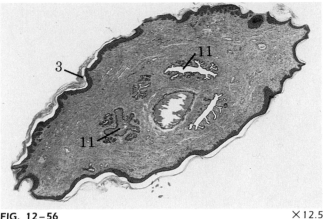

FIG. 12-56 ×12.5

KEY	
1. Connective tissue	**7.** Secretory cell, nucleus
2. Corpora amylacea	**8.** Secretory unit
3. Epidermis	**9.** Smooth muscle
4. Intralobular connective tissue	**10.** Sweat gland
5. Myoepithelial cell, nucleus	**11.** Teat sinus
6. Secretion	

FIG. 12-52. Mammary Gland, Active, Cow. A portion of a lobule containing numerous tubuloalveolar secretory units. Some of the alveoli contain round concretions of casein and cellular debris called corpora amylacea.

FIG. 12-53. Mammary Gland, Active, Cow. Many secretory cells have basally displaced nuclei and indistinct lateral cell borders. These cells appear pale because their cytoplasmic lipids have been extracted. Sloughed cells, whose dark nuclei are visible in the lumens, are part of the secretory product. Some of the flat nuclei surrounding the alveoli belong to myoepithelial cells.

FIG. 12-54. Teat, x.s., Dog. A portion of the teat shows numerous sinuses among intermingling bundles of smooth muscle and fibroelastic connective tissue. Nonruminants have multiple teat sinuses and teat canals. Some glands and hairs are associated with the skin of the teat of carnivores, horses, sheep, and goats.

FIG. 12-55. Teat Sinus, x.s., Dog. Detail of a teat sinus of Figure 12-54 reveals a highly folded lining. Glandular areas, composed of small secretory units, are associated with the wall of the sinus.

FIG. 12-56. Teat Sinus, x.s., Cat. This cross section through a teat reveals five teat sinuses. Some of these contain a pink-staining secretion.

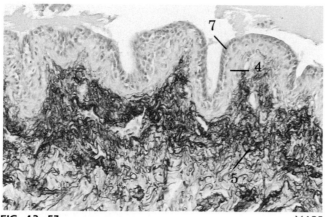

FIG. 12–57   ×125

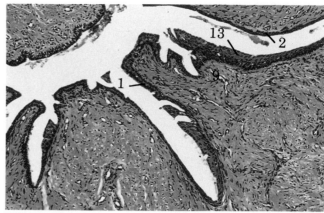

FIG. 12–61   ×62.5

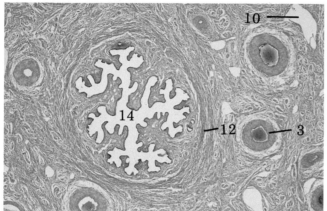

FIG. 12–58   ×12.5

FIG. 12–57. Teat Sinus, x.s., Horse, Orcein. A band of collagenous fibers lies between the epithelium and the underlying fibroelastic connective tissue.

FIG. 12–58. Teat Sinus, x.s., Cow. The mucosa of the teat sinus blends with the middle layer of the teat. The latter contains well developed, longitudinally oriented blood vessels (cut in x.s.), bundles of smooth muscle, fibroelastic tissue, and lymphatic vessels. The outer layer, the skin surface, is not shown.

FIG. 12–59. Teat Sinus, x.s., Cow. The teat sinus is lined by a bistratified cuboidal to columnar epithelium.

FIG. 12–60. Teat Sinus, x.s., Sheep, Male. The skin of the teat contains hairs, sebaceous glands, and sweat glands, except in the cow and pig (compare with Fig. 12–64).

FIG. 12–61. Teat Sinus and Canal, Junction, x.s., Horse. Patches of the bistratified epithelium (columnar and cuboidal) of the teat sinus intermingle with the stratified squamous epithelium of the teat canal.

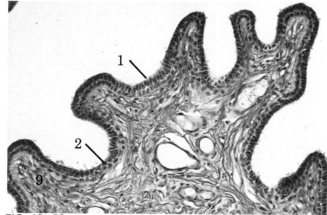

FIG. 12–59   ×125

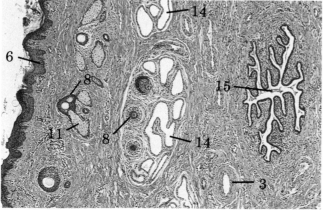

FIG. 12–60   ×25

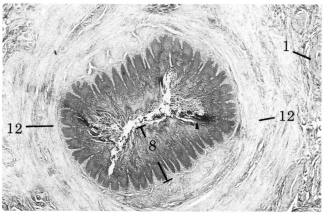

FIG. 12-62 ×12.5

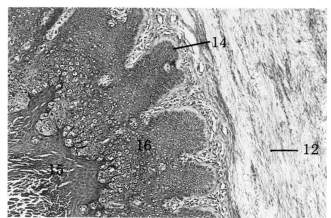

FIG. 12-63 ×62.5

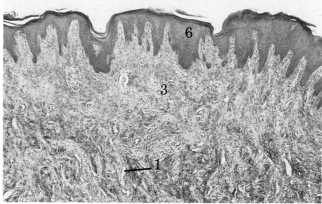

FIG. 12-64 ×25

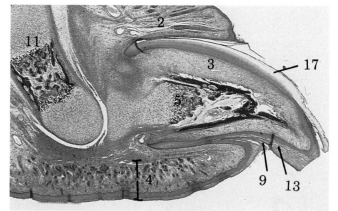

FIG. 12-65 ×12.5

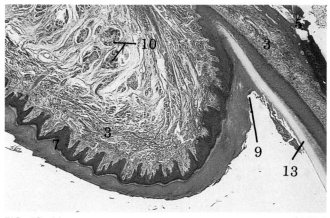

FIG. 12-66 ×12.5

KEY	
1. Blood vessel	**10.** Merocrine sweat glands
2. Claw fold	**11.** Middle phalanx
3. Dermis	**12.** Smooth muscle
4. Digital pad	**13.** Sole
5. Distal phalanx	**14.** Stratum basale
6. Epidermis	**15.** Stratum corneum
7. Epidermis, digital pad	**16.** Stratum spinosum
8. Epithelium	**17.** Wall
9. Limiting furrow	

FIG. 12-62. Teat Canal, x.s., Cow, Trichrome. The keratinized stratified squamous lining of the teat canal is encircled by a papillated connective tissue layer (green) and bundles of smooth muscle (pale orange).

FIG. 12-63. Teat Canal, x.s., Cow, Trichrome. Detail of the thick keratinized stratified squamous epithelium and the surrounding connective tissue and smooth muscle shown in Figure 12-62.

FIG. 12-64. Skin Surface, Teat, x.s., Cow, Trichrome. The skin surface of the teat of the cow and pig is hairless.

FIG. 12-65. Developing Claw, l.s., Fetus, Dog. The claw of carnivores consists of a dorsal and lateral wall (body, claw plate) and a ventral sole of hard keratin that cover the distal phalanx. The claw fold is the skin that covers the wall at the base of the claw. Endochondral bone formation has begun in the phalanges of this specimen.

FIG. 12-66. Sole of Claw and Digital Pad, Dog. The limiting furrow separates the digital pad from the sole of the claw.

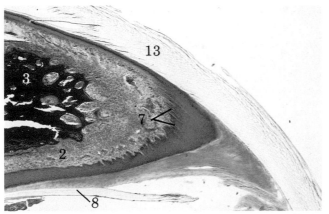

FIG. 12-67   ×12.5

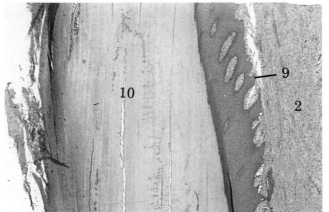

FIG. 12-68   ×12.5

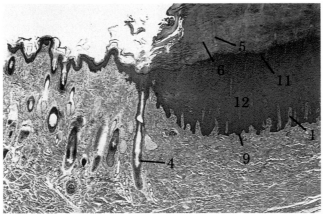

FIG. 12-69   ×12.5

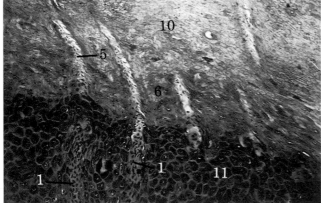

FIG. 12-70   ×62.5

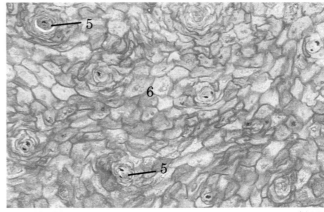

FIG. 12-71   ×125

KEY	
1. Dermal papilla	**8.** Sole
2. Dermis	**9.** Stratum basale
3. Distal phalanx	**10.** Stratum corneum
4. Hair follicle	**11.** Stratum granulosum
5. Horn tubule	**12.** Stratum spinosum
6. Intertubular horn	**13.** Wall
7. Laminae	

FIG. 12-67. Apex of Claw, l.s., Dog. The dermis of the wall bears laminae (lamellae) at the apex of the claw.

FIG. 12-68. Horn, Cow. Horns of ruminants are composed of bone of the cornual process covered by a dermis and epidermis. The epidermis with a thick stratum corneum of hard keratin (horn) and a portion of the underlying papillated dermis are shown here. *(Photograph of a histologic section borrowed from the College of Veterinary Medicine, Iowa State University.)*

FIG. 12-69. Chestnut, Horse. Junction of the hairy skin and chestnut. Chestnuts (and ergots) of horses are keratinized thickenings of the epidermis composed of horn tubules (tubular horn) and intertubular horn. Horn tubules arise from the cells of the stratum basale that cover the apex and sides of dermal papillae. Intertubular (interpapillary) horn arises from the cells of the stratum basale that are located between the bases of the dermal papillae. Only a small portion of the very thick stratum corneum of the chestnut is shown.

FIG. 12-70. Chestnut, Horse. Detail of a portion of the epidermis.

FIG. 12-71. Chestnut, Horse. The section was cut parallel to the surface of the chestnut at the level of the stratum corneum. Horn tubules appear in cross section between intertubular horn.

The equine **hoof** is the keratinized portion of the epidermis that covers the distal end of the digit. The various regions of the hoof are depicted in Figures 12–72 and 12–73. The **perioplic, coronary,** and **laminar** regions comprise the **wall** (the portion of the hoof that is visible when the digit is on the ground). The wall turns in ventrally at an acute angle to form the **bars.** The **sole,** which forms most of the ventral surface of the hoof, is attached to the bars and the adjacent, inner border of the wall. The **frog,** a caudal, wedge-shaped mass, lies between the bars. The apex of the frog merges with the sole cranially. The **bulbs** are the convex protuberances located above and behind the frog.

The keratinized tissue comprising the hoof is in the form of **tubular, intertubular,** and **laminar horn** (see Figs. 12–76, 12–77, 12–80, and 12–81). The underlying, living layers of the epidermis include the stratum spinosum, whose cells are undergoing keratinization, and the stratum basale. The stratum basale borders on the dermis (corium), which is rich in blood vessels and nerves. The dermis may be either papillated or laminated, depending on whether the overlying epidermis contains tubular or laminated horn, respectively. The dermis blends with underlying structures, such as the subcutaneous cushions and the periosteum of the third phalanx.

The **perioplic epidermis** forms a band of soft, nonpigmented tubular horn. It merges with the epidermis of the skin above, and extends downward as a thin, glossy, flaky layer of keratin that forms the outer coating of the wall of the hoof, called the **stratum tectorium** (stratum externum). This layer is well developed in young animals, but tends to be worn away in older horses. The perioplic epidermis widens at the heels to form the bulbs. The **perioplic dermis** is characterized by the presence of fine, short papillae (1 to 2 mm).

The germinal cells of the **coronary epidermis** form horn tubules (tubular horn) and intertubular horn that extend from the coronary region to the ground surface, forming the bulk of the wall of the hoof, the **stratum medium.** The horn tubules are oriented at an angle to the ground. They parallel the external surface of the hoof. The **coronary dermis** is marked by long dermal papillae (4 to 6 mm).

The **laminar epidermis** of the wall is in the form of **laminae** (lamellae) that are arranged parallel to the horn tubules of the stratum medium. They extend from the deep edge of the coronary region to the sole. Each **primary lamina** bears numerous **secondary laminae** (not present in the hooves of pigs and ruminants) that project at right angles along its length. The primary epidermal laminae are keratinized and fused with the inner portion of the stratum medium of the wall. The secondary epidermal laminae consist of a core of cells of the stratum spinosum bordered by cells of the stratum basale. The epidermal laminae form the **stratum internum** of the wall of the hoof. They interdigitate with primary and secondary dermal laminae of the **laminar dermis.** This extensive interdigitation serves to suspend the third phalanx from the hoof. At the ground surface, the junction of the epidermal laminae of the wall (unpigmented) with the sole is called the **white line.**

The tubular and intertubular horn of the bulbs, sole, and frog is softer than that of the wall of the hoof. The dermis of these regions, like that of the periople and coronary region, is papillated. The epidermis and dermis of the bars are laminated, being continuous with the laminar region of the wall.

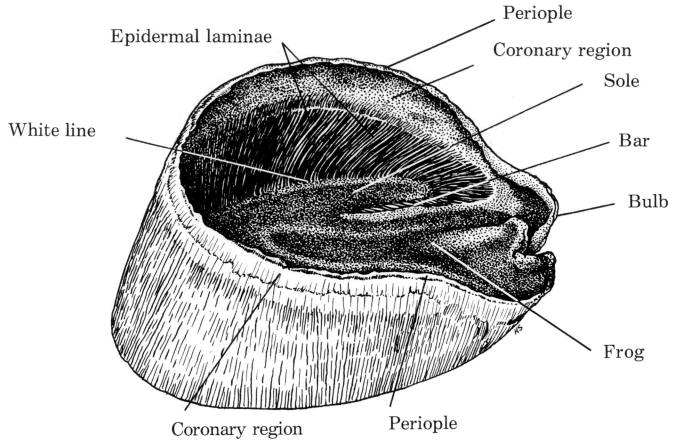

Epidermal laminae

Periople

Coronary region

Sole

Bar

Bulb

Frog

White line

Coronary region

Periople

FIG. 12–72. Hoof, Horse. The various regions of the hoof are shown. The inner surface of the periople and coronary region, and that of the sole, frog, and bulbs, are stippled in the drawing. In the intact toe, dermal papillae extend into the funnel-shaped depressions whose openings are represented by the stipples.

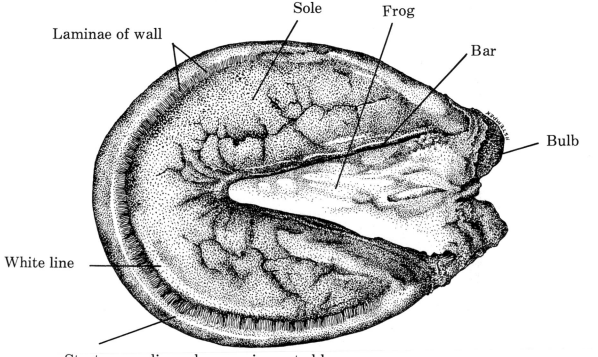

Laminae of wall

Sole

Frog

Bar

Bulb

White line

Stratum medium, deep unpigmented layer

FIG. 12–73. Sole, Hoof, Horse.

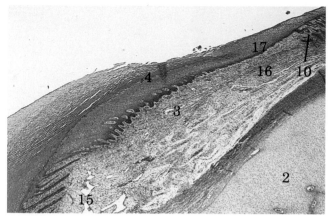

FIG. 12–74   ×12.5

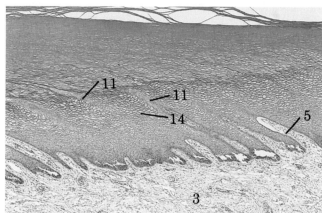

FIG. 12–75   ×25

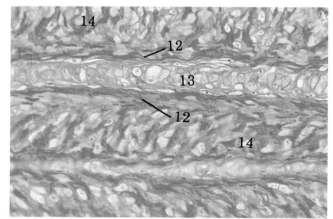

FIG. 12–76   ×125

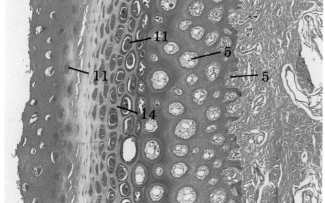

FIG. 12–77   ×12.5

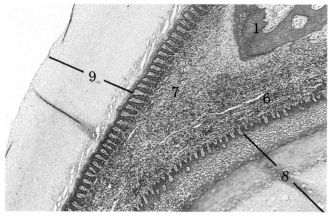

FIG. 12–78   ×25

KEY	
1. Bone, P₃	**10.** Hair follicle, developing
2. Cartilage, developing P₃	**11.** Horn tubule
3. Coronary dermis	**12.** Horn tubule, cortex
4. Coronary epidermis	**13.** Horn tubule, medulla
5. Dermal papilla	**14.** Intertubular horn
6. Dermis, sole	**15.** Laminar dermis
7. Dermis, wall	**16.** Perioplic dermis
8. Epidermis, sole	**17.** Perioplic epidermis
9. Epidermis, wall	

FIG. 12–74. Developing Hoof, l.s., Fetus, Horse. The regions that form the three layers of the hoof wall are apparent: the perioplic, coronary, and laminar regions.

FIG. 12–75. Developing Hoof, Coronary Region, l.s., Fetus, Horse. Portion of coronary epidermis and coronary dermis, later in development than in Figure 12–74, showing tubular and intertubular horn. The medulla and cortex of the horn tubules are formed from the cells of the stratum basale that cover the tip and the sides of dermal papillae, respectively. Intertubular horn is formed by cells of the stratum basale that are located between the bases of the dermal papillae. *(Photograph of a histologic section borrowed from the College of Veterinary Medicine, Iowa State University.)*

FIG. 12–76. Developing Hoof, Coronary Region, l.s., Fetus, Horse. Detail of Figure 12–75, showing two horn tubules in longitudinal section. *(Photograph of a histologic section borrowed from the College of Veterinary Medicine, Iowa State University.)*

FIG. 12–77. Hoof, Coronary Region, x.s., Horse. Dermal papillae and horn tubules of tubular horn. *(Photograph of a histologic section borrowed from the College of Veterinary Medicine, Iowa State University.)*

FIG. 12–78. Developing Hoof, Wall and Sole, x.s., Fetus, Horse. The dermis of the wall is laminated, while that of the sole is papillated.

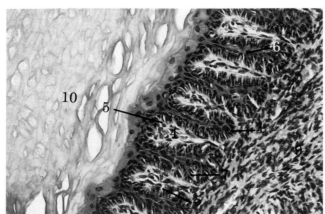

FIG. 12–79 ×125

FIG. 12–79. Developing Hoof, Wall, x.s., Fetus, Horse. Detail of Figure 12–78. The epidermal laminae, at this time, consist mainly of a layer of basal cells (stratum basale). Primary epidermal laminae have begun to form secondary laminae. The primary and secondary dermal laminae are extensions of the laminar dermis.

FIG. 12–80. Hoof, Laminar Region, x.s., Horse. Horn tubules of the stratum medium are seen in cross section. Primary and secondary epidermal laminae of the stratum internum interdigitate with the laminar dermis, which anchors the third phalanx to the wall of the hoof. Epidermal laminae, which are long ridges, appear featherlike in cross section. *(Photograph of a histologic section borrowed from the College of Veterinary Medicine, Iowa State University.)*

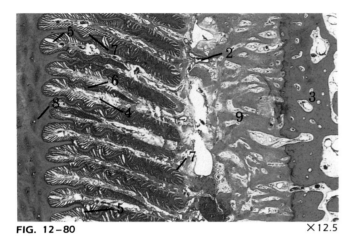

FIG. 12–80 ×12.5

FIG. 12–81. Hoof, Laminar Region, x.s., Horse. Primary epidermal laminae of the stratum internum, continuous with the stratum medium, bear secondary epidermal laminae. These interdigitate with primary and secondary dermal laminae. The secondary epidermal laminae and the dermal laminae comprise the sensitive laminae. Nuclei of the basal cells appear as small dark spots along the periphery of secondary epidermal laminae. *(Photograph of a histologic section borrowed from the College of Veterinary Medicine, Iowa State University.)*

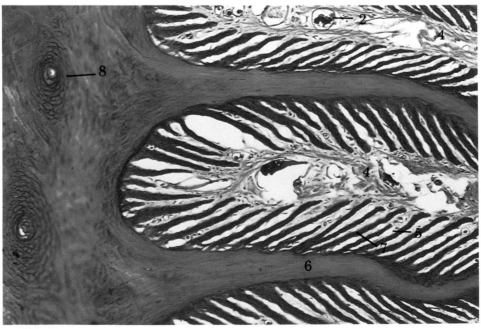

FIG. 12–81

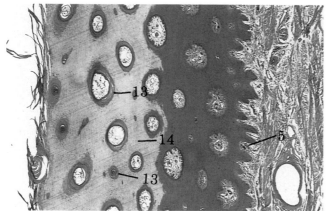

FIG. 12-82   ×25

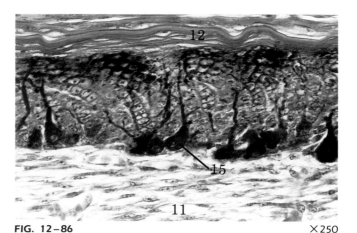

FIG. 12-86   ×250

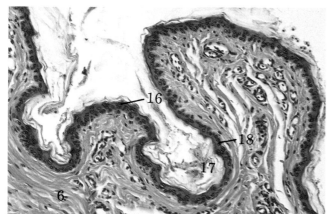

FIG. 12-83   ×125

KEY	
1. Axial blood vessel	**10.** Feather muscle
2. Barbs, pigmented	**11.** Feather pulp
3. Corneous cells	**12.** Feather sheath
4. Corneous connection	**13.** Horn tubule
5. Dermal papilla	**14.** Intertubular horn
6. Dermis	**15.** Melanocyte
7. Epidermal collar	**16.** Stack of nuclei
8. Epidermis	**17.** Stratum corneum
9. Feather follicle	**18.** Stratum germinativum

FIG. 12-82. Hoof, Sole, oblique section, Horse. Dermal papillae and horn tubules of the sole are shown. *(Photograph of a histologic section borrowed from the College of Veterinary Medicine, Iowa State University.)*

FIG. 12-83. Skin, Neck, Chicken. The epidermis of feathered skin is very thin and composed of a stratum germinativum and stratum corneum. The layers of the stratum germinativum are evident in Fig. 12-93. Nuclei of the epidermal cells are often organized into stacks perpendicular to the surface. Abundant small blood vessels appear in the superficial region of the dermis.

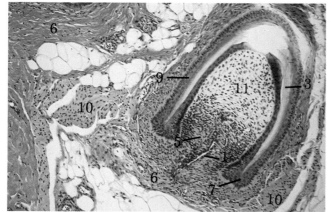

FIG. 12-84   ×62.5

FIG. 12-84. Feather Follicle, Skin, Neck, Chicken. Oblique section through the basal region of a follicle with a developing feather. An epidermal collar surrounds the dermal papilla. The upper portion of the dermal papilla blends with the feather pulp.

FIG. 12-85. Skin, Chicken. Oblique sections of developing contour feathers.

FIG. 12-86. Skin, Chicken. Oblique section of a developing contour feather. Melanocytes lie among cells of the barb. Barbule cells, beginning with the outermost ones, receive pigment from the processes of the melanocytes.

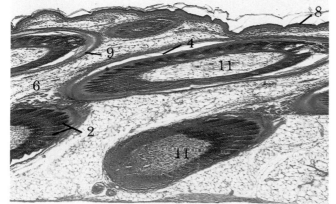

FIG. 12-85   ×25

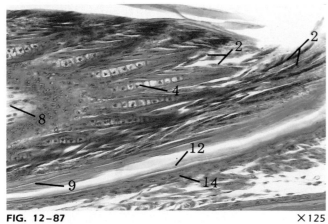

FIG. 12-87   ×125

KEY	
1. Air space	**10.** Follicle, contour feather
2. Barbules	**11.** Follicle, filoplume feather
3. Calamus	**12.** Stratum corneum, follicle
4. Cells of barb stem	**13.** Stratum corneum, skin
5. Dermis	**14.** Stratum germinativum,
6. Elastic tendon	follicle
7. Feather muscle	**15.** Stratum germinativum, skin
8. Feather pulp	
9. Feather sheath	

FIG. 12-87. Skin, Chicken. Longitudinal section of a contour feather showing several developing barbs, later in development than in Figure 12-86. The pale, cuboidal cells at the base of each barb form the stem of the barb.

FIG. 12-88. Skin, Chicken. Cross section of a contour feather showing numerous barbs.

FIG. 12-89. Skin, Chicken. Portion of contour feather follicle, x.s., at level of calamus (quill). Note that feather pulp has been replaced by an air space.

FIG. 12-90. Skin, Eyelid, Chicken. Feather follicles, x.s. The follicle wall of the tiny filoplume feather is relatively thick. A feather muscle attaches to the connective tissue sheath of the follicle of a contour feather by an elastic tendon.

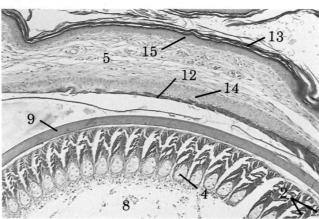

FIG. 12-88   ×62.5

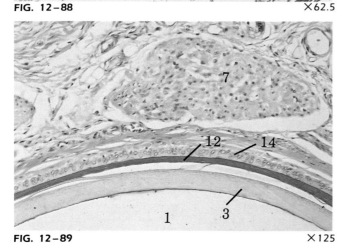

FIG. 12-89   ×125

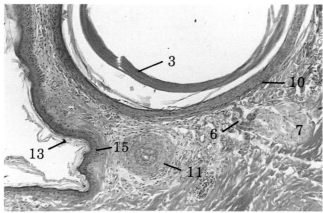

FIG. 12-90   ×62.5

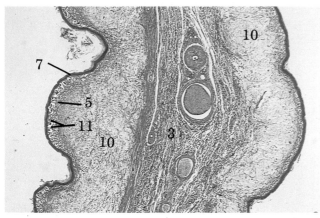

FIG. 12–91 ×12.5

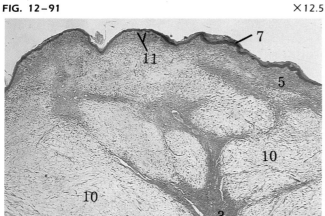

FIG. 12–92 ×12.5

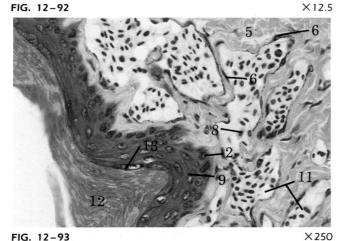

FIG. 12–93 ×250

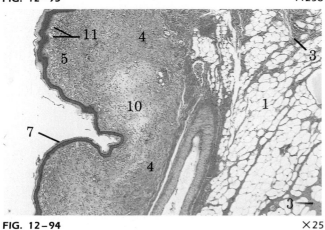

FIG. 12–94 ×25

KEY	
1. Adipose tissue	**8.** Erythrocyte
2. Basal layer	**9.** Intermediate layer
3. Dermis, central layer	**10.** Mucous connective tissue
4. Dermis, intermediate layer	**11.** Sinus capillaries
5. Dermis, superficial layer	**12.** Stratum corneum
6. Endothelial cell, nucleus	**13.** Transitional layer
7. Epidermis	

FIG. 12–91. Wattle, x.s., Rooster. Numerous sinus capillaries in the superficial layer of the dermis impart a red color to the wattle (and comb) when filled with blood. Mucous connective tissue of the intermediate layer of the dermis surrounds the central layer of dense connective tissue.

FIG. 12–92. Comb, Rooster. The point of a comb is similar in appearance to the wattle (Fig. 12–91). The collagenous fibers of the central layer of the dermis arise from the periosteum of the skull and carry vessels and nerves to the extremities of the comb.

FIG. 12–93. Comb, Rooster. Portion of epidermis and superficial dermis. The stratum corneum and layers of the stratum germinativum (basal, intermediate, and transitional layers) are evident. The lower ends of the cells of the basal layer bulge into the dermis, so that the epidermal-dermal boundary is uneven. Numerous anastomosing, blood-filled sinus capillaries in the superficial layer of the dermis are lined by pigment-laden endothelial cells.

FIG. 12–94. Comb, Hen. The comb of a laying hen, compared to that of a rooster, contains less mucous connective tissue and more dense connective tissue in the intermediate layer, as well as fewer and smaller sinus capillaries in the superficial layer of the dermis (see Fig. 12–95).

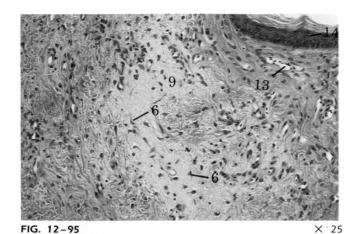

FIG. 12–95   ×·25

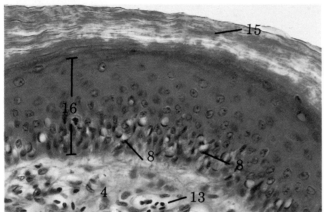

FIG. 12–96   ×250

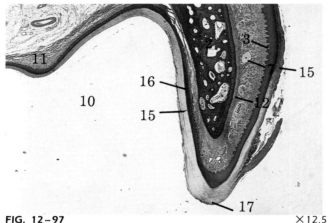

FIG. 12–97   ×12.5

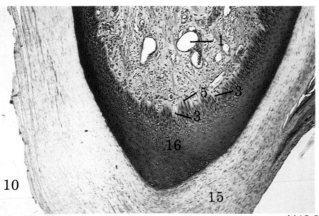

FIG. 12–98   ×62.5

KEY	
1. Blood vessel	**10.** Oral cavity
2. Bone	**11.** Palatine ridge
3. Dermal papilla	**12.** Periosteum
4. Dermis, superficial layer	**13.** Sinus capillary
5. Epidermal peg	**14.** Stack of nuclei
6. Fibroblast	**15.** Stratum corneum
7. Herbst corpuscle	**16.** Stratum germinativum
8. Merkel's cell	**17.** Tomial edge
9. Mucous connective tissue	

FIG. 12–95. Comb, Hen. Detail of the epidermis and a portion of the dermis in Figure 12–94. Fewer and smaller sinus capillaries are in the superficial layer of the dermis of the comb of the laying hen as compared to that of the rooster. Note the arrangement of the nuclei of epidermal cells into stacks.

FIG. 12–96. Comb, Hen. Numerous Merkel's cells are located along the inner surface of the epidermis. These cells are associated with tactile nerve endings.

FIG. 12–97. Upper Beak, x.s., Chicken. One side of the upper beak is shown. The bone of the premaxilla is covered by a periosteum, dermis, and epidermis with a thick layer of hard keratin. The dermis of the lateral surface of the upper beak often contains Herbst corpuscles; one corpuscle is shown here (see Fig. 9–34 for detail of this corpuscle). Dermal papillae of the lateral surface diminish medially. The lower beak slips inside the upper beak between the palatine ridge and the stratum corneum of the medial surface.

FIG. 12–98. Upper Beak, x.s., Chicken. Detail of dermis and epidermis of the tomial edge of Figure 12–97. Cells of the stratum basale vary in height and width, so that intermittent groups of tall slender cells form epidermal pegs, between which project dermal papillae.

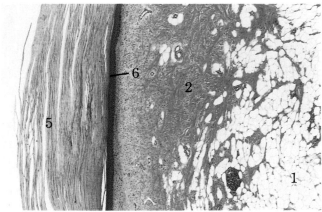

FIG. 12–99 ×25

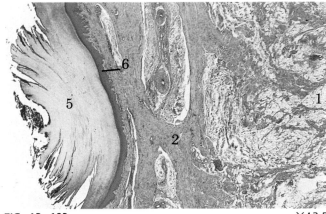

FIG. 12–103 ×12.5

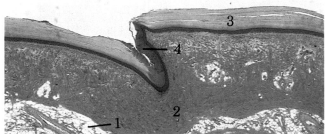

FIG. 12–100 ×12.5

FIG. 12–99. Spur, Hen. The spur cap consists of an extremely thick stratum corneum of hard keratin.

FIG. 12–100. Scutes, l.s., Anterior Metatarsus, Chicken. Scutes are large scales that are covered by hard keratin. Their region of overlap, shown here, forms a sulcus lined by soft keratin.

FIG. 12–101. Scutes, l.s., Anterior Metatarsus, Chicken. The region of overlap of two scutes shows the transition from the hard keratin to the deeper staining, soft keratin of the sulcus.

FIG. 12–102. Reticulate Scale, x.s., Digit, Chicken. The hard keratin of the stratum corneum covers the outer surface and lines the sulci of these small scales from the lateral metatarsus.

FIG. 12–103. Digital Pad, Chicken. A thick keratinized epithelium, a dermis, and a thick cushion of adipose tissue in the subcutis characterize the digital pad.

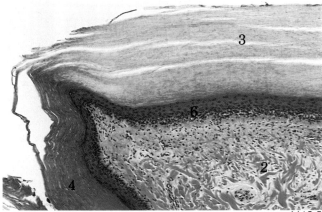

FIG. 12–101 ×62.5

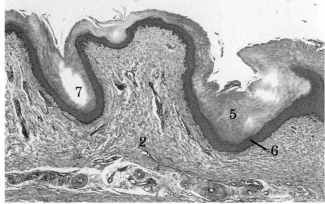

FIG. 12–102 ×25

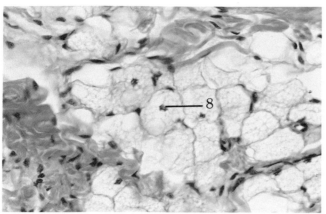

FIG. 12–104 ×250

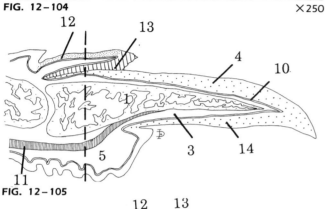

FIG. 12–105

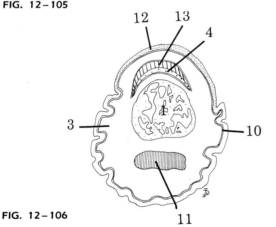

FIG. 12–106

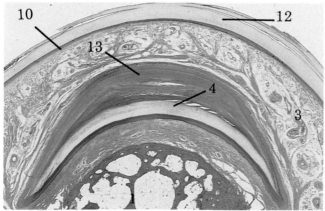

FIG. 12–107 ×12.5

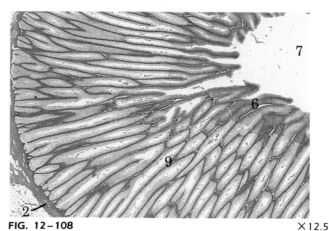

FIG. 12–108 ×12.5

KEY	
1. Bone, distal phalanx	**10.** Stratum germinativum
2. Connective tissue capsule	**11.** Tendon
3. Dermis	**12.** Unguinal scale, dorsal
4. Dorsal plate, claw	surface
5. Footpad	**13.** Unguinal scale, ventral
6. Glycogen zone	surface
7. Lobe, lumen	**14.** Ventral plate, claw
8. Multilocular fat cell, nucleus	
9. Sebaceous zone	

FIG. 12–104. Multilocular Fat, Digital Pad, Chicken. Multilocular fat cells, containing numerous lipid vacuoles and a central nucleus, are common in the subcutis of the chicken.

FIG. 12–105. Claw, l.s., Chicken. The dotted line indicates the approximate location of the drawing (cross section) of the claw shown in Figure 12–106.

FIG. 12–106. Claw, Base, x.s., Chicken.

FIG. 12–107. Claw, Base, x.s., Chicken. Compare this photomicrograph with Figures 12–105 and 12–106. The free edge of the dorsal, unguinal scale (scute type) overlaps the base of the claw, so that a cross section reveals a dorsal and ventral surface of the scale. The soft keratin of the ventral surface of the scale abuts the dorsal plate of hard keratin of the base of the claw. The dorsal plate curves ventrally over the bone of the distal phalanx.

FIG. 12–108. Uropygial Gland, l.s., Chicken. A portion of one lobe of this bilobed holocrine gland shows branched tubular glands surrounded by a connective tissue capsule. Each tubular gland is composed of a peripheral, sebaceous zone and an inner, glycogen zone. The latter communicates with the lumen of the lobe.

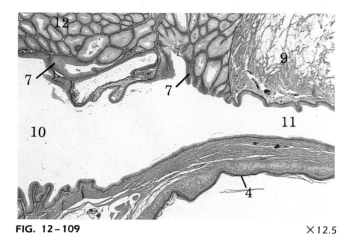

FIG. 12–109   ×12.5

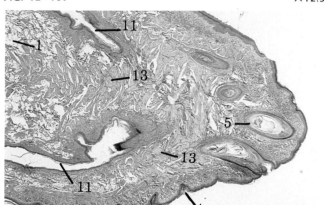

FIG. 12–110   ×12.5

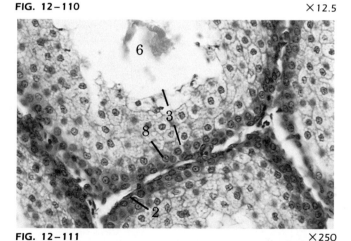

FIG. 12–111   ×250

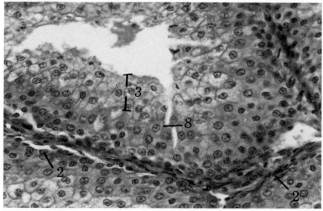

FIG. 12–112   ×250

KEY	
1. Adipose tissue	**8.** Intermediate cell
2. Basal cell, nucleus	**9.** Isthmus
3. Central layer	**10.** Lobe, lumen
4. Epidermis	**11.** Primary duct
5. Feather follicle	**12.** Sebaceous zone
6. Gland, lumen	**13.** Smooth muscle
7. Glycogen zone	

FIG. 12–109. Uropygial Gland, l.s., Chicken. The lumen of a lobe communicates with a primary duct, which passes through the isthmus toward the papilla of the gland.

FIG. 12–110. Uropygial Gland, l.s., Chicken. The two primary ducts pass through the papilla (nipple). Their openings (not shown) onto the surface are surrounded by feathers.

FIG. 12–111. Sebaceous Zone, Uropygial Gland, Chicken. Portions of tubular glands are shown in cross section. The basal layer of the glandular epithelium is represented by the oval to flat nuclei of the small basal cells. A single layer of acidophilic and grainy intermediate cells lies upon the basal layer. Cells of the thick, central (transitional) layer accumulate lipid, hypertrophy, and degenerate toward the luminal surface.

FIG. 12–112. Glycogen Zone, Uropygial Gland, Chicken. Portions of tubular glands are shown in cross section. Intermediate cells, with an acidophilic and grainy cytoplasm, form a thick layer in the glycogen zone. The pale cells of the central layer are less numerous (compare with Fig. 12–111).

109

DIGESTIVE SYSTEM

MAMMALS

The digestive tract extends from the mouth to the anus. Generally, its wall is composed of an outer **serosa** (or an **adventitia**), **muscularis externa, submucosa,** and inner **mucosa.** The mucosa consists of an inner **epithelium,** a middle **lamina propria,** and an outer **muscularis mucosae.** A muscularis mucosae is absent from the mouth, pharynx, portions of the esophagus, and the rumen. The mouth lacks a submucosa and muscularis externa.

From the lips through the nonglandular stomach, the epithelium of the mucosa is stratified squamous. Among other places, the epithelium is keratinized on the dental pad, surface of the tongue, hard palate, cheek, and the nonglandular stomach of ruminants, horses, and pigs. It is simple columnar in the glandular stomach and the intestine. In the anal canal it is stratified squamous.

From the mouth through the esophagus, the mucosa is moistened by the secretions (mucous or serous) of various glands, including the major salivary glands. Surface mucous cells and mucous neck cells of the stomach and goblet cells of the small and large intestines also contribute lubricating secretions.

The **tongue** has various small outgrowths, **papillae,** located primarily on its upper surface. These vary considerably in size and appearance. Some **(filiform)** have threadlike projections or bear spines. Some are cushion-shaped **(circumvallate, fungiform),** while others **(foliate)** take the form of a succession of folds. **Taste buds** occur in the epithelium of circumvallate, foliate, and fungiform papillae.

The **oropharynx** is lined by a stratified squamous epithelium and contains mucous glands, except in carnivores, in which the glands are mixed. A muscularis externa of skeletal muscle is surrounded by an adventitia.

Throughout most of its length, the **esophagus** is surrounded externally by an adventitia. The muscularis externa varies in composition. In the dog, it is composed of skeletal muscle throughout its length, except in the vicinity of the stomach, where skeletal muscle is replaced by smooth muscle. In ruminants, the entire muscularis externa is comprised of skeletal muscle. In the horse and cat, a switch from skeletal to smooth muscle occurs in the caudal third of the esophagus, whereas in the pig, the change occurs just cranial to the diaphragm.

The mucosa of the esophagus is lined by stratified squamous epithelium. The longitudinally arranged smooth muscle of the esophageal muscularis mucosae varies in amount from anterior to posterior. It is in the form of isolated bundles anteriorly and a continuous sheet posteriorly in the cat, horse, and ruminant. In the dog and pig, it is absent anteriorly and appears as a continuous sheet posteriorly.

Mucous or **mixed glands** occur in the submucosa of the esophagus. In the cat, horse, and ruminant, glands occur only at the junction of the pharynx and esophagus. In the pig they occur anteriorly, diminish in the mid-region, and are sparse caudally. In the dog, they occupy the entire length of the esophagus and extend into the stomach for a short distance.

The horse, ruminant, and pig have a nonglandular **forestomach** and a **glandular stomach.** In ruminants, the forestomach is divisible into a rumen, reticulum, and omasum. The glandular stomach of ruminants is the abomasum. The cat and dog have a glandular stomach but lack a forestomach. In all of these animals, the glandular stomach consists of **cardiac, fundic,** and **pyloric gland regions.** The cardiac gland region is relatively small in all but the pig.

The epithelium of the glandular stomach invaginates into the lamina propria, forming tubular structures called **gastric pits** (foveolae). Depressions of the mucosa known as **gastric furrows** are also present.

Various **tubular glands** empty into the bottom of the gastric pits. **Mucous glands** with occasional parietal cells are the principal type found in the cardiac gland region. In the fundic gland region, glands are constructed mostly of **parietal** and **chief cells,** which secrete hydrochloric acid and pepsinogen respectively.

The glands of the pyloric gland region are mainly of the mucous type with interspersed parietal cells.

In carnivores, the fundic gland region is separated into an adoral, narrow, thin **light zone** and an aboral, wider, thicker **dark zone.** These zones are readily visible on gross examination of the mucosa and are distinguishable histologically. The stomach of the cat has a thick layer of connective tissue between the base of the glands and the muscularis mucosae called the **stratum compactum.** This may be capped by a layer of fibroblasts, the **stratum granulosum.** The combination of these cells and the stratum compactum is called the **lamina subglandularis.** The latter may be absent in dogs. A submucosa, muscularis externa of smooth muscle, and serosa complete the wall of the stomach.

The intestines of mammals consist of a **small intestine** (duodenum, jejunum, and ileum) and a **large intestine** (cecum, colon, rectum, and anal canal). In both the small and large intestine, the epithelium is simple columnar with a **striated border. Goblet cells** occur among the columnar cells. The former increase in number from anterior to posterior, with the greatest number occurring in the large intestine.

Villi are confined to the small intestine in mammals. They are short and thick in ruminants, but long and slender in carnivores. At the bases of the villi are invaginations of the epithelium, the **crypts of Lieberkühn** (intestinal glands). Replacement of the mucosal epithelium occurs by cell division primarily within the crypts. A muscularis mucosae consisting of two layers of smooth muscle separates the crypts from the underlying submucosa. The latter is formed from loose connective tissue in the horse, ruminant, and pig. In contrast, it is composed of moderately dense connective tissue in carnivores. A **lamina subglandularis** may be present in the intestine of carnivores. The remainder of the wall of the intestine is comprised of a muscularis externa of smooth muscle and a serosa.

Compound, tubuloacinar **Brünner's glands** (duodenal glands, submucosal glands) occur within the submucosa and often extend into the lamina propria of the duodenum. In carnivores, sheep, and goats, they are limited to the initial or mid-region of the duodenum; in horses, pigs, and cows, they extend into the jejunum. Brünner's glands also project into the pyloric stomach for a short distance. Aggregations of lymphatic nodules, **Peyer's patches,** are present in the lamina propria and submucosa of the small intestine, especially the ileum.

The mucosa of the **large intestine** presents a flat surface. Villi are absent. Crypts are longer than in the small intestine. Flat bands, **taenia coli,** consisting of longitudinally arranged smooth muscle and elastic fibers, occur in the colon of horses and pigs. Similar structures, **taenia ceci,** occur in the cecum. The **rectum** terminates at the **anal canal** which is lined by a stratified squamous epithelium. The epithelium is nonkeratinized in the anterior portion of the canal and keratinized in the posterior portion, which is continuous with the hairy skin. Tubuloacinar **anal glands** occur in the submucosa and muscularis of the anal canal in carnivores and pigs. **Circumanal glands** occur in the subcutis around the anus of the dog. The upper portion of these glands is sebaceous, whereas the lower portion is nonsebaceous. The cells of the latter resemble hepatocytes. Accordingly, the nonsebaceous region is often called a hepatoid gland.

Paired **anal sacs** occur lateral to and below the anus of carnivores. Each is lined by a keratinized, stratified squamous epithelium and is located between the inner smooth muscle of the internal anal sphincter and the outer skeletal muscle of the external anal sphincter. The excretory duct of each gland opens into the keratinized portion of the anal canal. **Glands of the anal sac** are apocrine tubular in the dog. In the cat, both apocrine tubular glands and sebaceous glands surround the anal sac.

The **liver** is a large, lobed gland. Each lobe is covered by a mesothelium, beneath which is a thin connective tissue layer, the **capsule of Glisson.** Each lobe is divided into numerous **classic lobules.** These consist of **sinusoids** and of plates of parenchyma cells, **hepatocytes,** radially organized about a central vein. Lobules are indistinctly separated from one another in all animals but the pig, in which an abundance of connective tissue between lobules clearly identifies their boundaries. **Portal tracts** (areas) occur between three or more lobules. Each tract contains one or more branches of a portal vein, hepatic artery, bile ductule, and lymphatic vessel. These various components are supported by a connective tissue framework.

Bile, secreted by hepatocytes, enters tiny bile canaliculi, from which it flows into the canals of Hering, located close to each portal tract. The canals unite with the bile ductule of a tract. Bile ductules lead into bile ducts. The epithelium of bile ductules is simple cuboidal whereas that of the bile ducts is simple columnar. **Goblet cells** occur in the largest ducts.

The **gallbladder** is a storage depot for bile. Its mucosa is thrown into numerous folds. The simple columnar epithelial lining has a striated border. Goblet cells have been reported in the epithelium of the cow. We have observed them in the goat. Mucous, serous, or mixed glands are often seen in the wall of the gallbladder of ruminants. The smooth muscle of the muscularis is ar-

ranged circularly for the most part. The gallbladder is absent in the horse.

The **pancreas** consists of numerous tubuloacinar secretory units, which form the exocrine component of the organ. Clusters of epithelial cells, the endocrine **islets of Langerhans,** are scattered among the secretory units. Tubuloacinar units drain into long, narrow **intercalated ducts,** which are lined by elongated cells that present a cuboidal appearance in cross section. Intercalated ducts communicate directly with **interlobular ducts.** Striated (secretory) ducts are not present. Unlike salivary glands, myoepithelial cells are lacking around the secretory units. **Pacinian corpuscles** are commonly found within the connective tissue of the pancreas of dogs and cats.

CHICKEN

In the chicken, **salivary glands** are all of the mucous variety. They are located in the roof and floor of the oral cavity, tongue, and pharynx. **Taste buds** are present but sparse. They are associated with the ducts of salivary glands at the base of the tongue and the pharynx.

The **esophagus** has the usual seven layers. It is lined by a thick, nonkeratinized, stratified squamous epithelium. The muscularis externa is composed of smooth muscle along the entire length of the esophagus. Mucous glands occur in the lamina propria, but are lacking throughout most of the **crop,** which is a caudal diverticulum located approximately two thirds of the way down the esophagus. Except for the lack of mucous glands, the crop has a structure identical to the rest of the esophagus.

The **stomach** of the chicken consists of a glandular **proventriculus** and a muscular **ventriculus** (gizzard). The mucosa of the proventriculus is thrown into folds (plicae). Depressions between the folds are called sulci. The epithelium is simple columnar except at the base of the sulci, where it is cuboidal. The wall of the proventriculus consists of large compound tubular glands. The secretory cells, which are cuboidal to low columnar, produce both pepsinogen and hydrochloric acid, thus combining the function of mammalian chief and parietal cells. Each gland opens to the lumen of the stomach through a conical papilla.

The ventriculus is a highly muscular grinding organ. It is lined by an epithelium that invaginates into the lamina propria, forming elongated pits, each of which bears terminal secretory units. Cells of the latter secrete a thick, horny material. Although keratin-like, this substance, usually called keratinoid, is not chemically equivalent to keratin. It forms the tough inner lining, about one mm thick, of the ventriculus.

The **intestine** of the chicken is similar in structure throughout its length. It consists of a **duodenum, jejunum, ileum,** and **large intestine.** A pair of blind, elongated **ceca** join the intestine at the junction of the ileum and large intestine. The terminal end of the large intestine joins the coprodeum of the **cloaca.** Villi are present throughout the small and large intestine. They are longest in the duodenum but gradually shorten and thicken caudally. In the coprodeum they are stumpy and rounded. Villi are present in the ceca also, becoming flattened toward the blind end. **Crypts of Lieberkühn** are short and open between the villi, as in mammals. Although the wall of the intestine of the chicken is similar to that of the mammal, the absence of duodenal glands and an extremely thin submucosa in the chicken are notable differences.

As in mammals, the **liver** is covered by a mesothelium, beneath which is a layer of connective tissue, Glisson's capsule. Its lobes are subdivided into numerous lobules indistinctly separated from one another. The radiating plates of hepatocytes in each lobule are two cells wide in the chicken, contrasting with those of mammals, where they are one cell wide.

The **gallbladder** of the chicken is similar to that of the mammal. The mucosa is lined by a simple columnar epithelium and is strongly folded into villus-like projections when contracted.

The **pancreas** of the chicken resembles that of the mammal. The exocrine portion is tubuloacinar. Lobulation is indistinct because of the lack of interlobular connective tissue. Islets of Langerhans are abundant and two types of islets, alpha and beta, can be easily recognized. Columnar alpha cells characterize the alpha islet. Polygonal beta cells are the principal cells of the beta islets. Alpha islets produce glucagon, whereas beta islets form insulin.

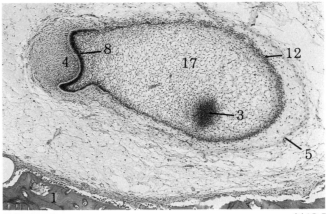

FIG. 13-1   ×25

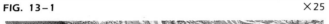

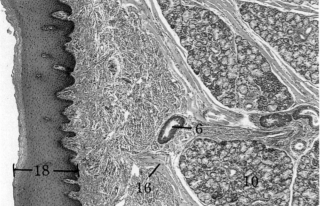

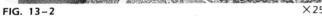

FIG. 13-2   ×25

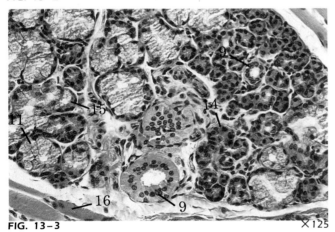

FIG. 13-3   ×125

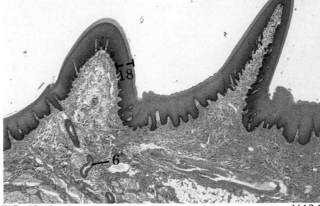

FIG. 13-4   ×12.5

FIG. 13-5   ×12.5

KEY	
1. Alveolar bone	**11.** Mucous acinus
2. Connective tissue papilla	**12.** Outer enamel epithelium
3. Dental lamina	**13.** Sebaceous gland
4. Dental papilla	**14.** Serous acinus
5. Dental sac	**15.** Serous demilune
6. Duct	**16.** Skeletal muscle
7. Hair follicle	**17.** Stellate reticulum
8. Inner enamel epithelium	**18.** Stratified squamous
9. Intralobular duct	epithelium, keratinized
10. Labial gland	**19.** Stratum granulosum

FIG. 13-1. Lip, Sheep. The section was taken through the junction of the hairy and nonhairy portions of the lip. The stratum granulosum is present in the epidermis of the hairy portion of the lip, but disappears at the junction with the nonhairy portion of the lip. Portions of hair follicles are present.

FIG. 13-2. Lip, Sheep. Oral surface of the lip with mixed labial glands among the skeletal muscle.

FIG. 13-3. Lip, Sheep. Mixed labial glands within the skeletal musculature.

FIG. 13-4. Cheek, Sheep. The mucous membrane of the cheek of ruminants is characterized by numerous, conical papillae. The apex and lateral surfaces of the papillae are highly keratinized.

FIG. 13-5. Developing Permanent Tooth, Dog. The ectodermally derived enamel organ has differentiated into the outer and inner enamel epithelium and the stellate reticulum. The dental papilla, derived from mesenchyme, is in contact with the inner enamel epithelium.

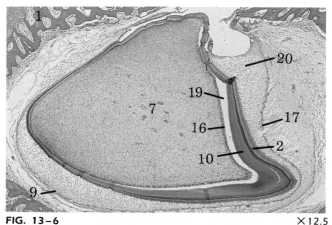

FIG. 13-6 ×12.5

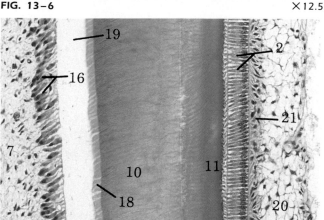

FIG. 13-7 ×125

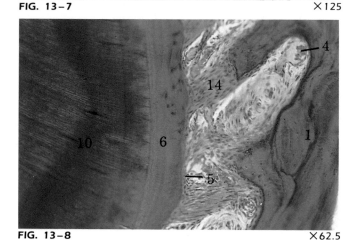

FIG. 13-8 ×62.5

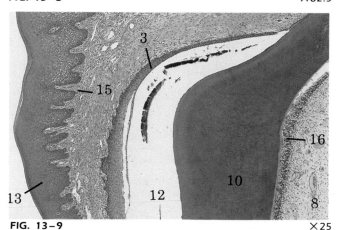

FIG. 13-9 ×25

KEY	
1. Alveolar bone	**12.** Enamel space
2. Ameloblasts	**13.** Epithelium, free gingiva
3. Attachment epithelium	**14.** Fiber bundle
4. Blood vessel	**15.** Lamina propria
5. Cementoid	**16.** Odontoblasts
6. Cementum	**17.** Outer enamel epithelium
7. Dental papilla	**18.** Predentin
8. Dental pulp	**19.** Space artifact
9. Dental sac	**20.** Stellate reticulum
10. Dentin	**21.** Stratum intermedium
11. Enamel	

FIG. 13-6. Developing Permanent Tooth, Dog. Dentin and enamel formation has begun (see Fig. 13-7).

FIG. 13-7. Dentinoenamel Junction, Developing Permanent Tooth, Dog. Odontoblasts cover the surface of the mesenchymal dental papilla. These cells produce predentin (uncalcified dentin). The pale layer of predentin abuts the recently calcified dentin. The enamel organ consists of tall columnar ameloblasts that produce enamel, a stratum intermedium, and the stellate reticulum.

FIG. 13-8. Root of Tooth, x.s., and Periodontal Ligament, Dog. The periodontal ligament consists of bundles of collagenous fibers, blood and lymphatic vessels, nerves, and cells (mostly fibroblasts). The fiber bundles extend between, and anchor to, the cementum of the tooth and the alveolar bone. The ends of the fibers that are embedded in either cementum or bone are called Sharpey's fibers. They are indistinct in this micrograph.

FIG. 13-9. Upper Deciduous Tooth, Decalcified, and Gingiva, l.s., Dog. The enamel space identifies the location of enamel before it was lost during decalcification. The attachment (junctional) epithelium of the gingiva is nonkeratinized stratified squamous and lacks connective tissue papillae. It abuts the enamel region and is continuous with the papillated, keratinized stratified squamous epithelium of the free gingiva.

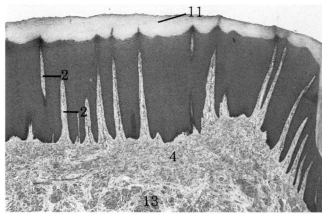

FIG. 13-10   ×12.5

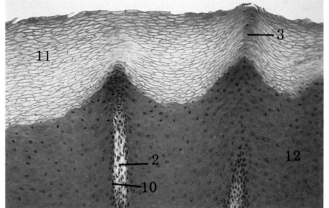

FIG. 13-11   ×62.5

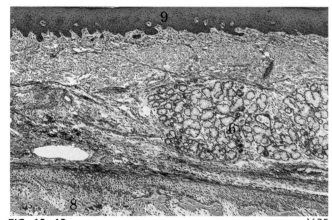

FIG. 13-12   ×25

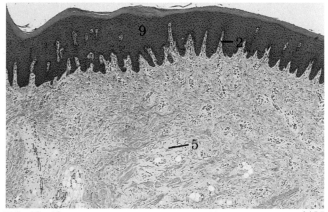

FIG. 13-13   ×25

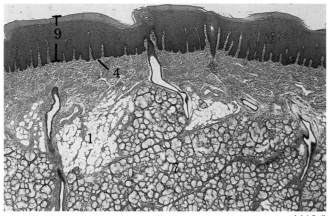

FIG. 13-14   ×12.5

KEY	
1. Adipose tissue	**8.** Palatine bone
2. Connective tissue papilla	**9.** Stratified squamous
3. Horn tubule-like structure	epithelium, keratinized
4. Lamina propria	**10.** Stratum basale
5. Loose connective tissue	**11.** Stratum corneum
6. Mixed gland	**12.** Stratum spinosum
7. Mucous gland	**13.** Submucosa

FIG. 13-10. Dental Pad, Cow. The dental pad of ruminants is distinguished by its thick stratum corneum and well developed connective tissue papillae.

FIG. 13-11. Epithelium, Dental Pad, Sheep. The section shows a thick stratum corneum and underlying stratum spinosum. A horn tubule-like structure extends through the stratum corneum.

FIG. 13-12. Hard Palate, Caudal, Dog, Masson's. All domestic mammals, except the pig, have glands (mucous or mixed) in the submucosa of the caudal portion of the hard palate. The cranial portion lacks glands in all of the domestic mammals.

FIG. 13-13. Hard Palate, Pig. Large irregular patches of pale, loose connective tissue are scattered throughout the submucosa.

FIG. 13-14. Soft Palate, Cow. Mucous glands and adipose tissue occupy portions of the lamina propria and submucosa. The epithelium is stratified squamous and keratinized.

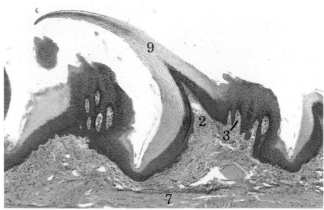

FIG. 13–15   ×25

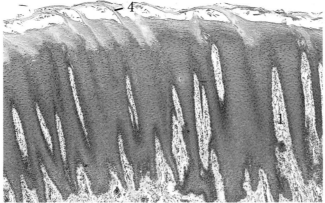

FIG. 13–16   ×25

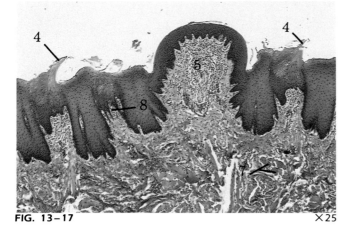

FIG. 13–17   ×25

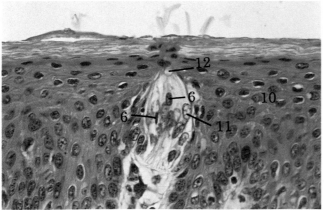

FIG. 13–18   ×250

KEY	
1. Connective tissue papilla	**6.** Sensory cell, nucleus
2. Connective tissue papilla, caudal	**7.** Skeletal muscle
3. Connective tissue papilla, rostral	**8.** Small papilla
4. Filiform papilla	**9.** Spine
5. Fungiform papilla, core	**10.** Stratum spinosum
	11. Supporting cell, nucleus
	12. Taste pore

FIG. 13–15. Filiform Papilla, Tongue, Cat. The filiform papilla of carnivores contains several small, rostral connective tissue papillae and a large, caudal connective tissue papilla. A large keratinized spine is associated with the caudal papilla.

FIG. 13–16. Filiform Papillae, Tongue, Horse. In horses and pigs, delicate, keratinized filiform papillae project from the upper surface of the tongue. The connective tissue papillae are long and unbranched.

FIG. 13–17. Fungiform and Filiform Papillae, Tongue, Goat. This section is from the tip of the tongue. The fungiform papilla is mound-like in section with a broad connective tissue core containing numerous nerves. Portions of keratinized filiform papillae appear on either side. In ruminants, the connective tissue papillae associated with the filiform papillae branch into several small papillae.

FIG. 13–18. Taste Bud, Fungiform Papilla, Tongue, Horse. The taste bud is embedded within the keratinized stratified squamous epithelium of a fungiform papilla. Supportive and sensory cells are visible within the bud. The nucleus and cytoplasm of the sensory cells are slightly darker than those of the supporting cells.

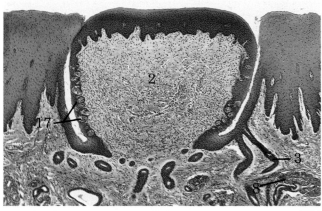

FIG. 13–19 ✕25

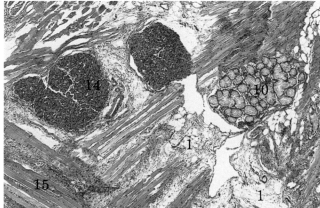

FIG. 13–20 ✕25

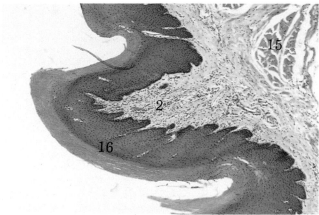

FIG. 13–21 ✕25

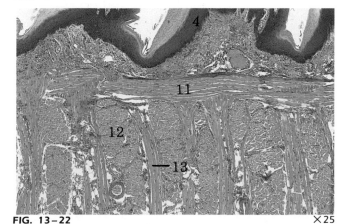

FIG. 13–22 ✕25

FIG. 13–23 ✕25

KEY	
1. Adipose tissue	**10.** Mucous gland
2. Connective tissue core	**11.** Muscle, longitudinal
3. Duct	**12.** Muscle, transverse
4. Filiform papilla	**13.** Muscle, vertical
5. Interlobular connective tissue	**14.** Serous gland
6. Interlobular duct	**15.** Skeletal muscle
7. Intralobular duct	**16.** Stratified squamous epithelium, keratinized
8. Lingual salivary gland	**17.** Taste buds
9. Lobule	

FIG. 13–19. Circumvallate Papilla, Tongue, Goat. This large papilla lies within a depression of the lingual epithelium. Taste buds occur within the epithelium of the papilla facing the cavity of the depression, but are usually absent from the upper surface of the papilla.

FIG. 13–20. Conical Papilla, Tongue, Goat. This highly keratinized papilla is located on the upper surface of the tongue.

FIG. 13–21. Lingual Salivary Glands, Horse. Both mucous and serous glands occur among the skeletal muscle of the tongue.

FIG. 13–22. Musculature, Tongue, l.s., Cat. The vertical, horizontal, and transverse arrangement of the lingual skeletal musculature can be seen below the mucosal papillae.

FIG. 13–23. Parotid Gland, Horse. Portions of several lobules are shown. Lobules are often delineated by space artifacts.

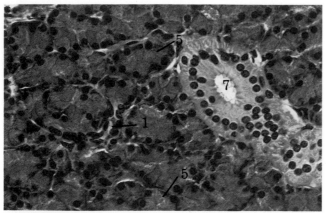

FIG. 13-24   ×250

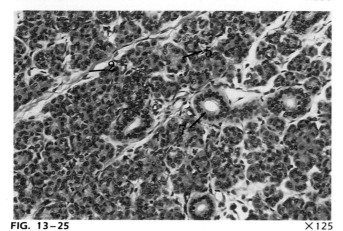

FIG. 13-25   ×125

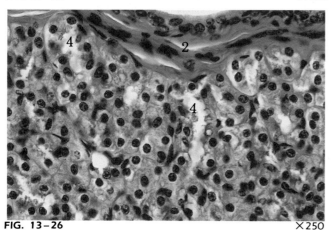

FIG. 13-26   ×250

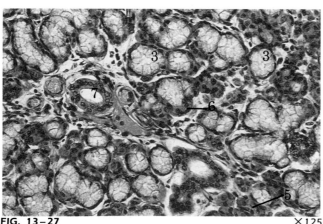

FIG. 13-27   ×125

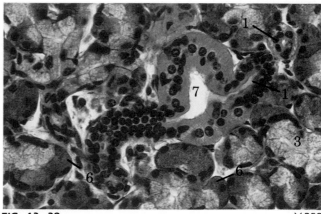

FIG. 13-28   ×250

KEY	
1. Intercalated duct	**4.** Secretory unit
2. Interlobular connective tissue	**5.** Serous acinus
	6. Serous demilune
3. Mucous acinus	**7.** Striated duct

FIG. 13-24. Parotid Gland, Horse. Serous acini, intercalated ducts, and striated (secretory) ducts are present. The latter show clearly defined basal striations.

FIG. 13-25. Parotid Gland, Dog. Serous acini and intralobular ducts are shown.

FIG. 13-26. Parotid Gland, Cow. The secretory units are lined by pale, acidophilic cells with large nuclei. The cells vary in height, giving the luminal surface a scalloped appearance. This feature is unique to the cow.

FIG. 13-27. Submandibular Gland, Dog. Mucous acini (some with serous demilunes) and serous acini characterize the parenchyma.

FIG. 13-28. Submandibular Gland, Sheep. Intercalated ducts branching from a striated duct.

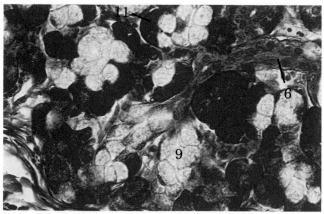

FIG. 13-29 ×250

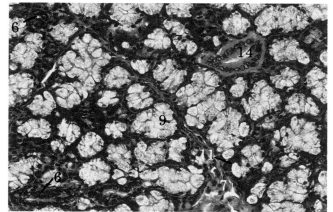

FIG. 13-30 ×62.5

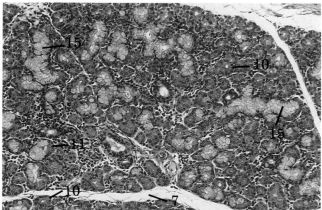

FIG. 13-31 ×125

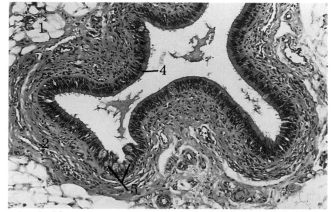

FIG. 13-32 ×62.5

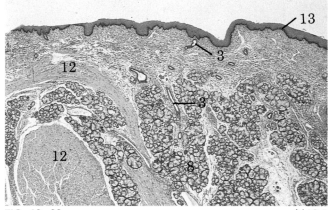

FIG. 13-33 ×12.5

KEY	
1. Adipose tissue	**9.** Mucous acinus
2. Connective tissue coat	**10.** Serous acinus
3. Duct	**11.** Serous demilune
4. Epithelium	**12.** Skeletal muscle
5. Goblet cells	**13.** Stratified squamous
6. Intercalated duct	epithelium
7. Interlobular connective	**14.** Striated duct
tissue	**15.** Tubular mucous unit
8. Mixed glands	

FIG. 13-29. Submandibular Gland, Sheep, Mallory's. The junction between a mucous acinus and an intercalated duct is illustrated.

FIG. 13-30. Sublingual Gland, Dog. In the cat, dog, and horse, the sublingual gland contains mucous secretory units, serous acini, and serous demilunes. Long tubular mucous units are a characteristic feature of the gland in the dog.

FIG. 13-31. Sublingual Gland, Pig. In the pig and ruminant, mucous tubuloacinar secretory units predominate. Serous demilunes are sparse.

FIG. 13-32. Interlobular Duct, Sublingual Gland, Pig. This large interlobular duct is lined by a columnar epithelium. In places the latter is bistratified. Goblet cells occur in the epithelium.

FIG. 13-33. Oropharynx, Dog. The section shows mixed glands among the skeletal muscle and within the submucosa. These glands are shown in detail in Figure 11-10.

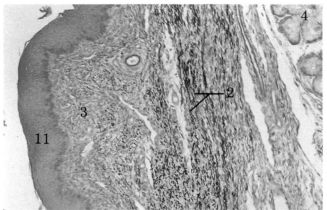

FIG. 13-34 ×62.5

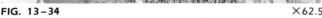

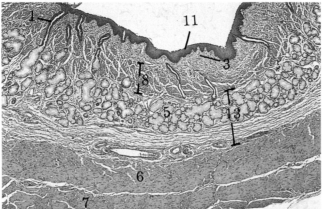

FIG. 13-35 ×25

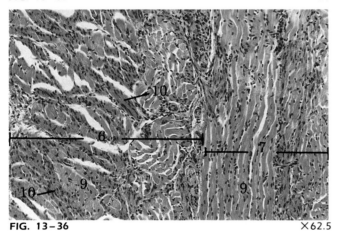

FIG. 13-36 ×62.5

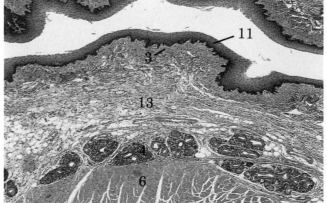

FIG. 13-37 ×25

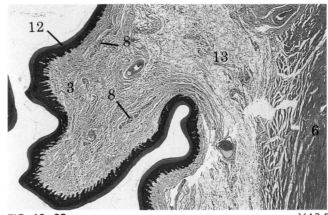

FIG. 13-38 ×12.5

KEY	
1. Duct	**8.** Muscularis mucosae
2. Elastic fibers	**9.** Skeletal muscle
3. Lamina propria	**10.** Smooth muscle
4. Mixed glands	**11.** Stratified squamous epithelium
5. Mucous glands	**12.** Stratified squamous epithelium, keratinized
6. Muscularis externa, inner circular	
7. Muscularis externa, outer longitudinal	**13.** Submucosa

FIG. 13-34. Oropharynx, Dog, Orcein. A thick band of connective tissue, containing numerous elastic fibers, parallels the mucosa.

FIG. 13-35. Esophagus, Mid-Region, x.s., Dog. The glands of the dog's esophagus are predominantly mucous. They are located in the submucosa throughout the length of the esophagus of the dog. The muscularis externa is skeletal muscle, except very near the stomach, see Figure 13-36.

FIG. 13-36. Esophagus, Near Stomach, l.s., Dog. The muscularis externa of the dog's esophagus is composed of skeletal muscle, except in the region caudal to the diaphragm, where the musculature is mixed.

FIG. 13-37. Esophagus, Cranial, l.s., Cat. A few mixed glands are present in the submucosa. In the cat, horse, and ruminant, esophageal glands occur only near the junction of the esophagus and pharynx. The stratified squamous lining of the esophagus of carnivores is typically nonkeratinized. In the cat and horse, the muscularis externa is skeletal muscle throughout much of the esophagus. The transition from skeletal to smooth occurs in the caudal 1/5 to 1/3 of the esophagus in these animals.

FIG. 13-38. Esophagus, Cranial, x.s., Horse. The papillated stratified squamous epithelium shows a distinct keratinized layer. The epithelium is also keratinized in pigs and ruminants. A sparse muscularis mucosae is present in the cranial esophagus in the horse, cat, and ruminant. The muscularis externa consists of skeletal muscle in this region.

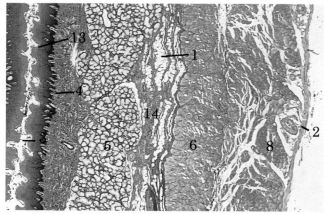

FIG. 13-39 ×12.5

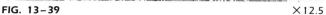

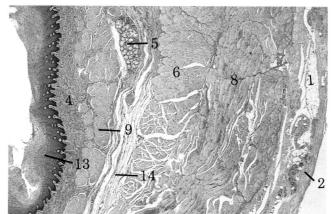

FIG. 13-40 ×12.5

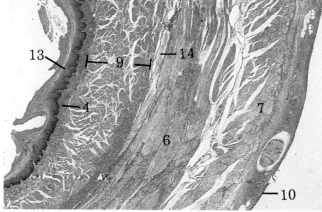

FIG. 13-41 ×12.5

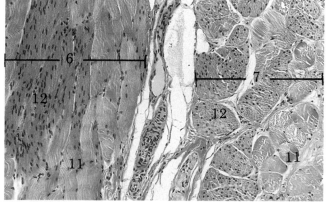

FIG. 13-42 ×62.5

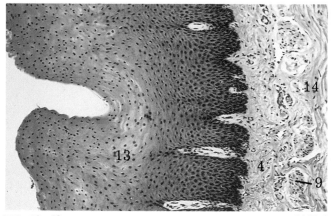

FIG. 13-43 ×62.5

KEY	
1. Adipose tissue	**8.** Muscularis externa, outer oblique
2. Adventitia	
3. Esophagus, lumen	**9.** Muscularis mucosae
4. Lamina propria	**10.** Serosa
5. Mucous gland	**11.** Skeletal muscle
6. Muscularis externa, inner circular	**12.** Smooth muscle
	13. Stratified squamous epithelium, keratinized
7. Muscularis externa, outer longitudinal	**14.** Submucosa

FIG. 13-39. Esophagus, Cranial, l.s., Pig. The stratified squamous epithelium is also keratinized in horses and ruminants. Note the abundance of mucous glands in the submucosa. In the cranial portion of the esophagus, a muscularis mucosae is absent in the pig and dog. The muscularis externa consists of skeletal muscle in this region.

FIG. 13-40. Esophagus, Mid-Region, l.s., Pig. Note the decrease in glandular tissue and the presence of a muscularis mucosae (compare with Fig. 13-39). The muscularis externa consists of skeletal muscle in this region.

FIG. 13-41. Esophagus, Caudal, x.s., Pig. The region of the pig's esophagus just cranial to the diaphragm shows the presence of smooth and skeletal muscle in the muscularis externa, a lack of glands, and a thick muscularis mucosae.

FIG. 13-42. Esophagus, Caudal, x.s., Pig. Detail of Figure 13-41 shows the smooth and skeletal musculature of the muscularis externa.

FIG. 13-43. Esophagus, Mid-Region, x.s., Sheep. The muscularis mucosae is less developed than in the pig (see Fig. 13-40).

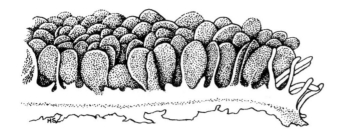

FIG. 13-44

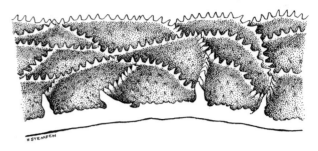

FIG. 13-48

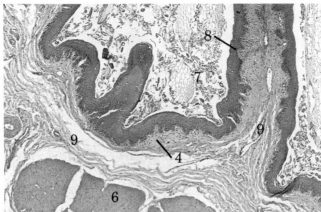

FIG. 13-45   ×25

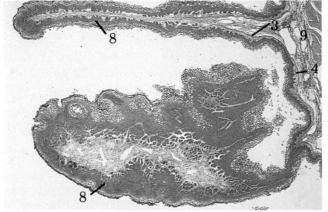

FIG. 13-46   ×12.5

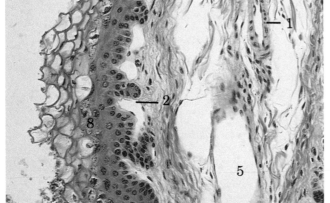

FIG. 13-47   ×125

KEY	
1. Arteriole	**6.** Muscularis externa
2. Capillary	**7.** Stomach contents
3. Connective tissue band	**8.** Stratified squamous
4. Lamina propria	epithelium, keratinized
5. Lymphatic vessel	**9.** Submucosa

FIG. 13-44. Rumen, Sheep. The mucosa of the rumen is differentiated into paddle-shaped papillae.

FIG. 13-45. Rumen, Cow. A part of the wall from the lumen to the beginning of the muscularis externa (smooth muscle). A complete short papilla and a portion of a long papilla are included. Note the submucosa entering the long papilla. A muscularis mucosae is not present in this part of the forestomach.

FIG. 13-46. Rumen, Sheep. Section shows two cuts through adjacent long papillae. These papillae are flat structures (see Fig. 13-44). The bottom one in the photograph was cut parallel to the flat surface, and the top one was cut perpendicular to the flat surface. A dense, more darkly stained band of connective tissue mimics a muscularis mucosae.

FIG. 13-47. Rumen, Sheep. Section illustrates the vacuolated, keratinized cells of the stratified squamous epithelium of a papilla. Numerous capillaries abut the epithelium.

FIG. 13-48. Reticulum, Sheep. The mucosa of the reticulum is extended into intersecting folds that subdivide the surface into distinct compartments suggesting a honeycomb. Conical papillae project from the crests of the folds and from the mucosa of the compartments.

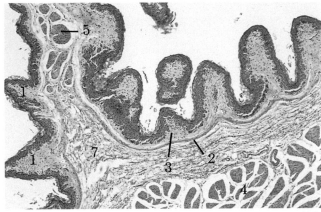

FIG. 13–49   ×25

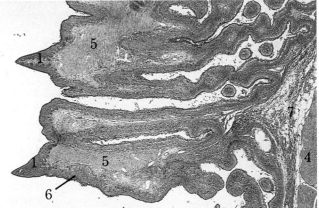

FIG. 13–50   ×12.5

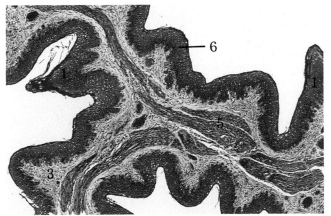

FIG. 13–51   ×25

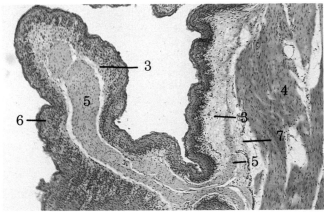

FIG. 13–53   ×25

KEY	
1. Conical papilla	**5.** Muscularis mucosae
2. Connective tissue band	**6.** Stratified squamous
3. Lamina propria	epithelium, keratinized
4. Muscularis externa	**7.** Submucosa

FIG. 13–49. Reticulum, Cow. Short folds and the base of a long fold are visible. A muscularis mucosae occurs in the upper segment of the long fold. This is a characteristic feature of the reticulum. Sides and crests of long folds have conical papillae with keratinized tips.

FIG. 13–50. Reticulum, Sheep. Section shows a long fold cut in a plane parallel to its flat surface. The apparent gaps are the result of undulations in the fold. Conical papillae are evident along the crest of the fold.

FIG. 13–51. Reticulum, Goat, Masson's. The section is parallel to the surface and through the region of intersection of three long folds. The muscularis mucosae passes from one fold to another at the intersection. Two conical papillae, with keratinized tips, project from the sides of two of the folds.

FIG. 13–52. Omasum, Sheep. Laminae (folds) of different sizes extend from the wall of the omasum somewhat like the pages of a book. The mucosal surfaces of the laminae are studded with numerous conical papillae.

FIG. 13–53. Omasum, Sheep. Small folds, such as the one shown, contain a lamina propria and muscularis mucosae, but lack an extension of smooth muscle from the muscularis externa.

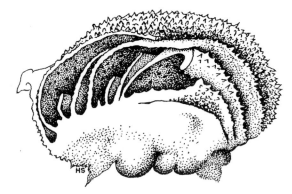

FIG. 13–52

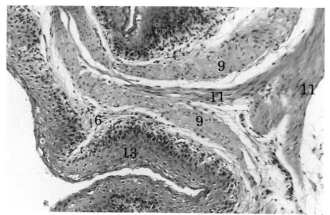

FIG. 13-54 ×62.5

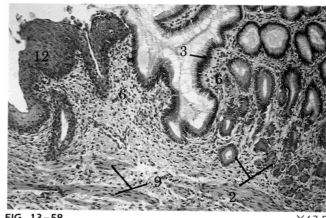

FIG. 13-58 ×62.5

KEY	
1. Cardiac gland region	**9.** Muscularis mucosae
2. Cardiac glands	**10.** Papilla
3. Columnar epithelium, stomach	**11.** Smooth muscle of muscularis externa
4. Elastic fiber	**12.** Stratified squamous epithelium, esophagus
5. Fundic gland region	
6. Lamina propria	**13.** Stratified squamous epithelium, keratinized
7. Lymphatic vessel	
8. Mixed glands	**14.** Vein

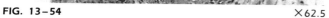

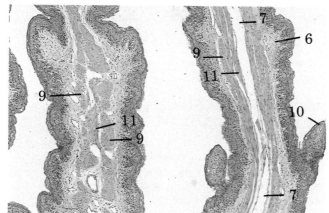

FIG. 13-55 ×25

FIG. 13-54. Omasum, Sheep. The base of a long fold is shown. In addition to the muscularis mucosae, smooth muscle from the muscularis externa projects into the center of the fold.

FIG. 13-55. Omasum, Sheep. Portions of two long folds are shown. Numerous small papillae cover the surface of the folds.

FIG. 13-56. Omasum, Goat, Orcein. The lamina propria of a portion of a small papilla contains an extensive network of elastic fibers.

FIG. 13-57. Junction, Esophagus and Cardiac Gland Region of Stomach, Dog. Numerous glands, predominantly mucous with a few serous demilunes, occupy the submucosa of the esophagus and extend into the cardiac gland region of the stomach of dogs.

FIG. 13-58. Junction, Esophagus and Cardiac Gland Region of Stomach, Dog. Detail of Figure 13-57. The stratified squamous epithelium of the esophagus ends abruptly where the columnar epithelium of the stomach begins.

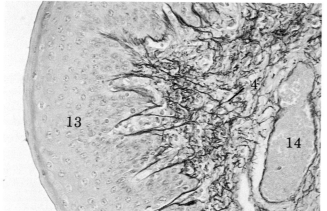

FIG. 13-56 ×125

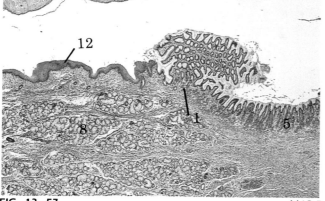

FIG. 13-57 ×12.5

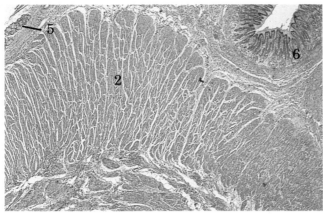

FIG. 13-59   ×12.5

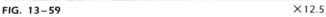

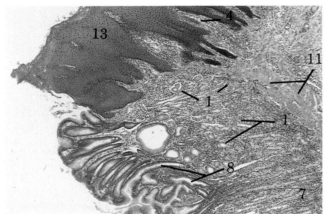

FIG. 13-60   ×25

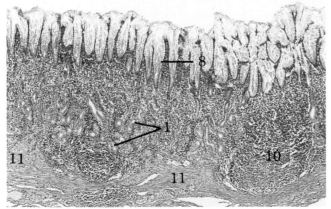

FIG. 13-61   ×25

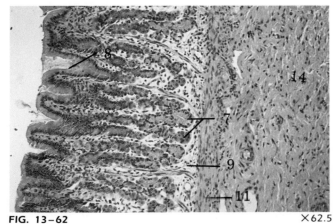

FIG. 13-62   ×62.5

FIG. 13-63   ×250

KEY	
1. Cardiac glands	**9.** Lamina propria
2. Cardiac sphincter	**10.** Lymphatic nodule
3. Chief cell	**11.** Muscularis mucosae
4. Connective tissue papilla	**12.** Parietal cell
5. Esophageal glands	**13.** Stratified squamous
6. Fundic gland region	epithelium, keratinized
7. Fundic glands	**14.** Submucosa
8. Gastric pit	

FIG. 13-59. Junction of Esophagus and Stomach, Dog. Section passes through the cardiac sphincter.

FIG. 13-60. Margo Plicatus, Horse. At the margo plicatus, the keratinized stratified squamous epithelium of the forestomach ends and the simple columnar epithelium of the cardiac gland region of the stomach begins.

FIG. 13-61. Cardiac Gland Region, Stomach, Pig. Numerous lymphatic nodules characterize the mucosa of the pig's cardiac gland region of the stomach.

FIG. 13-62. Light Zone, Fundic Gland Region, Stomach, Dog. The light zone of the carnivore's fundic stomach has a thinner mucosa than the more aboral dark zone. The gastric pits of the light zone are comparatively deep, extending, in some cases, to a depth equivalent to half the thickness of the mucosa. Compare to Figure 13-65. Smooth muscle cells of the muscularis mucosae of the stomach extend into the lamina propria.

FIG. 13-63. Light Zone, Fundic Gland Region, Stomach, Dog. Chief and parietal cells form the walls of the fundic glands. The glands are shown in cross section.

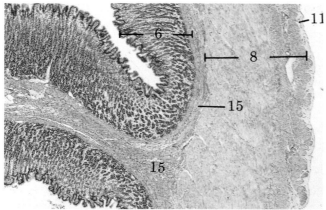

FIG. 13–64 ×12.5

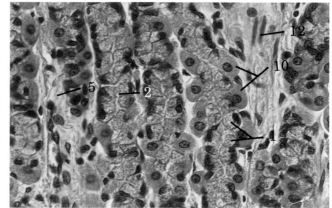

FIG. 13–68 ×250

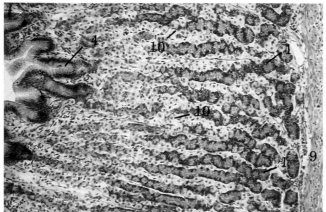

FIG. 13–65 ×62.5

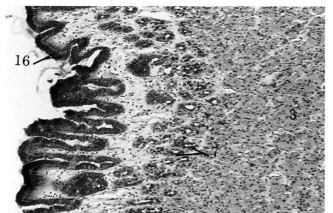

FIG. 13–66 ×62.5

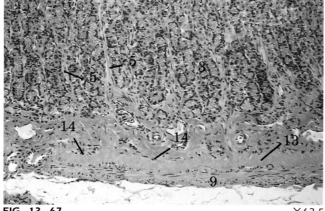

FIG. 13–67 ×62.5

KEY	
1. Chief cells	**9.** Muscularis mucosae
2. Fundic gland, lumen	**10.** Parietal cells
3. Fundic glands	**11.** Serosa
4. Gastric pit	**12.** Smooth muscle
5. Lamina propria	**13.** Stratum compactum
6. Mucosa	**14.** Stratum granulosum
7. Mucous neck cells	**15.** Submucosa
8. Muscularis externa	**16.** Surface mucous cells

FIG. 13–64. Dark Zone, Fundic Gland Region, Stomach, Dog. A portion of the stomach wall including the base of a fold is shown.

FIG. 13–65. Dark Zone, Fundic Gland Region, Stomach, Dog. The mucosa of the dark zone of the fundic stomach of carnivores is thicker than that of the light zone. The gastric pits are comparatively shallow, extending no farther into the mucosa than one third of its thickness. Compare to Figure 13–62.

FIG. 13–66. Dark Zone, Fundic Gland Region, Stomach, Dog, PAS. The surface mucous cells lining the lumen and the mucous neck cells of the glands both contain complex carbohydrates and are PAS positive (magenta stain).

FIG. 13–67. Lamina Subglandularis, Fundic Gland Region, Stomach, Cat (old). A thick layer of connective tissue, the stratum compactum, and an overlying layer of fibroblasts, the stratum granulosum, together form the lamina subglandularis, a structure seen consistently in cats and occasionally in dogs. Presumably, the lamina subglandularis protects the stomach from punctures by sharp objects.

FIG. 13–68. Fundic Gland Region, Stomach, Cat. The fundic glands have been cut longitudinally. They are formed largely from parietal and chief cells.

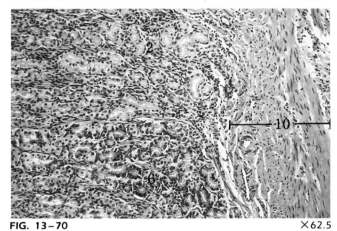

FIG. 13-69 ×12.5

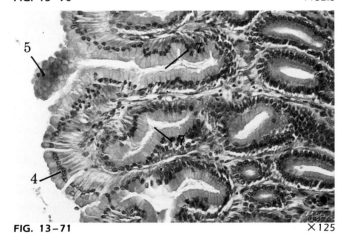

FIG. 13-70 ×62.5

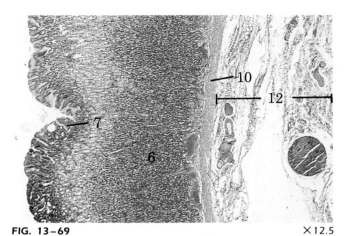

FIG. 13-71 ×125

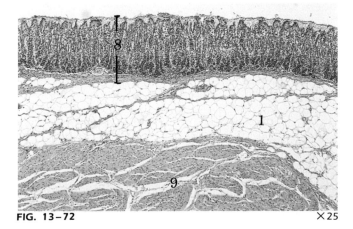

FIG. 13-72 ×25

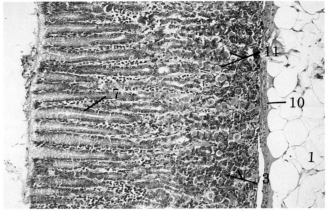

FIG. 13-73 ×62.5

KEY	
1. Adipose tissue	**7.** Gastric pit
2. Cardiac glands	**8.** Mucosa
3. Chief cells	**9.** Muscularis externa
4. Columnar epithelium	**10.** Muscularis mucosae
5. Epithelial cells, surface cut	**11.** Parietal cells
6. Fundic glands	**12.** Submucosa

FIG. 13-69. Fundic Gland Region, Stomach, Horse. Note the thick mucosa and submucosa.

FIG. 13-70. Junction of the Cardiac and Fundic Gland Regions, Stomach, Horse. The mucous glands of the cardiac gland region are distinct from the parietal and chief cells of the fundic gland region of the stomach.

FIG. 13-71. Fundic Gland Region, Stomach, Horse. A unique feature of the surface epithelium of the glandular stomach is the presence of a mucous precursor that fills the apical region of the cells.

FIG. 13-72. Fundic Gland Region, Abomasum, Sheep. The submucosa shows extensive infiltration by adipose tissue.

FIG. 13-73. Fundic Gland Region, Abomasum, Goat. Parietal and chief cells of the glands are evident. Note the deep gastric pits.

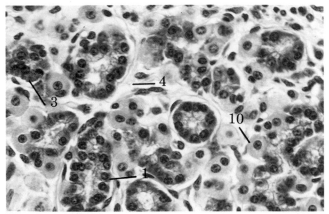

FIG. 13-74   ×250

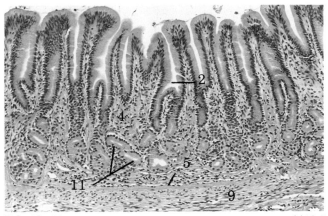

FIG. 13-78   ×62.5

KEY	
1. Chief cell	**8.** Muscularis externa
2. Gastric pit	**9.** Muscularis mucosae
3. Globular leukocyte	**10.** Parietal cell
4. Lamina propria	**11.** Pyloric gland
5. Lamina subglandularis	**12.** Serosa
6. Lymphocytes	**13.** Submucosa
7. Mucous precursor	**14.** Surface mucous cells

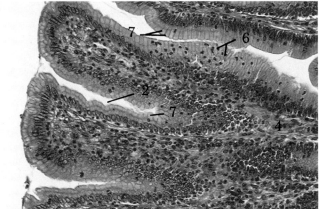

FIG. 13-75   ×62.5

FIG. 13-74. Fundic Gland Region, Abomasum, Cow. Parietal and chief cells of the fundic glands.

FIG. 13-75. Mucosa, Pyloric Gland Region, Stomach, Dog, PAS. The content of the surface mucous cells and that of the secretory units of the pyloric glands are PAS positive (magenta color).

FIG. 13-76. Surface Mucous Cells, Pyloric Gland Region, Stomach, Dog. Columnar cells lining the gastric pits and bordering the gastric lumen show typical cup-shaped concentrations of mucous precursor in their apical ends. The epithelium contains many migrating lymphocytes.

FIG. 13-77. Pyloric Gland Region, Stomach, Cat. Note the deep gastric pits. Some extend halfway through the thickness of the mucosa.

FIG. 13-78. Mucosa, Pyloric Gland Region, Stomach, Cat. Note the presence of deep gastric pits. Some extend to about half the depth of the mucosa.

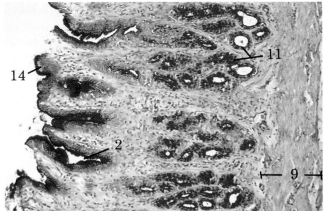

FIG. 13-76   ×125

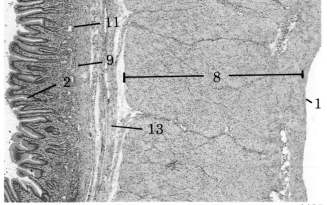

FIG. 13-77   ×25

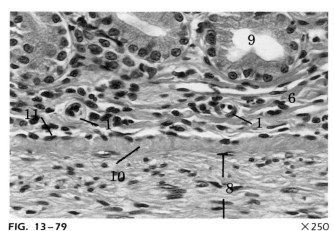

FIG. 13–79   ×250

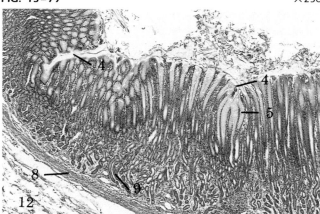

FIG. 13–82   ×25

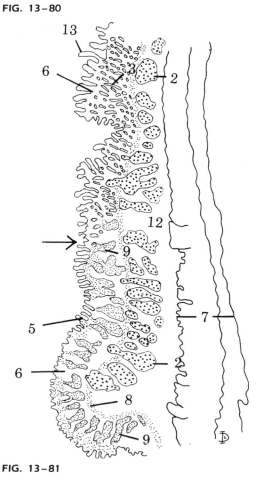

FIG. 13–80   ×25

KEY	
← Junction, pyloric gland region and duodenum	**7.** Muscularis externa
1. Arteriole	**8.** Muscularis mucosae
2. Brünner's gland	**9.** Pyloric gland
3. Crypt of Lieberkühn	**10.** Stratum compactum
4. Gastric furrow	**11.** Stratum granulosum
5. Gastric pit	**12.** Submucosa
6. Lamina propria	**13.** Villus

FIG. 13–79. Pyloric Gland Region, Stomach, Cat. Basal ends of pyloric glands and the stratum granulosum and stratum compactum of the lamina subglandularis are present in this section.

FIG. 13–80. Pyloric Gland Region, Abomasum, Goat. Gastric furrows and gastric pits can be seen.

FIG. 13–81. Junction, Pyloric Gland Region and Duodenum, l.s., Dog. Brünner's glands are located primarily in the submucosa of the duodenum. They also extend a short distance into the pyloric gland region of the stomach. They occasionally break through the muscularis mucosae and extend into the lamina propria.

FIG. 13–82. Junction, Pyloric Gland Region and Duodenum, l.s., Dog. Gastric pits and mucous glands of the pyloric gland region of the stomach can be seen. Brünner's glands (mucous) occur below the interrupted muscularis mucosae.

FIG. 13–81

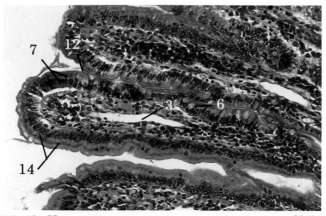

FIG. 13-83 ×125

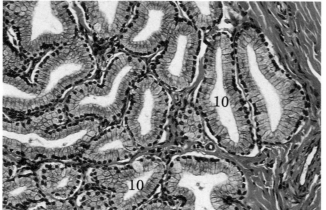

FIG. 13-84 ×125

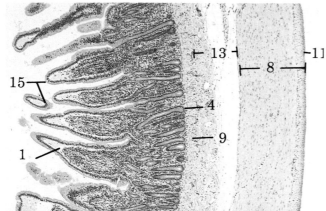

FIG. 13-85 ×25

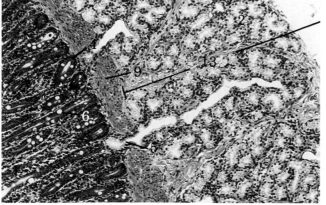

FIG. 13-86 ×62.5

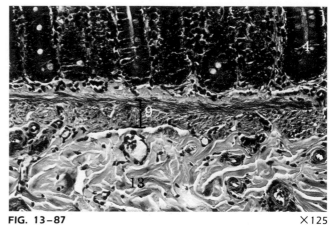

FIG. 13-87 ×125

KEY	
1. Artifact	**9.** Muscularis mucosae
2. Brünner's gland	**10.** Secretory unit
3. Central lacteal	**11.** Serosa
4. Crypt of Lieberkühn	**12.** Striated border
5. Duct	**13.** Submucosa
6. Goblet cell	**14.** Surface mucous cells
7. Intestinal absorptive cells	**15.** Villus
8. Muscularis externa	

FIG. 13-83. Junction, Pyloric Gland Region and Duodenum, Dog. Note the change in the epithelium when it passes from the stomach to the duodenum. Typical columnar surface mucous cells of the pyloric gland region of the stomach contrast with the columnar absorptive cells and goblet cells of the duodenum.

FIG. 13-84. Brünner's Gland, Duodenum, l.s., Dog. Detail of mucous secretory units. The latter, in the dog, are lined by tall columnar cells and have large lumens.

FIG. 13-85. Duodenum, x.s., Cat. A segment of the wall of the duodenum is shown. The intestinal villi of carnivores tend to be longer than those of noncarnivores. Note the shrinkage artifact at the apical ends of the villi.

FIG. 13-86. Duodenum, Proximal, x.s., Cat, Masson's. Ducts of Brünner's glands penetrate the muscularis mucosae. Brünner's glands are marked off into distinct lobules in the cat.

FIG. 13-87. Duodenum, x.s., Cat, Masson's. The submucosa in the cat and dog is a moderately dense irregular connective tissue. In other domestic mammals, it is a loose connective tissue.

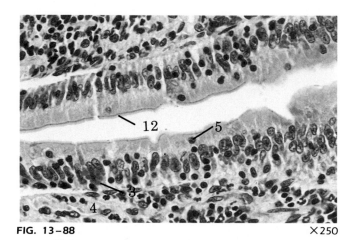

FIG. 13-88   ×250

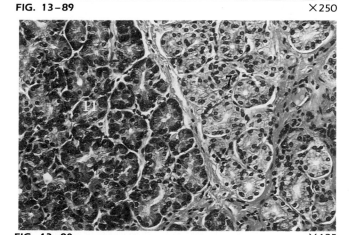

FIG. 13-89   ×250

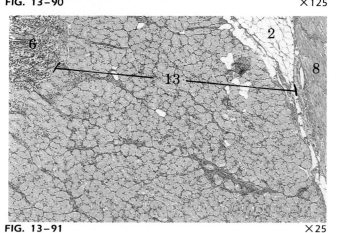

FIG. 13-90   ×125

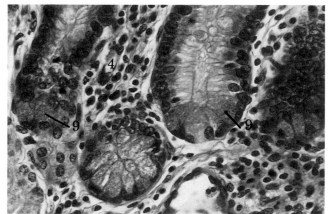

FIG. 13-91   ×25

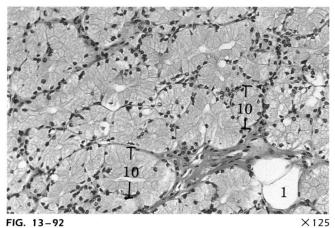

FIG. 13-92   ×125

KEY	
1. Adipose cell	**8.** Muscularis externa
2. Adipose tissue	**9.** Paneth cell
3. Globular leukocyte	**10.** Secretory unit
4. Lamina propria	**11.** Serous gland
5. Lymphocyte	**12.** Striated border
6. Mucosa	**13.** Submucosa
7. Mucous gland	

FIG. 13-88. Epithelium of Villus, Duodenum, Cat. Lymphocytes can be seen migrating through the simple columnar epithelium.

FIG. 13-89. Duodenum, Horse. Paneth cells are visible in the basal portions of the crypts of Lieberkühn in the small intestine of the horse.

FIG. 13-90. Duodenum, Horse. In the horse, Brünner's glands have both mucous and serous components. Note that the lumens of the secretory units are small.

FIG. 13-91. Duodenum, Pig. Brünner's glands fill the entire submucosa.

FIG. 13-92. Duodenum, Pig. In the pig, the lumens of the secretory units of Brünner's glands are very small.

DIGESTIVE SYSTEM   **133**

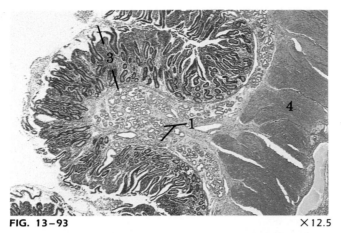

FIG. 13-93   ×12.5

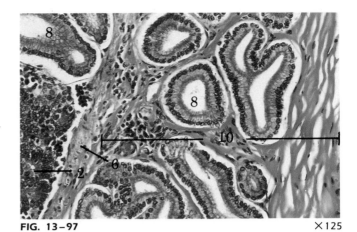

FIG. 13-97   ×125

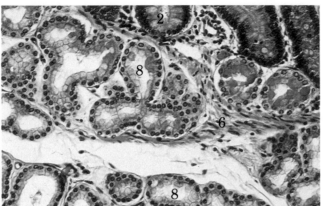

FIG. 13-94   ×125

FIG. 13-93. Duodenum, l.s., Cow. Brünner's glands are present throughout much of the submucosa of an intestinal fold (plica).

FIG. 13-94. Duodenum, Cow. Detail of Brünner's gland. In the cow, some gland cells have an acidophilic cytoplasm. The lumens of secretory units are large.

FIG. 13-95. Duodenum, x.s., Sheep. The muscularis externa of the intestine is arranged into an inner circular and an outer longitudinal layer of smooth muscle. Compare the appearance of the muscle layers seen in this cross section with that of the longitudinal section of the intestine in Figure 13-96.

FIG. 13-96. Duodenum, l.s., Sheep. This section is through the muscularis externa. Compare the appearance of the muscle layers in this preparation with that in Figure 13-95.

FIG. 13-97. Duodenum, Goat. Portions of the mucosa and submucosa. The lumens of the secretory units of Brünner's glands are large in the goat.

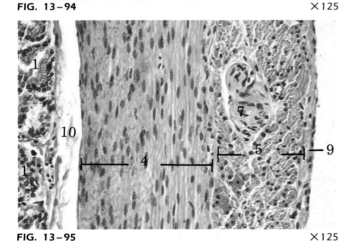

FIG. 13-95   ×125

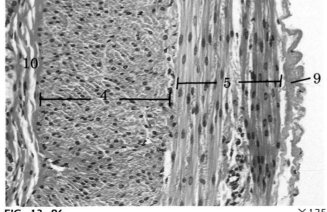

FIG. 13-96   ×125

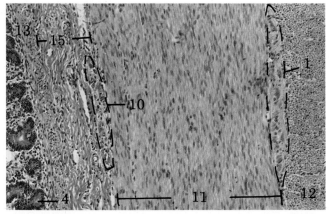

FIG. 13-98 ×62.5

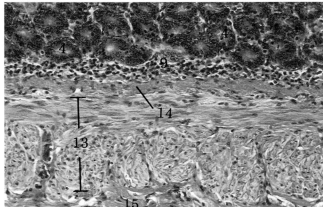

FIG. 13-99 ×125

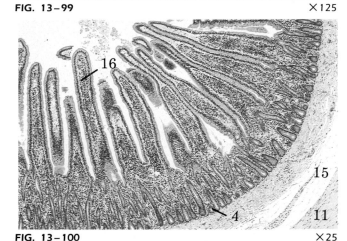

FIG. 13-100 ×25

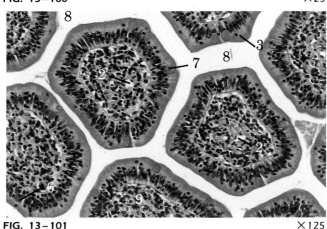

FIG. 13-101 ×125

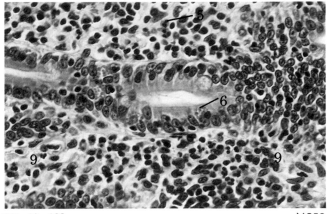

FIG. 13-102 ×250

KEY	
1. Auerbach's plexus	**10.** Meissner's plexus
2. Central lacteal, x.s.	**11.** Muscularis externa, inner
3. Columnar epithelium	circular
4. Crypt of Lieberkühn	**12.** Muscularis externa, outer
5. Eosinophil	longitudinal
6. Globular leukocyte	**13.** Muscularis mucosae
7. Goblet cell	**14.** Stratum compactum
8. Intestinal lumen	**15.** Submucosa
9. Lamina propria	**16.** Villus

FIG. 13-98. Jejunum, x.s., Dog. A Meissner's plexus is present in the periphery of the submucosa. An Auerbach's plexus is wedged between the inner circular and outer longitudinal layers of the muscularis externa.

FIG. 13-99. Jejunum, Dog. A well developed stratum compactum is present between the lamina propria and muscularis mucosae of the small intestine in some cats and dogs.

FIG. 13-100. Jejunum, x.s., Cat. Slender villi and well defined crypts of Lieberkühn are evident.

FIG. 13-101. Jejunum, Cat. Transverse sections of villi. Central lacteals are evident in two of them. Migrating lymphocytes are visible within the epithelium.

FIG. 13-102. Jejunum, Cat. Globular leukocytes are present among the columnar cells lining a crypt of Lieberkühn. Numerous eosinophils are scattered through the lamina propria.

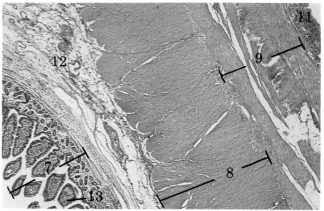

FIG. 13–103 ×12.5

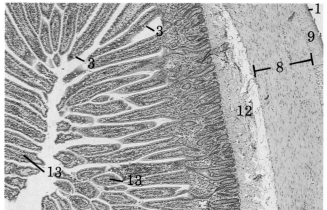

FIG. 13–104 ×25

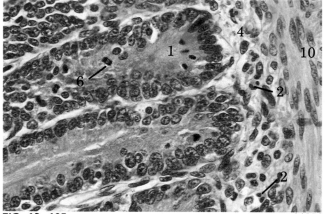

FIG. 13–105 ×250

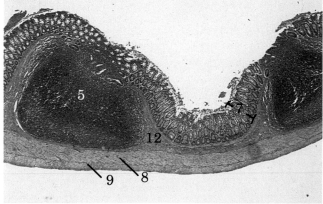

FIG. 13–106 ×12.5

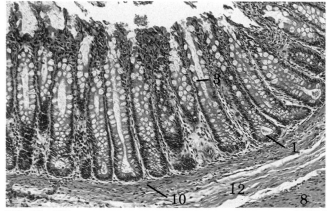

FIG. 13–107 ×62.5

KEY	
1. Crypt of Lieberkühn	**9.** Muscularis externa, outer
2. Eosinophil	longitudinal
3. Goblet cell	**10.** Muscularis mucosae
4. Lamina propria	**11.** Serosa
5. Lymphatic nodule	**12.** Submucosa
6. Mitotic figure	**13.** Villus
7. Mucosa	
8. Muscularis externa, inner	
circular	

FIG. 13–103. Jejunum, l.s., Horse. All layers of the wall are included in this section. Note that the villi are shorter than those of carnivores (see Fig. 13–100).

FIG. 13–104. Ileum, x.s., Cat. A portion of the wall from the lumen to the serosa is shown. The epithelium of the villi contain numerous goblet cells.

FIG. 13–105. Ileum, Dog. Mitotic figures can be seen in the crypts.

FIG. 13–106. Cecum, Tip, Dog. Large lymphatic nodules are present in the submucosa.

FIG. 13–107. Cecum, Dog. Numerous goblet cells in the lining of the crypts of Lieberkühn are characteristic of the organ. The epithelial cells bordering the lumen in this preparation have undergone some autolysis and look tattered.

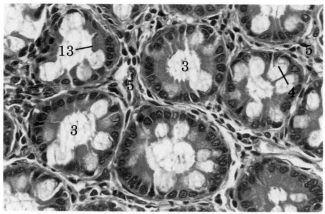

FIG. 13–108 ×250

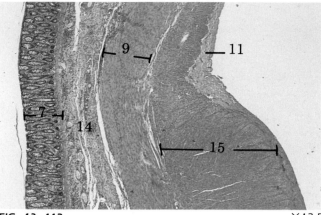

FIG. 13–112 ×12.5

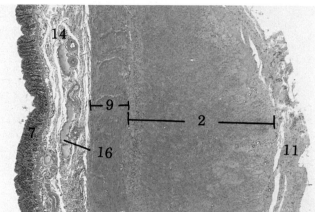

FIG. 13–109 ×12.5

FIG. 13–108. Cecum, Dog. Several crypts of Lieberkühn appear in cross section. A striated border is present on the columnar cells. Goblet cells are numerous.

FIG. 13–109. Cecal Band, x.s., Horse. A cecal band consists of an admixture of smooth muscle (thickened outer longitudinal layer of the muscularis externa) and elastic fibers. Elastic fibers are predominant in the bands of both the cecum and the ventral large colon of the horse. Compare with Figure 13–112.

FIG. 13–110. Cecum, Horse. Veins with bands of smooth muscle in their walls are common in the submucosa throughout the digestive tract of the horse. Similar vessels are shown at low magnification in Figure 13–109.

FIG. 13–111. Cecum, Cow. In the large intestine of ruminants, the crypts of Lieberkühn are usually tortuous. Adipose tissue is abundant in the submucosa.

FIG. 13–112. Taenia Coli, Small Colon, x.s., Horse. The taenia coli are thickenings of the outer longitudinal layer of the muscularis externa. In contrast to the bands of the cecum and ventral large colon, where elastic fibers are predominant, smooth muscle predominates in the bands of the small colon and dorsal large colon. Compare with Figure 13–109.

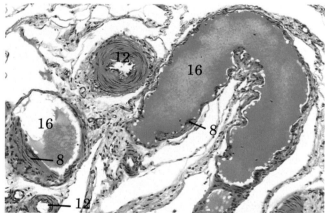

FIG. 13–110 ×62.5

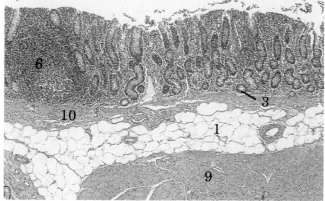

FIG. 13–111 ×25

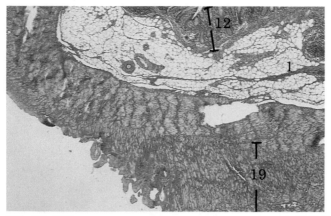

FIG. 13-113   ×12.5

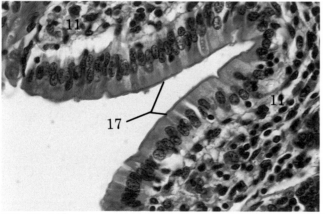

FIG. 13-114   ×25

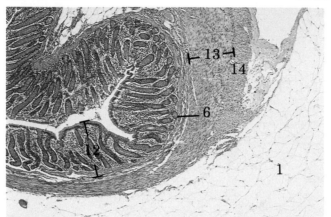

FIG. 13-115   ×250

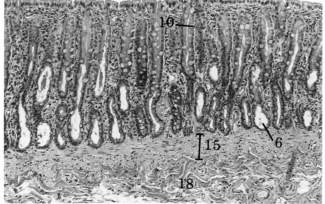

FIG. 13-116   ×62.5

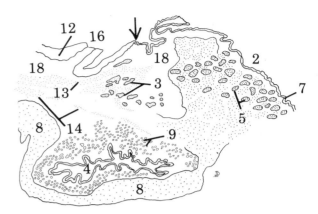

FIG. 13-117

KEY	
← Rectoanal junction	**11.** Lamina propria
1. Adipose tissue	**12.** Mucosa
2. Anal canal	**13.** Muscularis externa, inner
3. Anal glands	circular
4. Anal sac	**14.** Muscularis externa, outer
5. Circumanal glands	longitudinal
6. Crypt of Lieberkühn	**15.** Muscularis mucosae
7. Epidermis	**16.** Rectum
8. External anal sphincter	**17.** Striated border
9. Glands of anal sac	**18.** Submucosa
10. Goblet cell	**19.** Taenia coli

FIG. 13-113. Taenia Coli, Colon, x.s., Pig. The muscular taenia coli is formed from the outer longitudinal layer of the muscularis externa. The submucosa is infiltrated with fat.

FIG. 13-114. Spiral Colon. x.s., Goat. The mucosa contains both tortuous and straight crypts of Lieberkühn. The muscularis externa shows an abrupt thickening of its inner circular layer and outer longitudinal layer.

FIG. 13-115. Spiral Colon, x.s., Goat. The columnar epithelial cells have a distinct striated border.

FIG. 13-116. Rectum, x.s., Cat. The epithelium of the rectum presents a flat, uniform surface.

FIG. 13-117. Rectoanal Junction, l.s., Dog. Note that the anal glands mark the junction (arrow) of the rectum and anal canal.

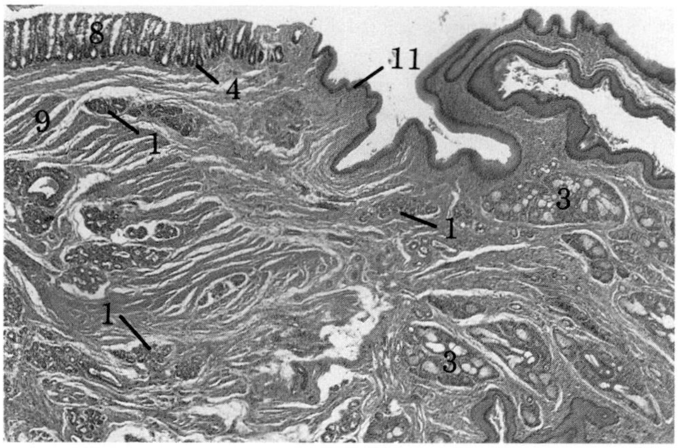

FIG. 13–118 ×12.5

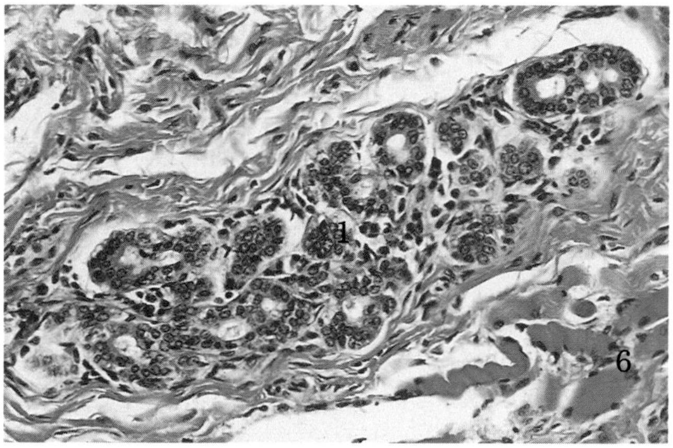

FIG. 13–119 ×125

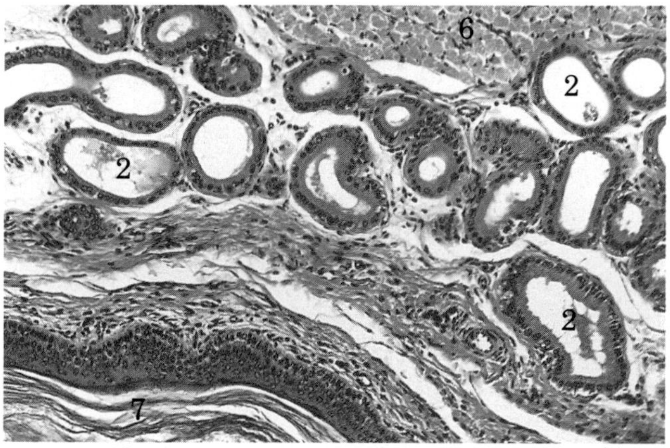

FIG. 13–120 ×62.5

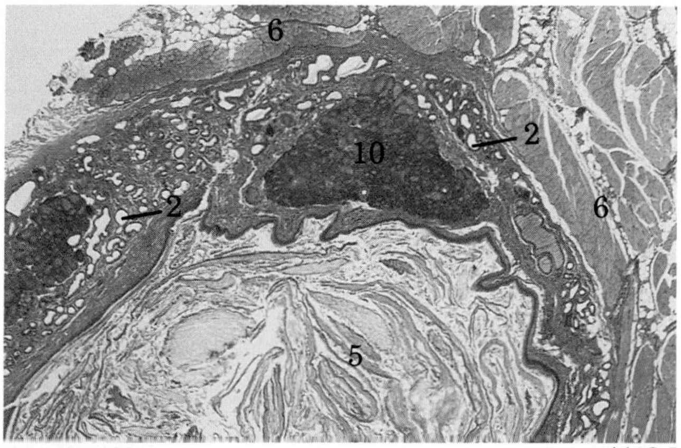

FIG. 13–121 ×12.5

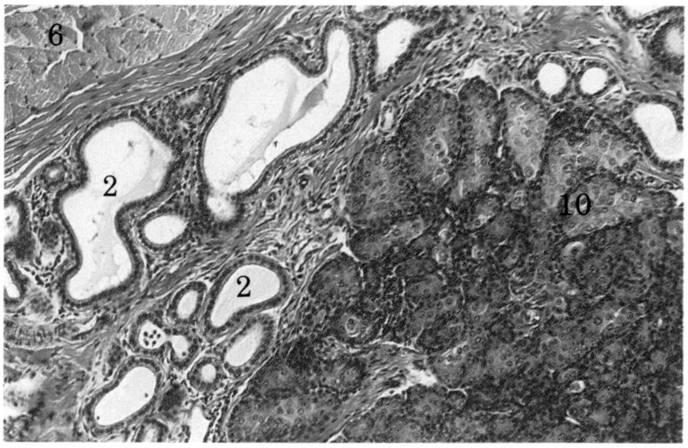

FIG. 13–122 ×62.5

KEY

1. Anal gland	**8.** Mucosa
2. Apocrine tubular gland	**9.** Muscularis externa, inner circular
3. Circumanal glands	**10.** Sebaceous gland
4. Crypt of Lieberkühn	**11.** Stratified squamous epithelium
5. Debris in anal sac	
6. External anal sphincter	
7. Keratinized epithelium of anal sac	

FIG. 13–118. Rectoanal Junction, l.s., Dog. Note the change between the stratified squamous epithelium of the anal canal and the crypts of Lieberkühn of the rectal mucosa. Note also that anal glands are located in the submucosa and are scattered among the smooth muscle of the internal anal sphincter (inner circular layer of the muscularis externa).

FIG. 13–119. Anal Glands, Dog. Section is through the secretory units of an anal gland.

FIG. 13–120. Glands of the Anal Sac, Dog. A small portion of the wall of an anal sac and the secretory units of some of the glands of the anal sac are shown.

FIG. 13–121. Anal Sac, Cat. About one half of the wall of an anal sac is shown.

FIG. 13–122. Glands of the Anal Sac, Cat. Portions of these glands are shown adjacent to the skeletal muscle of the external anal sphincter. The presence of sebaceous glands in this location is a characteristic of the cat.

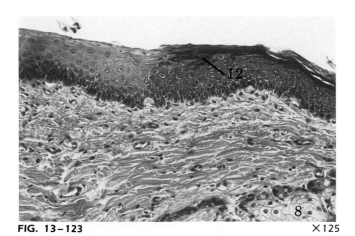

FIG. 13–123 ×125

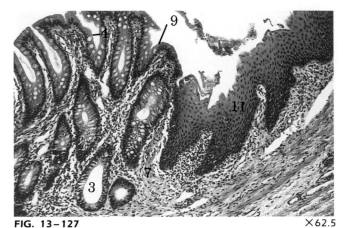

FIG. 13–127 ×62.5

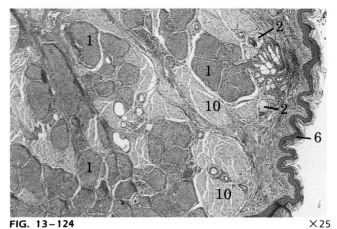

FIG. 13–124 ×25

KEY	
1. Circumanal gland, nonsebaceous	**7.** Lamina propria
2. Circumanal gland, sebaceous	**8.** Sebaceous gland
3. Crypt of Lieberkühn	**9.** Simple columnar epithelium
4. Goblet cell	**10.** Skeletal muscle
5. Hair follicle	**11.** Stratified squamous epithelium
6. Keratinized epidermis	**12.** Stratum granulosum

FIG. 13–123. Anal Canal, l.s., Dog. Junction of the keratinized and nonkeratinized regions of the anal canal. The stratum granulosum of the keratinized region stops abruptly at the junction.

FIG. 13–124. Circumanal Glands, Dog. Numerous nonsebaceous portions of circumanal glands are present subcutaneously among the skeletal muscle of the anal sphincter. These nonsebaceous portions are often called hepatoid glands because their cells resemble hepatocytes.

FIG. 13–125. Circumanal Gland, Dog. Detail of a part of one of the glands. The lower, nonsebaceous portion of these glands is more acidophilic than the upper, sebaceous portion.

FIG. 13–126. Rectoanal Junction, l.s., Horse. The stratified squamous epithelium of the anal canal contrasts with the rectal mucosa.

FIG. 13–127. Rectoanal Junction, Horse. The abrupt change between the stratified squamous epithelium of the anal canal and the simple columnar epithelium of the rectal mucosa is apparent.

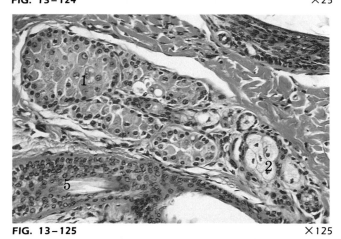

FIG. 13–125 ×125

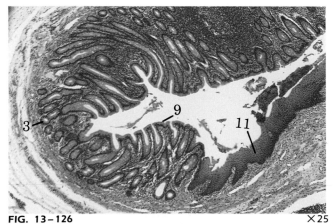

FIG. 13–126 ×25

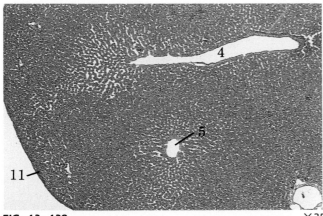

FIG. 13–128 ×25

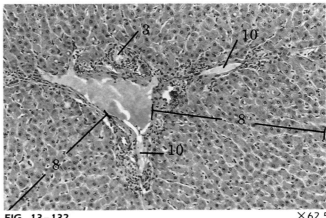

FIG. 13–132 ×62.5

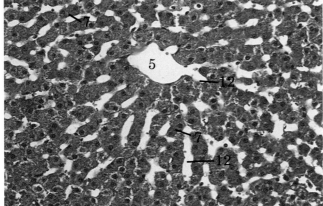

FIG. 13–129 ×125

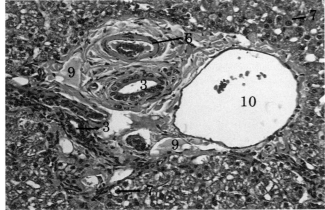

FIG. 13–130 ×125

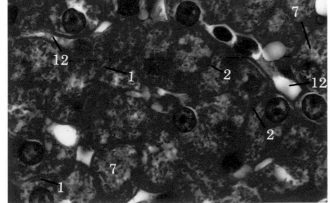

FIG. 13–131 ×625

KEY	
1. Bile canaliculus, l.s.	**7.** Hepatocyte
2. Bile canaliculus, x.s.	**8.** Lobule
3. Bile ductule	**9.** Lymphatic vessel
4. Central vein, l.s.	**10.** Portal vein, branch
5. Central vein, x.s.	**11.** Serosa
6. Hepatic artery, branch	**12.** Sinusoid

FIG. 13–128. Liver, Cat. Transverse and longitudinal sections through the central veins of two classic lobules.

FIG. 13–129. Liver, Cat. Transverse section through a classic lobule. Sinusoids empty into the central vein. Hepatocytes radiate as hepatic plates from the central vein.

FIG. 13–130. Liver, Cat. The portal tract in this section includes a branch of the hepatic portal vein and hepatic artery, bile ductule, and lymphatic vessel.

FIG. 13–131. Liver, Cat, Masson's. Sections through various bile canaliculi are evident in this section.

FIG. 13–132. Liver, Horse. A portal tract is at the intersection of three classic lobules. Branches of the portal vein can be seen extending between the lobules.

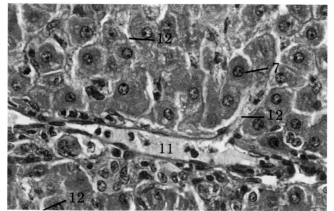

FIG. 13-133 ×250

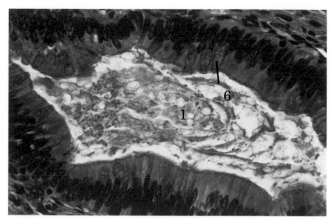

FIG. 13-137 ×250

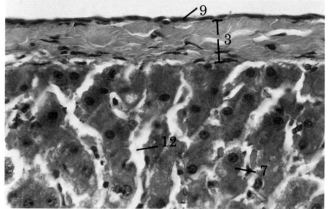

FIG. 13-134 ×250

FIG. 13-133. Liver, Horse. A sinusoid joins with a branch of the portal vein.

FIG. 13-134. Liver, Horse. Section is through mesothelial cells and connective tissue of the capsule of Glisson surrounding the liver. Together, the mesothelial cells and the capsule of Glisson comprise the serosa.

FIG. 13-135. Liver, Pig. Classic lobules are clearly separated from one another by connective tissue partitions in the pig.

FIG. 13-136. Liver, Pig. Particulate-laden Kupffer cells within sinusoids of a classic lobule are evident in this section. Binucleate hepatocytes can also be seen.

FIG. 13-137. Liver, Goat. A large bile duct with columnar epithelium and goblet cells.

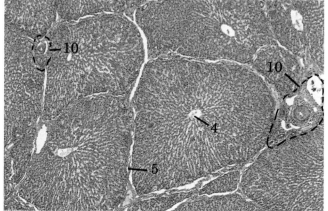

FIG. 13-135 ×25

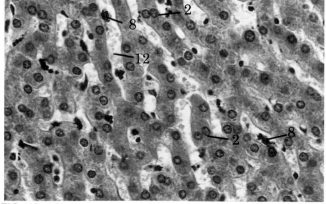

FIG. 13-136 ×250

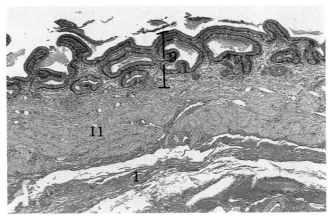

FIG. 13–138   ×25

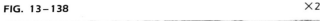

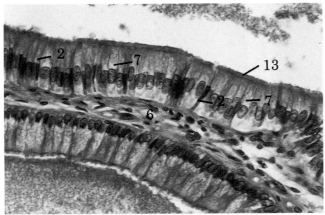

FIG. 13–139   ×250

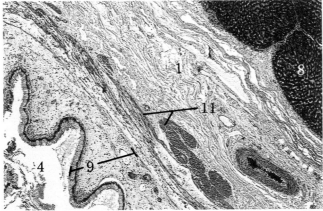

FIG. 13–140   ×25

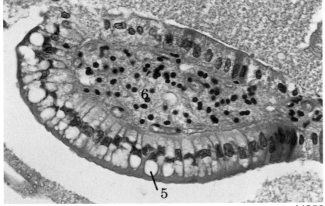

FIG. 13–141   ×250

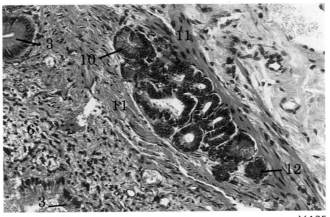

FIG. 13–142   ×125

KEY	
1. Adventitia	**8.** Liver
2. Dark cell	**9.** Mucosa
3. Epithelium	**10.** Mucous acinus
4. Gallbladder, lumen	**11.** Muscularis
5. Goblet cell	**12.** Serous acinus
6. Lamina propria	**13.** Striated border
7. Light cell	

FIG. 13–138. Gallbladder, Dog. A portion of the wall showing the highly folded mucosa.

FIG. 13–139. Gallbladder, Dog. Epithelial lining with light and dark columnar cells.

FIG. 13–140. Gallbladder and Liver, Pig, Masson's. Section shows a portion of the liver and gallbladder.

FIG. 13–141. Gallbladder, Goat. Portion of a mucosal fold showing goblet cells in the epithelium.

FIG. 13–142. Gallbladder, Goat. Mixed glands occur within the wall of the gallbladder of ruminants.

DIGESTIVE SYSTEM   **143**

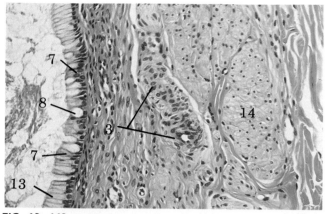

FIG. 13–143 ×125

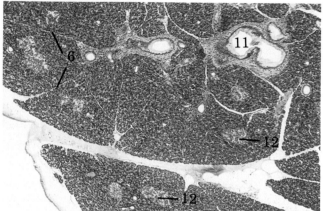

FIG. 13–144 ×25

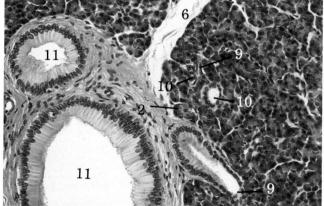

FIG. 13–145 ×125

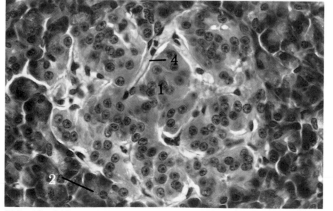

FIG. 13–146 ×250

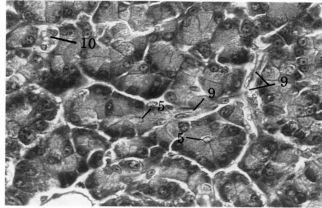

FIG. 13–147 ×250

KEY	
1. A cells	**8.** Goblet cell
2. Acinus	**9.** Intercalated duct, l.s.
3. Anastomotic artery	**10.** Intercalated duct, x.s.
4. Capillary	**11.** Interlobular duct
5. Centroacinar cell	**12.** Islet of Langerhans
6. Connective tissue septum	**13.** Light cell
7. Dark cell	**14.** Muscularis

FIG. 13–143. Cystic Duct, Pig. The epithelium is composed of light cells, dark cells, and goblet cells.

FIG. 13–144. Pancreas, Horse. The organ is divided into lobules by connective tissue septa. Most of the pancreas is formed from exocrine acinar cells. Islets of Langerhans are scattered through the exocrine region of the gland.

FIG. 13–145. Pancreas, Horse. Portions of two lobules showing acinar cells, interlobular ducts, and intercalated ducts.

FIG. 13–146. Pancreas, Horse. An islet of Langerhans with some surrounding exocrine acini. In the horse, the darker, A cells are located in the center of the islet, while the lighter B cells are positioned in the periphery. Compare with Figure 13–150. Note the numerous capillaries among cords of islet cells.

FIG. 13–147. Pancreas, Dog. Detail of acini and intercalated ducts. Note acidophilic apical regions and basophilic basal regions of the acinar cells.

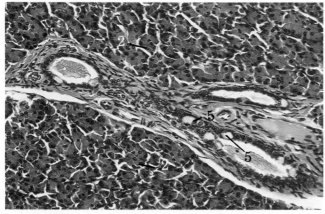

FIG. 13–148   ×125

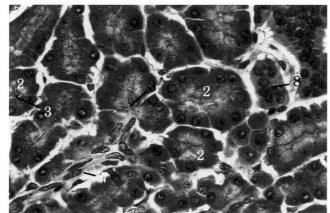

FIG. 13–149   ×250

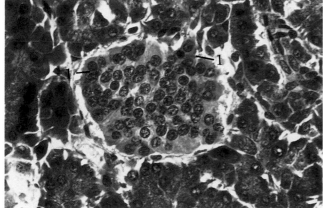

FIG. 13–150   ×250

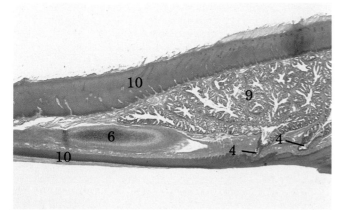

FIG. 13–151   ×12.5

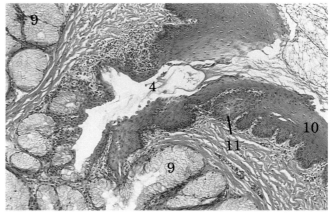

FIG. 13–152   ×62.5

KEY	
1. A cell	**7.** Intercalated duct
2. Acinus	**8.** Islet of Langerhans
3. Centroacinar cell	**9.** Salivary gland
4. Duct	**10.** Stratified squamous
5. Goblet cell	epithelium
6. Hyaline cartilage	**11.** Taste bud

FIG. 13–148. Pancreas, Pig. An interlobular duct with goblet cells in the epithelium.

FIG. 13–149. Pancreas, Cow, Masson's. An intercalated duct enters an acinus.

FIG. 13–150. Pancreas, Sheep, Masson's. In ruminants, darkly stained A cells are located at the periphery of the islets of Langerhans, while light-staining B cells are centrally located. Compare with Figure 13–146.

FIG. 13–151. Tongue, Tip, l.s., Chicken. The upper surface of the tongue is covered by a thick stratified squamous epithelium, which is keratinized near the tip. The stratified squamous epithelium of the lower surface is thinner and also keratinized rostrally. Anteriorly, the tongue is supported by hyaline cartilage. The ducts of salivary glands (mucous) open at the ventral surface.

FIG. 13–152. Taste Bud, Tongue, Base, Chicken. A taste bud (characteristically large and scarce in the chicken) can be seen closely associated with the duct of a salivary gland.

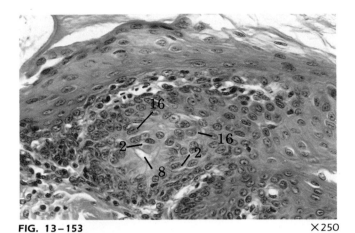

FIG. 13–153 ×250

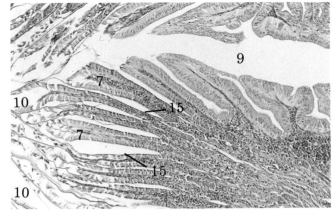

FIG. 13–157 ×62.5

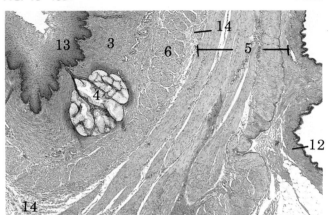

FIG. 13–154 ×25

KEY	
1. Gland	**10.** Proventriculus, lumen
2. Intercellular space	**11.** Secondary duct
3. Lamina propria	**12.** Serosa
4. Mucous gland	**13.** Stratified squamous
5. Muscularis externa	epithelium
6. Muscularis mucosae	**14.** Submucosa
7. Plica	**15.** Sulcus
8. Pore	**16.** Taste bud cell
9. Primary duct	**17.** Tertiary duct

FIG. 13–153. Taste Bud, Chicken. Detail of the taste bud seen in Figure 13–152. Its cells stain lightly with eosin. Numerous spaces occur between cells. A taste bud pore is visible.

FIG. 13–154. Esophagus, x.s., Chicken. The esophagus is lined by a thick nonkeratinized stratified squamous epithelium. Mucous glands occur in the lamina propria. The submucosa is sparse.

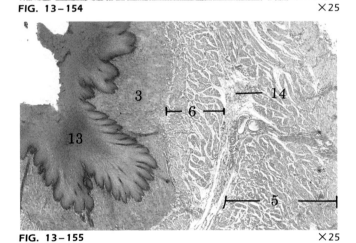

FIG. 13–155 ×25

FIG. 13–155. Crop, Chicken. The crop is a diverticulum of the esophagus. Unlike the latter, it lacks mucous glands, except close to its junction with the esophagus.

FIG. 13–156. Proventriculus (Glandular Stomach), x.s., Chicken. The submucosa contains lobules of compound tubular glands that are arranged around a central, secondary duct. A primary duct, which drains several lobules, opens through a raised mucosal papilla.

FIG. 13–157. Proventriculus, x.s., Chicken. A magnified view of Figure 13–156 shows that the mucosa of the papilla is arranged into folds (plicae) covered by columnar cells, and depressions (sulci) lined by shorter cells. A primary duct, lined by columnar cells, joins the lumen of the proventriculus.

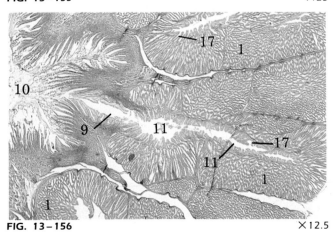

FIG. 13–156 ×12.5

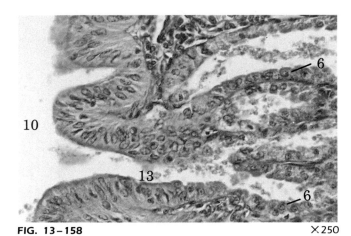

FIG. 13-158   ×250

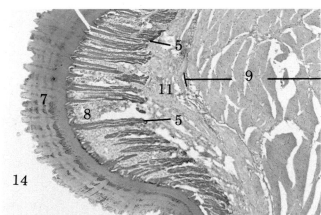

FIG. 13-159   ×25

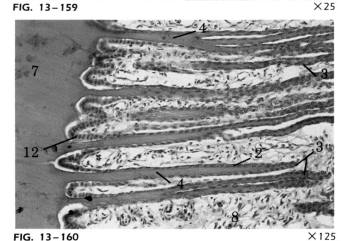

FIG. 13-160   ×125

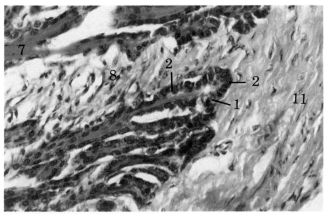

FIG. 13-161   ×250

KEY	
1. Basal cell	**8.** Lamina propria
2. Chief cell	**9.** Muscularis externa
3. Gastric gland	**10.** Secondary duct
4. Gastric pit	**11.** Submucosa
5. Gland	**12.** Surface epithelium
6. Gland cell	**13.** Tertiary duct
7. Keratinoid	**14.** Ventriculus, lumen

FIG. 13-158. Proventriculus, x.s., Chicken. A tertiary duct branching from the secondary duct leads into a glandular unit. The glandular epithelial cells vary from simple cuboidal to low columnar and appear grainy with secretory material. These cells secrete both pepsinogen and HCl.

FIG. 13-159. Ventriculus (Gizzard), Chicken. The pink, thick layer of keratinoid that lines the ventriculus is produced by branched tubular glands in the lamina propria. The submucosa and a portion of the smooth muscle layers of a thick muscularis externa are shown.

FIG. 13-160. Ventriculus, Chicken. Keratinoid lines the mucosal surface and fills the lumen of the gastric pits and glands. The epithelial cells of the surface are low to tall columnar. The cells decrease in height as they extend into the gastric pits. Flattened cells (chief cells) line the upper and mid-regions of the tubular gastric glands seen in this micrograph. Branching of some of the glands is evident.

FIG. 13-161. Ventriculus, Chicken. The flattened chief cells lining the mid-portion of the glands become cuboidal to low columnar in the fundus of the gland. A few large basal cells with pale nuclei and pale cytoplasm occur in the fundus of the glands.

DIGESTIVE SYSTEM   **147**

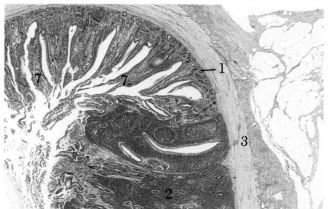

FIG. 13–162 ×12.5

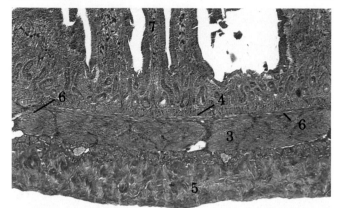

FIG. 13–163 ×25

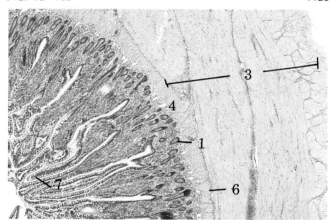

FIG. 13–164 ×25

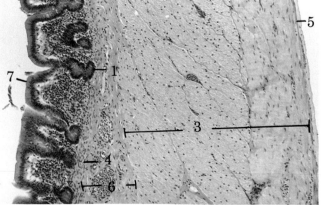

FIG. 13–165 ×62.5

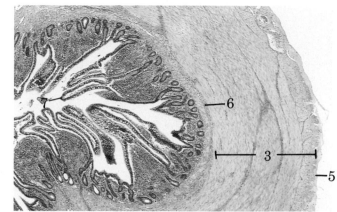

FIG. 13–166 ×25

KEY	
1. Crypt of Lieberkühn	**5.** Serosa
2. Lymphatic tissue	**6.** Submucosa
3. Muscularis externa	**7.** Villus
4. Muscularis mucosae	

FIG. 13–162. Duodenum, x.s., Chicken. Lymphatic tissue (diffuse and nodular) in the duodenum close to the stomach.

FIG. 13–163. Duodenum, x.s., Chicken, Mallory's. The serosa is thick. The submucosa is characteristically sparse.

FIG. 13–164. Ileum, x.s., Chicken. Villi are long and slender, with numerous goblet cells. The submucosa is thin.

FIG. 13–165. Cecum, Tip, l.s., Chicken. In the tip of the cecum, villi are short and broad. Compare with Figure 11–51 of the cecal tonsil.

FIG. 13–166. Large Intestine, x.s., Chicken. Villi are present in the chicken's large intestine.

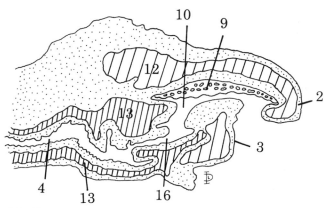

FIG. 13–167

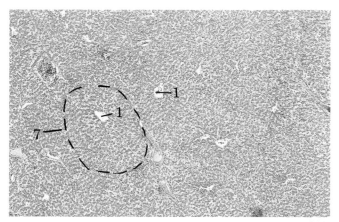

FIG. 13–171   ×25

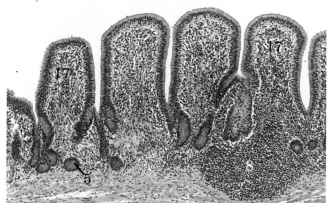

FIG. 13–168   ×62.5

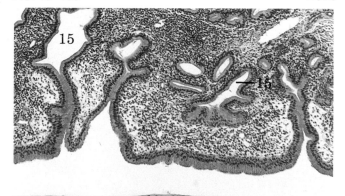

FIG. 13–169   ×62.5

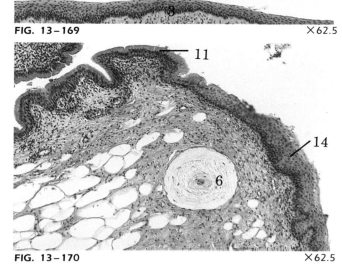

FIG. 13–170   ×62.5

KEY	
1. Central vein	**10.** Proctodeum
2. Cloacal lip, dorsal	**11.** Simple columnar epithelium
3. Cloacal lip, ventral	**12.** Skeletal muscle
4. Coprodeum	**13.** Smooth muscle
5. Crypt of Lieberkühn	**14.** Stratified squamous epithelium
6. Herbst corpuscle	
7. Lobule, parenchyma	**15.** Tubular glands
8. Lymphatic nodule	**16.** Urodeum
9. Lymphoglandular ridge	**17.** Villus

FIG. 13–167. Cloaca, l.s., Chicken. The cloaca is subdivided into three regions: the coprodeum, urodeum, and proctodeum. The large intestine is continuous with the coprodeum. The ureters and genital ducts terminate in the urodeum. The terminal proctodeum opens to the exterior through the cloacal lips.

FIG. 13–168. Coprodeum, Cloaca, Chicken. The mucosa of the coprodeum is thrown into short, flat villi. Shallow crypts of Lieberkühn open at their bases. Simple columnar epithelium covers their surface.

FIG. 13–169. Cloaca, l.s., Chicken. Branched tubular glands (modified crypts) form a part of the lymphoglandular ridge of Jolly located in the dorsal proctodeum. The epithelium of the ridge consists of tall columnar cells. A portion of the stratified squamous epithelium of the inner surface of the ventral cloacal lip can be seen.

FIG. 13–170. Cloaca, l.s., Chicken. A large Herbst corpuscle lies beneath the stratified squamous epithelium of the cloacal lip. These corpuscles occur, typically, close to the latter's point of juncture with the simple columnar epithelium of the proctodeum.

FIG. 13–171. Liver, Chicken. Central veins of several lobules are evident. One lobule is indicated by a dashed line.

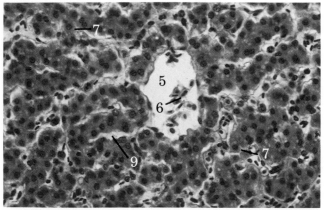
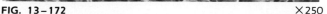

FIG. 13-172 ×250

KEY	
1. A cells	**6.** Erythrocytes
2. Acinus	**7.** Hepatocyte
3. B cells	**8.** Reticular fibers
4. Capillary	**9.** Sinusoid
5. Central vein	

FIG. 13-172. Liver, Chicken. Sinusoids can be seen entering a central vein. Radiating plates of hepatocytes are two cells thick in the chicken.

FIG. 13-173. Liver, Chicken, Silver. The wall of a central vein and surrounding cords of hepatocytes (whose celluar features are indistinct in this preparation) are supported by a network of reticular fibers that have been blackened with silver.

FIG. 13-174. Pancreas, Chicken. Numerous portions of tubuloacinar serous glands surround an alpha islet of Langerhans. Alpha islets consist primarily of columnar A cells, and a few D cells, and are larger than beta islets. Erythrocytes in capillaries can be seen between cords of islet cells.

FIG. 13-175. Pancreas, Chicken. Beta islets contain polygonal B cells and some D cells and are smaller than alpha islets.

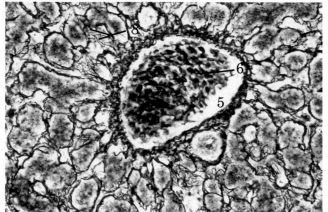

FIG. 13-173 ×250

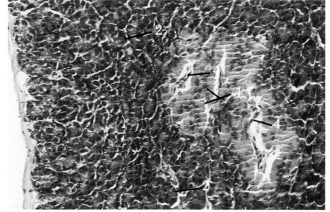

FIG. 13-174 ×125

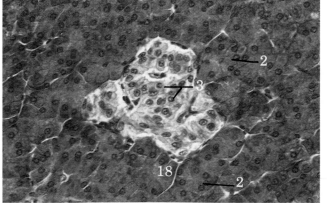

FIG. 13-175 ×250

URINARY SYSTEM

MAMMALS

The urinary system of mammals is comprised of the paired kidneys, renal pelvises, ureters, urinary bladder, and urethra.

The **kidneys** are highly vascularized, compound tubular glands, which function to maintain the composition of body fluids at a constant level and to remove excretory wastes. Each kidney is surrounded by a connective tissue **capsule,** which may contain a distinct layer of smooth muscle in its deepest portion, as in the cow, sheep, and goat. Both the cortex and medullary regions of the kidney are formed principally of numerous, closely packed uriniferous tubules. The spaces between tubules are mainly occupied by an extensive capillary network. In the **cortex,** groups of radially arranged tubules form the **pars radiata** (cortical ray or medullary rays), consisting of collecting tubules and straight portions of nephrons. The **pars convoluta** (cortical labyrinth) are located between the rays and consist of renal corpuscles and numerous proximal and distal convoluted tubules. The **proximal convoluted tubules** are longer than the **distal convoluted tubules** and comprise the major portion of the cortex. Proximal convoluted tubules are distinguished by the **brush borders** of their epithelial cells, and the somewhat scalloped appearance of the apical surface of their cells when the latter are seen in profile. Distal convoluted tubules have a smooth internal surface, and their cells lack a brush border.

Filtrate processed by the nephrons is passed to **col-**

lecting tubules, which open either directly or indirectly via calyces into the **renal pelvis** through **papillary ducts** at the tip of a **renal papilla**. The epithelial cells of the collecting tubules are pale and vary from cuboidal near the distal tubules to columnar close to the papilla. Cell boundaries are normally clearly defined compared to the cells of the proximal and distal convoluted tubules. As they progress toward the renal papilla, the collecting tubules become wider. The terminal portion of these tubules is lined by a columnar or pseudostratified epithelium and is called the papillary duct.

Each **renal corpuscle** consists of a **Bowman's capsule** and **glomerulus**. The outer layer of Bowman's capsule is the **capsular** (parietal) **epithelium,** a simple squamous layer. The inner layer is the **glomerular** (visceral) **epithelium.** It is formed from highly branched podocytes that surround the capillary loops of the glomerulus. In most histologic preparations made for light microscopy, it is not possible to distinguish podocytes from the adjacent endothelial cells of the capillary loops. The cavity between the capsular and glomerular layers is the **urinary space.** The latter is continuous with the lumen of a proximal convoluted tubule at the urinary pole of each corpuscle. At the opposite, vascular pole, an afferent and efferent arteriole unite with the capillaries of the glomerulus. A portion of the distal convoluted tubule is positioned between the afferent and efferent arterioles. The **macula densa** of the **juxtaglomerular apparatus** forms a part of the wall of the distal convoluted tubule in this region. Each macula is composed of closely grouped epithelial cells and is easily identified by the tightly packed nuclei of these cells. **Juxtaglomerular cells** are modified smooth muscle cells in the walls of afferent arterioles close to the glomerulus. They have an epithelioid appearance when seen in cross section.

The **medulla** of each kidney is formed from collecting tubules, thick and thin segments of the **loops of Henle,** and numerous **vasa rectae. Thick descending portions** of Henle's loop are continuations of the proximal convoluted tubules and are located close to the corticomedullary junction. They are straight tubules whose cells are lined by a brush border. Each thick descending tubule joins abruptly with a **thin segment** whose wall is formed from flattened cells with round, bulging nuclei. The straight, **thick ascending portion** of each loop resembles the distal convoluted tubule with which it is continuous.

The walls of the renal pelvis, ureter, urinary bladder, and urethra include a mucosa, muscularis of smooth muscle, and adventitia. A submucosa may be present. The lining of the mucosa is almost exclusively transitional epithelium. The hilus region, between the capsule of the kidney and the outer wall of the renal pelvis, contains loose connective tissue and adipose tissue.

The mucosa of the **ureter** presents a folded appearance. Its transitional epithelium is separated from the muscularis by a lamina propria. Tubuloalveolar mucous glands occur in the lamina propria of the first several centimeters of the ureter of the horse. A submucosa is lacking in the ureter. The muscularis consists of inner longitudinal, middle circular, and outer longitudinal layers. An adventitia of loose connective tissue surrounds the muscularis.

The transitional epithelial cells of the **urinary bladder** become flattened when the bladder is distended with urine. A lamina propria and submucosa are present. Usually there is a thin muscularis mucosae between these layers. The muscularis, external to the submucosa, is composed of an outer and inner longitudinal and a thick middle circular layer. The inner and outer longitudinal layers may be incomplete in some areas. Much of the bladder (body and apex) is covered by a serosa. An adventitia of loose connective tissue is present at the neck of the bladder.

CHICKEN

The urinary system of the chicken consists of large, elongated paired kidneys. Ureters drain each kidney and open into the urodeum of the cloaca. There is no renal pelvis or urinary bladder in the bird. Each kidney is composed of three divisions called cranial, middle, and caudal. Each division is comprised of lobules consisting of a large cortical and smaller medullary component. All of the lobules that drain into a single branch of the ureter constitute a lobe.

There are two types of nephrons. The **cortical** (reptilian) **type** is more numerous and lacks a loop of Henle. It is located entirely within the cortex. The other is the less numerous **medullary** (mammalian) **type.** It has a loop of Henle (also called a medullary loop), which extends into the medulla. Cortical nephrons are arranged radially around **central** (intralobular) **veins** of the cortex. Their renal corpuscles lie approximately midway between the intralobular vein and a peripheral interlobular vein. The cortical nephron has a smaller renal corpuscle than the medullary nephron. The large renal corpuscles of medullary nephrons lie close to the medulla. Other than size, there is no structural difference between small and large renal corpuscles. Each glomerulus contains a compact mass of **mesangial cells** (small cells with large nuclei) at its center. The mass appears basophilic because of the relatively high concentration of nuclear material. A layer of podocytes, with large round or oval nuclei, covers the surface of the glomerular capillaries, forming the **glomerular epithelium** of Bowman's capsule. The **capsular** (parietal) **layer** of

Bowman's capsule consists of a simple squamous epithelium. **Juxtaglomerular cells** and a **macula densa** are associated with the renal corpuscle at its vascular pole.

Generally, cortical tissue that is located between renal corpuscles and interlobular veins consists mainly of proximal convoluted tubules, and that between renal corpuscles and intralobular veins is comprised of distal convoluted tubules. Cells of proximal convoluted tubules are low columnar and have a well developed brush border. Distal convoluted tubules are shorter than proximal convoluted tubules. Their cuboidal cells lack a brush border, but the apex may form a projecting bleb of clear cytoplasm that fills much of the lumen. In cortical nephrons, a short intermediate tubule (without a brush border, and about half the diameter of a distal convoluted tubule) connects proximal convoluted tubules to distal convoluted tubules. In medullary nephrons, long or short medullary loops connect proximal convoluted tubules to distal convoluted tubules. The thin segment of a medullary loop forms only a part of the descending limb. Hence, thin segments are less numerous than either thick descending or thick ascending portions of the loop. The diameter of a thin segment is about one half that of a thick segment. The cells of the thin segment are cuboidal and do not stain as deeply as the cuboidal cells of the thick segments. Apical cytoplasmic blebs of the cells of the thick segments project into the lumen.
Collecting tubules occur in the more peripheral parts of the cortex. They are lined by pale cells with cuboidal to low columnar shape and are intermediate in size between proximal convoluted and distal convoluted tubules. Collecting tubules join distal convoluted tubules to **perilobular collecting ducts.** The latter unite with those of other lobules to form **medullary tracts,** each of which is surrounded by a thin connective tissue capsule. Tracts group together to form a **medullary cone.** Each cone terminates in a single branch of the ureter. Cones and tracts contain thin and thick segments of medullary loops in addition to collecting ducts. The lining epithelium of the smallest collecting ducts is simple cuboidal. It gradually becomes simple columnar and finally changes to pseudostratified columnar in the proximity of the ureteral branch.

The **ureter** of the chicken is a muscular duct about 2 mm in diameter. Its wall consists of a mucosa, muscularis, and adventitia. It is generally lined by a pseudostratified columnar epithelium. The majority of cells are tall, with a lesser number of cuboidal cells lying close to the basement membrane. The apices of the columnar cells contain numerous vacuoles filled with mucus. Beneath the epithelium is a thick layer of loose connective tissue containing varying amounts of diffuse lymphatic tissue and, sometimes, a lymphatic nodule. The muscularis consists of an inner longitudinal and outer circular layer of smooth muscle. A third outer longitudinal layer is present near the cloaca. The adventitia consists of a layer of loose connective tissue.

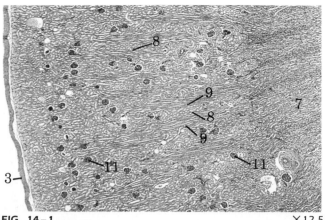

FIG. 14-1 ×12.5

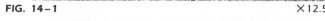

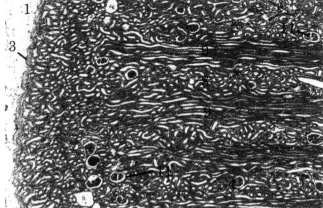

FIG. 14-2 ×25

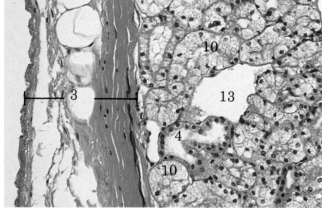

FIG. 14-3 ×125

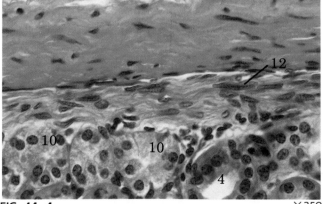

FIG. 14-4 ×250

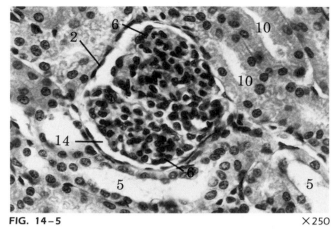

FIG. 14-5 ×250

FIG. 14-1. Cortex and Portion of Medulla, Kidney, Dog.
Renal corpuscles are limited to the cortex.

FIG. 14-2. Cortex, Kidney, Dog, Masson's. Pars radiata alternate with the pars convoluta.

FIG. 14-3. Capsule and Superficial Cortex, Kidney, Cat. The capsule consists entirely of connective tissue in the cat. cat.

FIG. 14-4. Capsule, Kidney, Sheep. The inner portion of the capsule of ruminants contains a distinct layer of smooth muscle. Smooth muscle cells are also present in the capsule of the dog, horse, and pig.

FIG. 14-5. Renal Corpuscle, Kidney, Puppy. In young animals, the podocytes of the glomerular epithelium have round to oval nuclei.

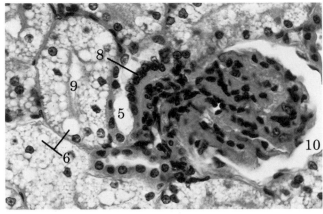

FIG. 14-6   ×250

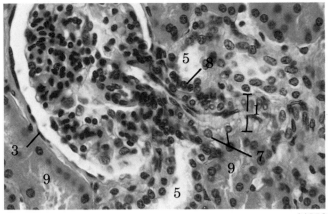

FIG. 14-10   ×250

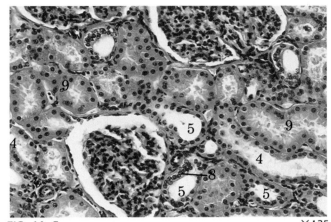

FIG. 14-7   ×125

KEY		
1. Afferent arteriole		**6.** Fat vacuole
2. Brush border		**7.** Juxtaglomerular cells
3. Capsular epithelium		**8.** Macula densa
4. Collecting tubule		**9.** Proximal convoluted tubule
5. Distal convoluted tubule		**10.** Urinary space

FIG. 14-6. Renal Corpuscle, Kidney, Cat. Cells of the proximal convoluted tubules of the cat contain numerous fat vacuoles. A macula densa, consisting of closely packed cells, forms a portion of the wall of the distal convoluted tubule adjacent to the vascular pole of the renal corpuscle.

FIG. 14-7. Cortex, Kidney, Horse. Portions of three renal corpuscles, each with an accompanying macula densa, are present. In the horse, the macula densa commonly consists of a stratified layer of cells.

FIG. 14-8. Cortex, Kidney, Horse. A collecting tubule with clearly defined cells and a smooth lining can be contrasted with proximal convoluted tubules whose cells possess a brush border of microvilli.

FIG. 14-9. Cortex, Kidney, Pig. The junction of a proximal convoluted tubule with the capsule of a renal corpuscle is shown.

FIG. 14-10. Afferent Arteriole, Kidney, Pig. An afferent arteriole, with juxtaglomerular cells, is entering a glomerulus. The juxtaglomerular cells are epithelioid. Note that a macula densa borders the afferent arteriole.

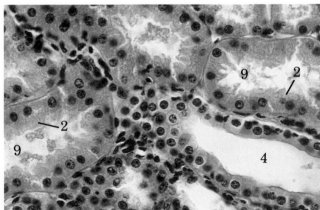

FIG. 14-8   ×250

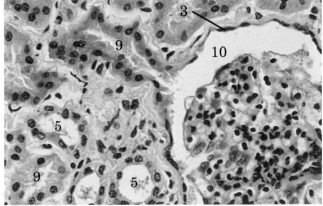

FIG. 14-9   ×250

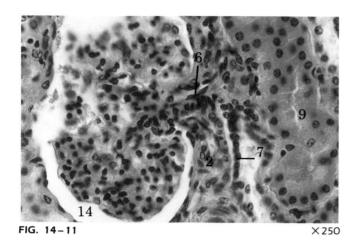

FIG. 14–11 ×250

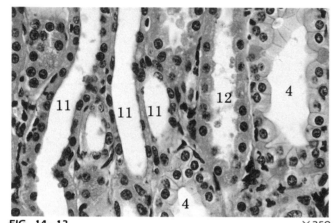

FIG. 14–12 ×250

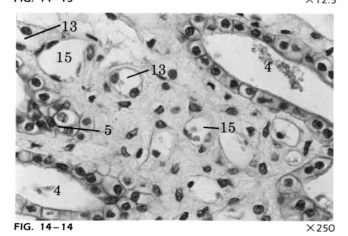

FIG. 14–13 ×12.5

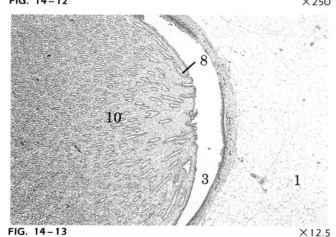

FIG. 14–14 ×250

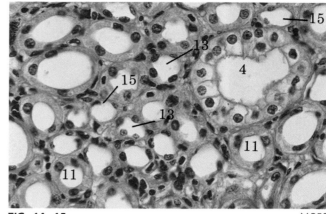

FIG. 14–15 ×250

KEY	
1. Adipose tissue	**9.** Proximal convoluted tubule
2. Afferent arteriole	**10.** Renal papilla
3. Cavity of renal pelvis	**11.** Thick ascending, Henle's
4. Collecting tubule	loop
5. Collecting tubule, surface	**12.** Thick descending, Henle's
cut	loop
6. Efferent arteriole	**13.** Thin segment, Henle's loop
7. Macula densa	**14.** Urinary space
8. Papillary duct	**15.** Vasa recta

FIG. 14–11. Afferent and Efferent Arterioles, Kidney, Pig. Junction of a glomerulus with an afferent arteriole. A macula densa parallels the afferent arteriole.

FIG. 14–12. Pars Radiata, l.s., Cortex, Kidney, Horse. The component tubules of a medullary ray include collecting tubules as well as thick descending and thick ascending portions of the loop of Henle.

FIG. 14–13. Renal Papilla, Kidney, Dog. Papillary ducts open onto the tip of a renal papilla.

FIG. 14–14. Medulla, Kidney, Dog. Nuclei of the cells lining the thin segment of Henle's loop are rounded; those of endothelial cells of the vasa recta are flattened and more darkly stained.

FIG. 14–15. Medulla, Kidney, Horse. Various portions of uriniferous tubules appear in transverse section.

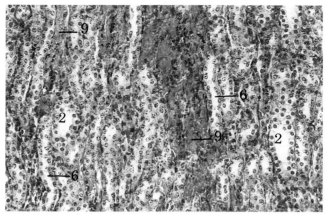

FIG. 14-16   ×125

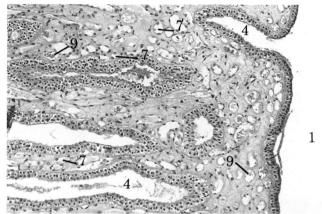

FIG. 14-17   ×62.5

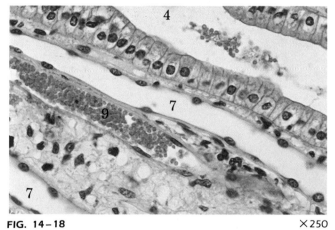

FIG. 14-18   ×250

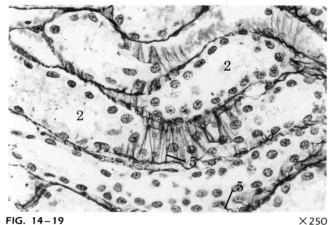

FIG. 14-19   ×250

FIG. 14-20   ×125

KEY	
1. Cavity of renal pelvis	**6.** Thick ascending, Henle's loop
2. Collecting tubule	
3. Mucous connective tissue	**7.** Thin segment, Henle's loop
4. Papillary duct	**8.** Transitional epithelium
5. Reticular fiber	**9.** Vasa recta

FIG. 14-16. Medulla, Kidney, Cow, Trichrome. Longitudinal sections of vasa rectae and portions of uriniferous tubules. The vasa rectae are filled with red blood cells (stained orange).

FIG. 14-17. Renal Papilla, Kidney, Goat. Papillary ducts near the tip of a renal papilla are lined by transitional epithelium.

FIG. 14-18. Medulla, Kidney, Goat. A papillary duct, l.s., some distance away from the apex of the papilla, is lined by columnar cells. A thin segment of Henle's loop parallels the duct.

FIG. 14-19. Medulla, Kidney, Goat, Silver. The collecting tubules are encircled by reticular fibers (stained black). The fibers provide a supportive framework for other portions of the uriniferous tubules as well.

FIG. 14-20. Urachus, Umbilical Cord, Cow. The urachus (allantoic stalk) is lined by a transitional epithelium. A portion of the lining is shown.

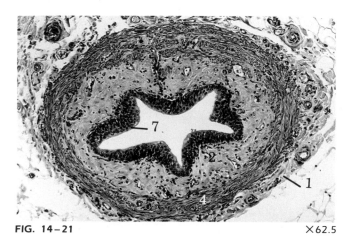

FIG. 14-21　　　　　　　　　　　　　　　　×62.5

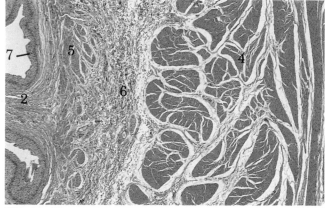

FIG. 14-25　　　　　　　　　　　　　　　　×12.5

KEY	
1. Adventitia	**5.** Muscularis mucosae
2. Lamina propria	**6.** Submucosa
3. Mucous gland	**7.** Transitional epithelium
4. Muscularis	

FIG. 14-21. Ureter, x.s., Cat, Masson's. The middle circular layer of smooth muscle of the muscularis is most evident. Inner and outer longitudinal layers are present but sparse in this section.

FIG. 14-22. Ureter, x.s., Horse, Masson's. The proximal (anterior) portion of the horse's ureter contains tubuloalveolar mucous glands.

FIG. 14-23. Ureter, x.s., Horse. Distally (posteriorly), the horse's ureter lacks mucous glands. The muscularis consists of an inner longitudinal, middle circular, and outer longitudinal layer of smooth muscle.

FIG. 14-24. Urinary Bladder, Pig. The mucosa to a portion of the muscularis is shown. Scattered fibers of the muscularis mucosae are located adjacent to the lamina propria.

FIG. 14-25. Urinary Bladder, Cow. The bladder contains a muscularis mucosae between the lamina propria and submucosa. Only a portion of the thick muscularis is shown.

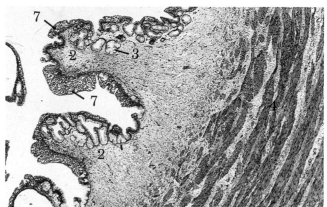

FIG. 14-22　　　　　　　　　　　　　　　　×25

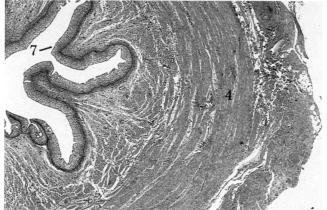

FIG. 14-23　　　　　　　　　　　　　　　　×12.5

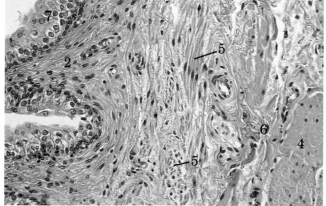

FIG. 14-24　　　　　　　　　　　　　　　　×125

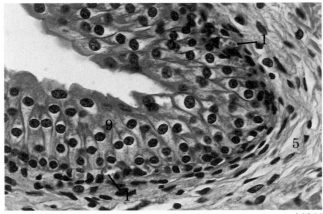

FIG. 14-26 ×250

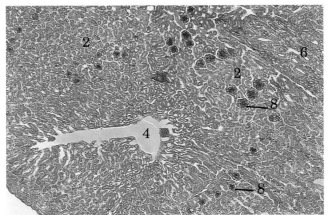

FIG. 14-27 ×25

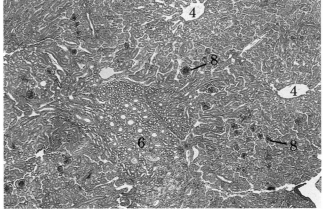

FIG. 14-28 ×25

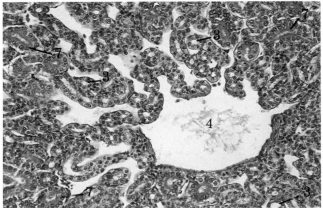

FIG. 14-29 ×125

FIG. 14-26. Urinary Bladder, Goat. Numerous capillaries are located beneath the transitional epithelial lining of the bladder of ruminants.

FIG. 14-27. Kidney, Chicken. Cortical parenchyma and portion of a medullary cone are shown. An intralobular vein and both cortical (small) and medullary (large) renal corpuscles are apparent.

FIG. 14-28. Kidney, Chicken. A portion of a medullary cone is surrounded by cortical lobules. The intralobular veins of two cortical lobules are clearly represented.

FIG. 14-29. Cortex, Kidney, Chicken. An intralobular vein is surrounded by cortical tissue. Distal convoluted tubules are located mainly in the region of the intralobular vein.

URINARY SYSTEM **159**

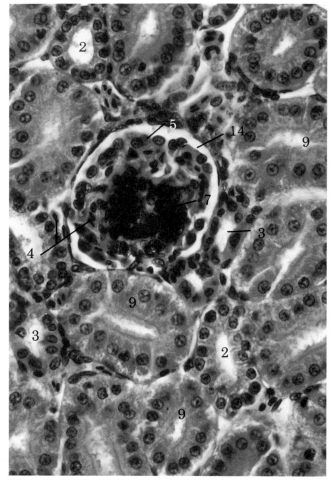

FIG. 14-30   ×360

FIG. 14–30. Cortex, Kidney, Chicken. In the chicken, the glomerular epithelium is composed of podocytes that have large round or oval nuclei. The center of the glomerulus contains a compact mass of mesangial cells.

FIG. 14–31. Medullary Cone, Kidney, Chicken. Various portions of uriniferous tubules (medullary type) are evident. Cells lining the thick ascending portions of Henle's loop show characteristic clear cytoplasmic blebs. A small portion of the cortex containing a proximal convoluted tubule can be seen on the upper right side.

FIG. 14–32. Ureter, x.s., Chicken. The lamina propria is infiltrated with lymphocytes. Outer circular and inner longitudinal layers of the muscularis are distinguishable. The epithelium is pseudostratified columnar.

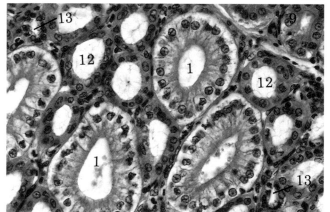

FIG. 14–31   ×250

FIG. 14–32   ×62.5

15

RESPIRATORY SYSTEM

MAMMALS

From the nostrils, air flows through a system of passages to the respiratory surfaces of the lungs. As it progresses, it becomes warmed, humidified, and cleansed of some of its particulate matter. Dust, which finds its way to the alveoli, is ultimately consumed by macrophages patrolling the tiny cul-de-sacs. The major components of the air-passage system are the **nasal cavity, pharynx, larynx, trachea, bronchi,** and the various smaller subdivisions of the bronchial tree leading to the alveoli.

From the naris, air enters the **vestibule,** the first part of the nasal cavity. The vestibule is lined by a stratified squamous epithelium, which is continuous with the skin externally and with the respiratory portion of the nasal cavity internally. In the horse, hairy skin continues into the vestibule. A lamina propria and underlying submucosa support the vestibular epithelium.

The **respiratory portion** of the nasal cavity is lined by a ciliated, pseudostratified columnar epithelium with goblet cells. The lamina propria contains tubuloalveolar glands. The latter are mainly serous, but mucous and mixed glands do occur. Glands are sparse in carnivores. A submucosa supports the lamina propria.

The **olfactory epithelium** (pseudostratified columnar) is composed of olfactory (sensory) cells, supporting cells, and basal cells. Bowman's glands, tubular and mucoserous, occur within the lamina propria. They open to the surface through ducts lined by cuboidal or flattened cells. A submucosa lies below the lamina propria.

The **nasopharynx** and **oropharynx** are subdivisions of the pharynx. The former is lined by a ciliated, pseudostratified columnar epithelium with goblet cells, whereas the latter is covered by a stratified squamous epithelium. The lamina propria contains tubular mixed glands in the nasopharynx and mucous glands in the oropharynx. In carnivores, the glands of the oropharynx are mixed. A network of elastic fibers separates the mucosa from an underlying sheet of skeletal muscle consisting of circularly and longitudinally arranged cells. The musculature is separated from an adventitia of loose connective tissue by a layer of connective tissue containing elastic networks.

The **larynx** is lined in part by a stratified squamous epithelium and partly by a ciliated, pseudostratified columnar epithelium. Numerous elastic fibers are present in the lamina propria. Glands (serous, mucous, and mixed) occur in the lamina propria and submucosa, but are lacking in the vocal and vestibular folds. Hyaline and elastic cartilage provide support for the laryngeal wall. The elastic cartilage of the **epiglottis** may be partially or completely replaced by adipose tissue, as in carnivores. Skeletal muscles are an integral part of the laryngeal structure.

The **trachea** is lined by a ciliated, pseudostratified columnar epithelium with goblet cells. A lamina propria and submucosa lie below the epithelium, but are not clearly demarcated from one another. Glands, mostly mixed, occur in the deeper layers of the lamina propria and within the submucosa. Rings of hyaline cartilage, which are incomplete dorsally, support the tracheal wall. A layer of smooth muscle, the **trachealis muscle,** is located dorsally in the trachea. It is positioned internal to the gap in the tracheal cartilages in the horse, pig, and ruminants. In the cat and dog, it lies external to the gap. A connective tissue adventitia completes the wall of the trachea.

The trachea bifurcates into bronchi, which enter the **lungs,** where they branch extensively. The lungs are covered by a **visceral pleura,** which is thick in large mammals and thinner in carnivores. Connective tissue and some smooth muscle form a part of the visceral pleura. The interior of the lungs contains a connective tissue framework, rich in elastic fibers, which supports the bronchial tree and divides the lungs into lobules. The interlobular connective tissue is sparse in carnivores.

A ciliated, pseudostratified columnar epithelium with goblet cells lines the **bronchi.** The epithelium becomes reduced in height as the caliber of the bronchi diminishes. The lamina propria is surrounded by a layer of obliquely arranged smooth muscle. The connective tissue external to the musculature contains mixed glands and plates of hyaline cartilage. In the cat, the bronchial cartilages may contain elastic fibers. When seen in histologic sections, the mucosa of large bronchi has few folds. Folds increase as the bronchi decrease in diameter.

The smallest bronchi give rise to suborders of **bronchioles.** The smallest of the latter, terminal bronchioles, branch into two or more respiratory bronchioles. The latter divide into alveolar ducts which, in turn, empty into alveolar sacs.

Bronchioles lack cartilage and glands. Glands, however, may extend into bronchioles from bronchi in cats. Spirally or obliquely arranged smooth muscle forms part of the wall of a bronchiole. The amount of smooth muscle is proportional to the size of the bronchiole. Large bronchioles are lined by ciliated columnar cells, whereas the smallest (terminal) bronchioles are lined by ciliated cuboidal cells and, distally, by noncilated cells. The mucosa of the bronchioles is folded, unless the lungs were inflated at the time when the tissue was processed.

Respiratory bronchioles branch from the ends of terminal bronchioles. They are lined by a cuboidal epithelium, which becomes flattened distally, and their wall contains some smooth muscle. Alveoli occur within the epithelium. Respiratory bronchioles are best developed in the cat and dog.

Alveolar ducts branch from respiratory bronchioles. Their thin walls are constructed entirely of alveoli. The edge surrounding the opening of each alveolus of an alveolar duct contains smooth muscle cells. The presence of the muscle gives the lip of the alveolus a knoblike appearance in sections.

Ultimately, each alveolar duct branches into three or more **alveolar sacs.** No smooth muscle is present in the sacs. Therefore, the alveoli, which form the walls of the sacs, do not have lips with knoblike expansions.

Alveoli are lined mainly by exceedingly thin squamous epithelial cells (type I cells). Alveoli are separated from one another by a thin, highly vascularized layer of fine collagenous and elastic fibers. This layer, together with the squamous cells lining the adjacent alveoli, forms an alveolar septum.

CHICKEN

The nostrils, nasal cavity, pharynx, trachea, syrinx, bronchi, air capillaries, and air sacs comprise the respiratory system of the bird. The skin enters the nostrils to the first part of the nasal cavity, the **vestibule**, which is lined by a modified, keratinized, stratified squamous epithelium. It is characterized by epithelial cells that are organized into columns, giving the surface a wavy appearance. The **respiratory region** of the nasal cavity is lined by a ciliated, pseudostratified columnar epithelium. Mucous glands occur within the respiratory epithelium. The **olfactory epithelium** is pseudostratified columnar. It is located in the upper portions of the nasal cavities. Its structure, like that of mammals, is composed of basal, sensory, and supporting cells. Bowman's glands are present.

The **pharynx** is lined by a stratified squamous epithelium. A dense lamina propria and less dense submucosa lie below the epithelium. Salivary glands (mucous) occur within the lamina propria or submucosa. Bundles of skeletal muscle occur below the floor of the pharynx.

At the anterior end of the trachea is a cranial larynx, which is reinforced by a cartilaginous ring. A caudal larynx (syrinx) is located at the posterior end of the trachea. The **trachea** is supported by overlapping, complete cartilaginous rings. It is lined by a ciliated, pseudostratified columnar epithelium containing numerous, simple alveolar mucous glands. In the posterior portion of the trachea, the glands are replaced by goblet cells. A lamina propria and submucosa are present. Each consists of dense connective tissue. The submucosa is rich in elastic fibers.

The **syrinx,** or voice box, is located in the thoracic cavity at the point of tracheal bifurcation into two bronchi. Internal and external **tympanic membranes,** located in the region of the tracheal bifurcation, characterize the wall of the syrinx. **Intersyringeal cartilages** and a bony wedge, the **pessulus,** provide support in the region of the syrinx.

Each **extrapulmonary primary bronchus** enters a lung as an **intrapulmonary primary bronchus** (meso-bronchus). **Secondary bronchi stem** from the primary bronchi and branch into numerous **parabronchi** (tertiary bronchi) within the lung. The latter anastomose with each other. Tiny, respiratory **air capillaries** form extensive networks interconnecting the tertiary bronchi.

Primary bronchi are lined by a ciliated pseudostratified columnar epithelium with mucous glands and goblet cells. Extrapulmonary primary bronchi have C-shaped cartilages, while the walls of intrapulmonary primary bronchi contain cartilaginous plates, which become scarce distally. Bundles of smooth muscle, mainly circular, occur below the lamina propria. Numerous elastic fibers are found throughout the connective tissue of the bronchi.

Secondary bronchi are lined by a ciliated, columnar epithelium with mucous cells. There is a lamina propria and a well-developed muscularis.

Parabronchi are lined by a cuboidal epithelium. A thin layer of connective tissue lies below the epithelium. Bundles of smooth muscle cells lie below the connective tissue layer. The inner wall of each tertiary bronchus is pierced by numerous openings, each of which leads into a cavity called an **atrium** (air vesicle). Atria are lined by a squamous to cuboidal epithelium. **Air capillaries,** lined by squamous cells, open into atria and form the respiratory surface. Numerous vascular capillaries surround the air capillaries and are separated from the latter by a basement membrane.

Air sacs are paired or unpaired, thin-walled structures occurring in the cervical, clavicular, thoracic, and abdominal regions of the body. They connect to the lungs by bronchi. Many of the hollow bones of the fowl contain extensions of the air sacs. Among others, these include the sternum, humerus, pelvic girdle, and most of the thoracic and cervical vertebrae. The air sacs are lined by squamous, ciliated cuboidal, and ciliated columnar cells. The epithelium is supported by a thin connective tissue layer consisting of collagenous and elastic fibers. The sacs are poorly vascularized and do not participate in gas exchange.

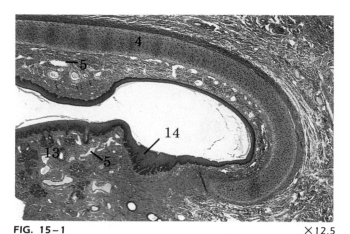

FIG. 15-1 ×12.5

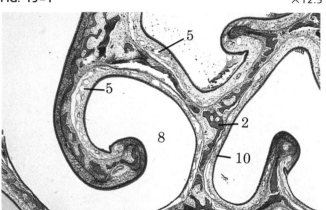

FIG. 15-2 ×12.5

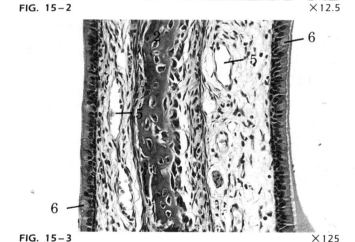

FIG. 15-3 ×125

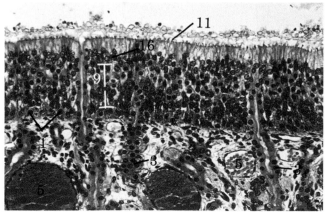

FIG. 15-4 ×125

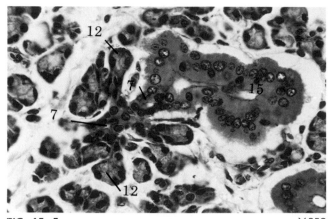

FIG. 15-5 ×250

KEY	
1. Basal cells	**10.** Pseudostratified epithelium
2. Bone	**11.** Sensory hairs
3. Bowman's gland	**12.** Serous acinus
4. Cartilage	**13.** Serous gland
5. Cavernous vein	**14.** Stratified squamous
6. Goblet cell	epithelium
7. Intercalated duct	**15.** Striated duct
8. Nasal cavity	**16.** Supporting cells, nuclei
9. Olfactory cells, nuclei	

FIG. 15-1. Nasal Cavity, Vestibule, Dog. This portion of the vestibule is supported by hyaline cartilage and lined by a stratified squamous epithelium. Numerous cavernous veins occur throughout the connective tissue of the mucosa. In addition, there are tubular serous glands within the connective tissue.

FIG. 15-2. Portion of Nasal Concha, Dog. The scroll-like nasal conchae are supported by spongy bone and are lined by a mucous membrane with a ciliated, pseudostratified columnar epithelium.

FIG. 15-3. Respiratory Epithelium, Nasal Concha, Dog. Ciliated, pseudostratified columnar epithelium with goblet cells and underlying vascular loose connective tissue and bone.

FIG. 15-4. Olfactory Epithelium, Nasal Cavity, Dog, Masson's. This thick, pseudostratified columnar epithelium is composed of three types of cells. Basal cells are located at the level of the basement membrane. The nuclei of olfactory cells form a broad band in the central portion of the epithelium. The nuclei of supporting cells are pale and form the uppermost level of nuclei. The apices of olfactory cells bear sensory hairs.

FIG. 15-5. Lateral Nasal Gland, Dog, Masson's. This serous gland is located in the maxillary sinus in carnivores.

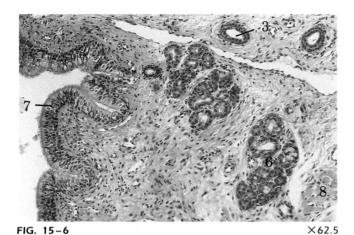

FIG. 15-6   ×62.5

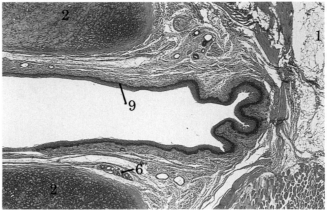

FIG. 15-10   ×12.5

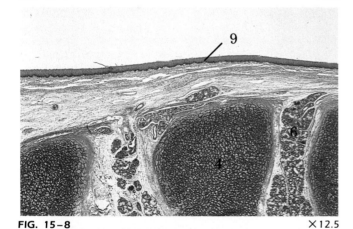

FIG. 15-7   ×25

KEY	
1. Adipose tissue	**7.** Pseudostratified epithelium
2. Arytenoid cartilage	**8.** Skeletal muscle
3. Duct	**9.** Stratified squamous
4. Elastic cartilage	epithelium, nonkeratinized
5. Lamina propria	**10.** Submucosa
6. Mixed gland	**11.** Taste bud

FIG. 15-6. Nasopharynx, Dog. This portion of the pharynx is lined by a ciliated, pseudostratified columnar epithelium with goblet cells. Mixed glands are present in the mucosal connective tissue. The muscularis consists of skeletal muscle, a portion of which is visible.

FIG. 15-7. Epiglottis, Dog. The supporting elastic cartilage of the epiglottis is heavily infiltrated, in its midregion, by adipose tissue in carnivores.

FIG. 15-8. Epiglottis, l.s., Sheep. Block-like chunks of elastic cartilage, without infiltrating adipose tissue, are found in the epiglottis of the sheep and goat.

FIG. 15-9. Epiglottis, Sheep. Occasionally, taste buds are found in the epithelium of the laryngeal surface of the epiglottis.

FIG. 15-10. Glottis, x.s., Goat. The glottis is supported by the arytenoid cartilages (elastic) and is lined by a nonkeratinized stratified squamous epithelium.

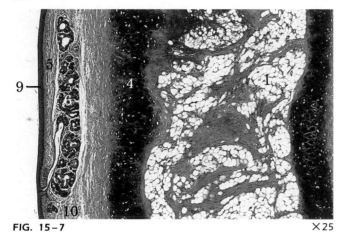

FIG. 15-8   ×12.5

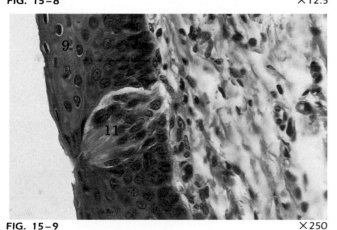

FIG. 15-9   ×250

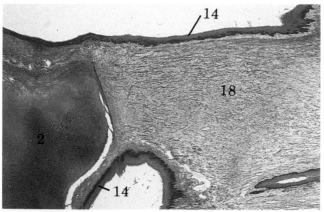

FIG. 15-11   ×12.5

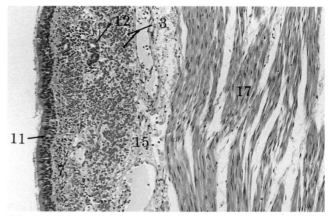

FIG. 15-15   ×62.5

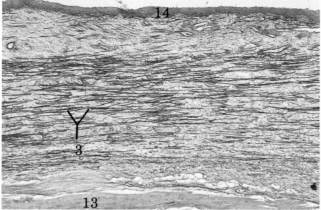

FIG. 15-12   ×25

KEY	
1. Adipose tissue	**11.** Pseudostratified epithelium
2. Arytenoid cartilage	**12.** Serous gland
3. Elastic fibers	**13.** Skeletal muscle
4. Esophagus	**14.** Stratified squamous
5. Goblet cell	epithelium
6. Hyaline cartilage	**15.** Submucosa
7. Lamina propria	**16.** Trachea
8. Mixed gland	**17.** Trachealis muscle
9. Muscularis externa	**18.** Vocal ligament
10. Plasma cell	

FIG. 15-11. Vocal Fold, l.s., Cat. Junction of the vocal fold with the arytenoid cartilage.

FIG. 15-12. Vocal Fold, Goat, Orcein. The vocal fold consists of a fold of the mucous membrane. The vocal fold encloses the vocal ligament, which is a band of elastic fibers.

FIG. 15-13. Trachea and Esophagus, x.s., Cat. Note that the trachealis muscle (smooth) lies external to the gap in the C-shaped cartilage in carnivores.

FIG. 15-14. Trachea, x.s., Cat. The trachea is lined by a ciliated, pseudostratified columnar epithelium with goblet cells. The lamina propria contains a band of longitudinally oriented elastic fibers.

FIG. 15-15. Trachea, x.s., Horse. A thick band of longitudinally arranged elastic fibers extends from the lamina propria into the submucosa.

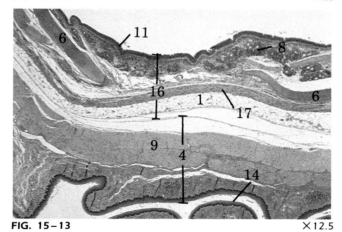

FIG. 15-13   ×12.5

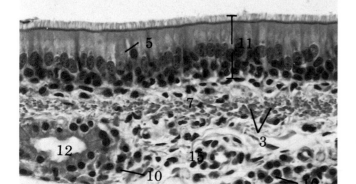

FIG. 15-14   ×250

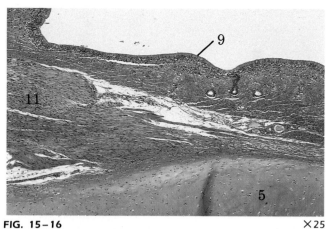

FIG. 15–16   ×25

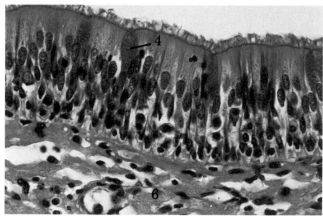

FIG. 15–17   ×250

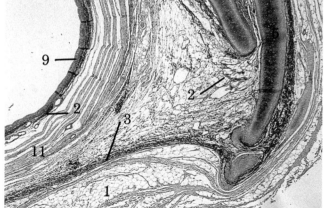

FIG. 15–18   ×12.5

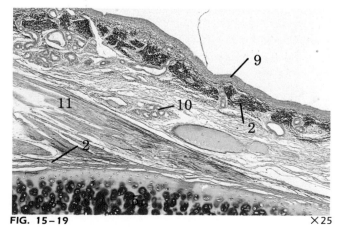

FIG. 15–19   ×25

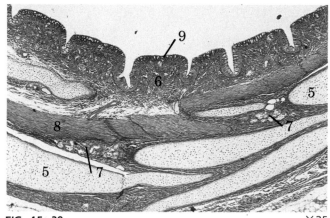

FIG. 15–20   ×25

KEY		
1. Adipose tissue	**7.** Mixed glands	
2. Elastic fibers	**8.** Muscularis	
3. Fibroelastic membrane	**9.** Pseudostratified epithelium	
4. Goblet cell	**10.** Tracheal glands	
5. Hyaline cartilage	**11.** Trachealis muscle	
6. Lamina propria		

FIG. 15–16. Trachea, x.s., Cow. In noncarnivores, the trachealis muscle attaches to the perichondrium on the inside of the tracheal cartilage. The lamina propria and submucosa are both very rich in elastic fibers.

FIG. 15–17. Trachea, x.s., Cow. Ciliated, pseudostratified columnar epithelium with goblet cells.

FIG. 15–18. Trachea, x.s., Sheep, Orcein. A fibroelastic membrane surrounds the C-shaped tracheal cartilage, and also spans the gap in the cartilage.

FIG. 15–19. Trachea, x.s., Goat, Orcein. Numerous elastic fibers occur below the epithelium. Elastic fibers are also present where the trachealis muscle joins with the perichondrium.

FIG. 15–20. Primary Bronchus, Extrapulmonary, x.s., Dog, Mallory's. Plates of hyaline cartilage support the wall of the bronchus. Smooth muscle bundles of the muscularis occur between the plates and internal to them.

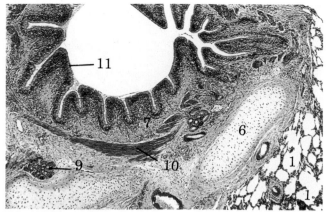

FIG. 15–21 ×25

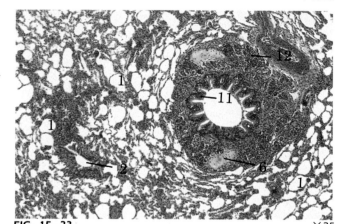

FIG. 15–22 ×62.5

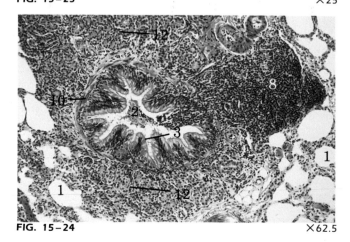

FIG. 15–23 ×25

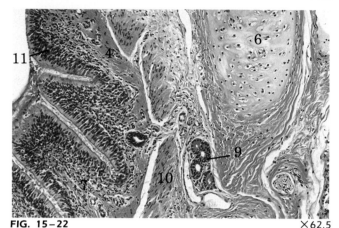

FIG. 15–24 ×62.5

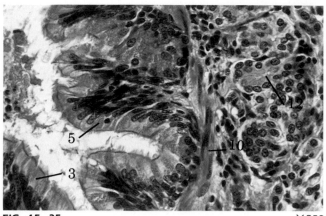

FIG. 15–25 ×250

KEY	
1. Alveolus	**7.** Lamina propria
2. Bronchiole	**8.** Lymphatic nodule
3. Columnar epithelium, ciliated	**9.** Mixed gland
4. Elastic band	**10.** Muscularis
5. Goblet cell	**11.** Pseudostratified epithelium
6. Hyaline cartilage	**12.** Serous gland

FIG. 15–21. Bronchus, x.s., Cow, Masson's.

FIG. 15–22. Bronchus, x.s., Cow. Detail of the wall of a bronchus. Numerous lymphocytes are present below the epithelium.

FIG. 15–23. Small Bronchus, x.s., and Bronchioles, Cat. Bronchioles lack cartilaginous plates and possess a simple epithelium.

FIG. 15–24. Large Bronchiole, x.s., Cat. In cats, submucosal serous glands extend from bronchi into the bronchioles.

FIG. 15–25. Large Bronchiole, x.s., Cat. Detail of a portion of the bronchiole shown in Fig. 15–24.

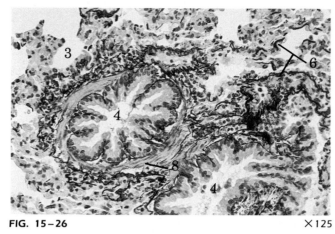

FIG. 15-26 ×125

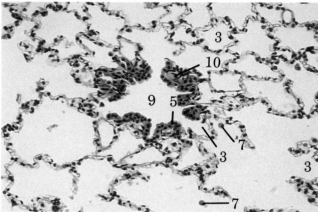

FIG. 15-27 ×125

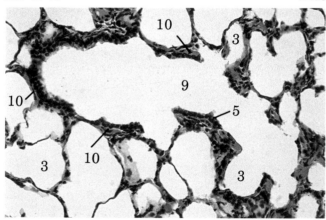

FIG. 15-28 ×125

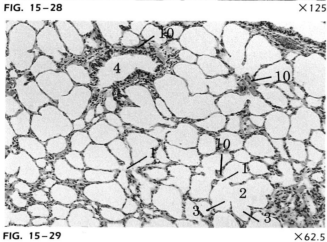

FIG. 15-29 ×62.5

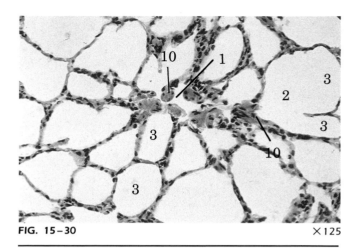

FIG. 15-30 ×125

KEY	
1. Alveolar duct	**6.** Elastic fibers
2. Alveolar sac	**7.** Macrophage
3. Alveolus	**8.** Muscularis
4. Bronchiole	**9.** Respiratory bronchiole
5. Cuboidal epithelium	**10.** Smooth muscle

FIG. 15-26. Bronchioles, Pig, Orcein. The tissues of the lung are heavily infiltrated with elastic fibers.

FIG. 15-27. Respiratory Bronchiole, x.s., Cat. Respiratory bronchioles are lined by a cuboidal epithelium, and have alveoli in their walls.

FIG. 15-28. Respiratory Bronchiole, l.s., Sheep.

FIG. 15-29. Alveolar Ducts and Alveolar Sacs, Sheep. An alveolar duct is characterized by the presence of circumferentially disposed smooth muscle at the entrance of the alveoli that form its wall. Conversely, the alveoli of alveolar sacs lack smooth muscle.

FIG. 15-30. Alveolar Duct, x.s., Sheep. Detail of an alveolar duct. The smooth muscle associated with the entrance of the alveoli forming the wall of the duct is evident.

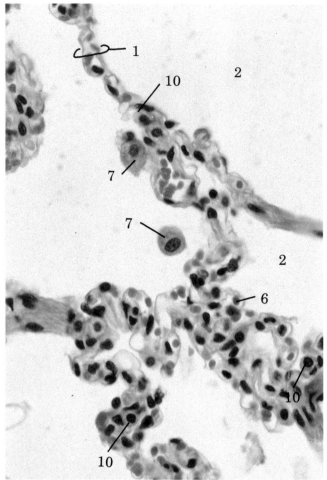

FIG. 15-31   ×360

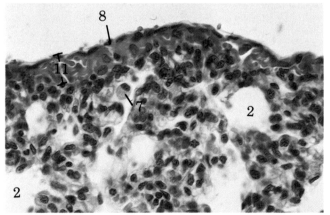

FIG. 15-32   ×250

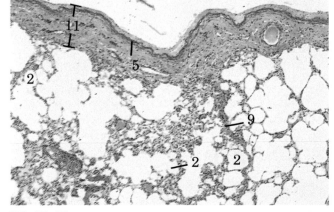

FIG. 15-33   ×25

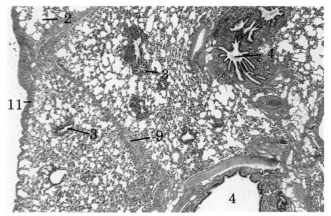

FIG. 15-34   ×12.5

KEY	
1. Alveolar septum	**7.** Macrophage
2. Alveolus	**8.** Mesothelium
3. Bronchiole	**9.** Septum
4. Bronchus	**10.** Type II alveolar cell
5. Elastic band	**11.** Visceral pleura
6. Erythrocyte in capillary	

FIG. 15-31. Alveoli, Cat. Detail of alveolar septa.

FIG. 15-32. Visceral Pleura, Dog. The visceral pleura of carnivores is relatively thin.

FIG. 15-33. Visceral Pleura, Horse. The visceral pleura of domestic mammals, except carnivores, is thick. Incomplete septa extend inward from the visceral pleura in the horse.

FIG. 15-34. Visceral Pleura, Pig. Lungs are highly lobulated in the pig and ruminants. Unlike those of the horse, the septa are complete.

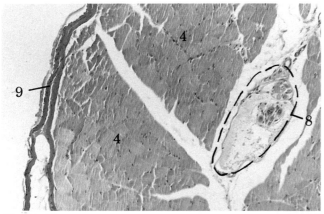

FIG. 15–35   ×62.5

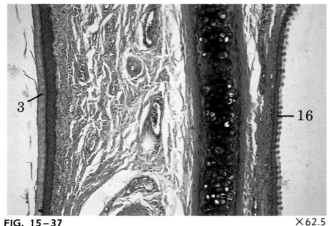

FIG. 15–36   ×125

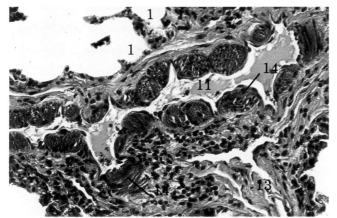

FIG. 15–37   ×62.5

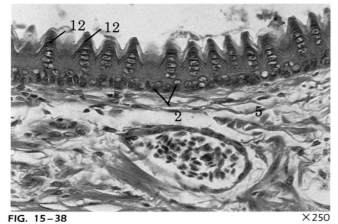

FIG. 15–38   ×250

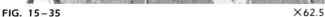

FIG. 15–39   ×125

KEY	
1. Alveolus	**9.** Parietal pleura
2. Basal cells	**10.** Pseudostratified epithelium
3. Epidermis	**11.** Pulmonary vein
4. Intercostal muscle	**12.** Pyknotic nucleus
5. Lamina propria	**13.** Septum
6. Mucous gland	**14.** Smooth muscle
7. Nerve	**15.** Turbinate cartilage
8. Neuromuscular spindle	**16.** Vestibular epithelium

FIG. 15–35. Parietal Pleura, Cat. Parietal pleura and intercostal muscle. The parietal pleura lines the wall of the pleural cavity. It consists of a mesothelium and underlying connective tissue.

FIG. 15–36. Lung, Cow, Masson's. In the cow and pig, pulmonary veins have thick bands of circularly arranged smooth muscle.

FIG. 15–37. Nasal Cavity, Chicken. The vestibule is lined by a uniquely structured, keratinized, stratified squamous epithelium (see Fig. 15–38). The vestibular epithelium blends with the epidermis on the inner side of each nostril. In this micrograph, these epithelia lie to either side of a turbinate cartilage.

FIG. 15–38. Vestibular Epithelium, Chicken. This keratinized, stratified squamous epithelium is characterized by the presence of columns of cells. The uppermost cells in each column have pyknotic nuclei. One or two layers of basal cells are present. The outer surface of the epithelium presents a corrugated appearance.

FIG. 15–39. Respiratory Epithelium, Chicken, Masson's. This ciliated, pseudostratified columnar epithelium is interrupted by simple, branched, alveolar mucous glands.

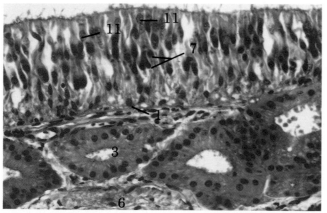

FIG. 15-40 ×250

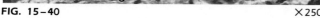

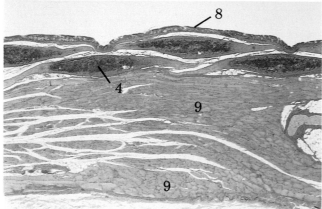

FIG. 15-41 ×12.5

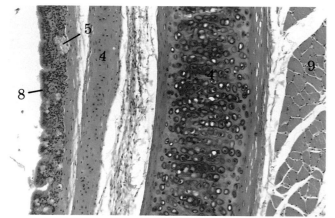

FIG. 15-42 ×62.5

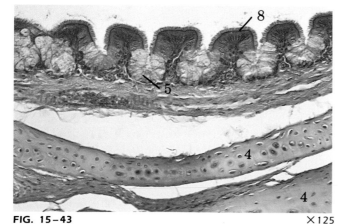

FIG. 15-43 ×125

172   COLOR ATLAS OF VETERINARY HISTOLOGY

FIG. 15-44 ×25

KEY	
1. Basal cell	**7.** Olfactory cells, nuclei
2. Bony tracheal ring	**8.** Pseudostratified epithelium
3. Bowman's gland	**9.** Skeletal muscle
4. Cartilaginous tracheal ring	**10.** Stratified squamous epithelium
5. Mucous gland	
6. Nerve	**11.** Supporting cell, nucleus

FIG. 15-40. Olfactory Epithelium, Chicken, Masson's.
This pseudostratified columnar epithelium is similar to that found in mammals (see Fig. 15-4). It is composed of basal, olfactory, and supporting cells.

FIG. 15-41. Trachea, l.s., Chicken. Cartilaginous tracheal rings are complete and overlap each other. When the trachea is cut longitudinally, as in this preparation, the rings present a lenticular profile.

FIG. 15-42. Trachea, x.s., Chicken. Simple alveolar mucous glands occur in the ciliated, pseudostratified columnar epithelium. Portions of two overlapping tracheal rings are present. The inner ring was cut through its thin edge, while the outer one was cut through its thick middle region.

FIG. 15-43. Trachea, x.s., Chicken. Intraepithelial mucous glands are abundant in the trachea of the chicken.

FIG. 15-44. Trachea, Near Syrinx, Chicken. The majority of the posterior, complete rings of the trachea shown here are bony. The ciliated pseudostratified columnar epithelium of the trachea is followed in the syrinx by a stratified squamous epithelium.

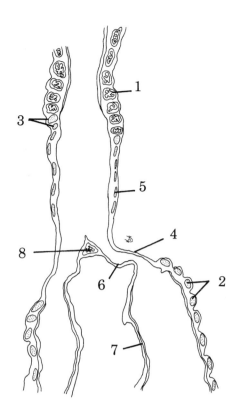

FIG. 15–45. Trachea, Syrinx and Primary Bronchi, l.s., Chicken.

FIG. 15–46. Syrinx, l.s., Chicken.

FIG. 15–47. Syrinx, l.s., Chicken. A portion of the external tympanic membrane and intermediate syringeal cartilage.

FIG. 15–45

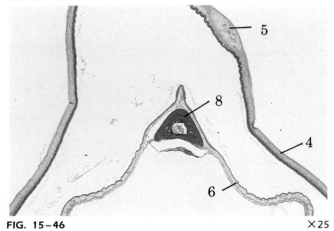

FIG. 15–46 ×25

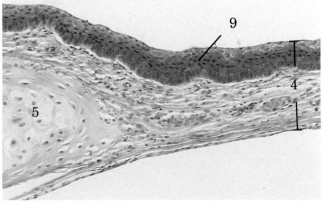

FIG. 15–47 ×125

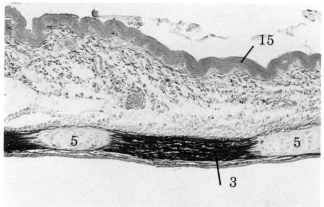

FIG. 15-48   ×62.5

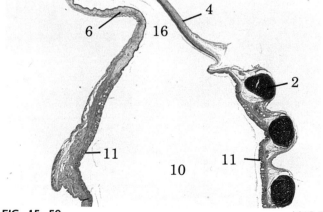

FIG. 15-49   ×125

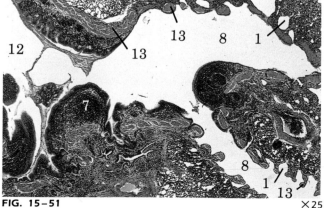

FIG. 15-50   ×12.5

FIG. 15-51   ×25

KEY	
1. Atrium	**9.** Pessulus
2. Bronchial cartilage	**10.** Primary bronchus
3. Elastic fibers	**11.** Pseudostratified epithelium
4. External tympanic membrane	**12.** Secondary bronchus
5. Intermediate syringeal cartilage	**13.** Smooth muscle
6. Internal tympanic membrane	**14.** Stratified columnar epithelium
7. Lymphatic tissue	**15.** Stratified squamous epithelium
8. Parabronchus	**16.** Syrinx

FIG. 15-48. Syrinx, l.s., Chicken, Orcein. Intermediate syringeal cartilages are connected by numerous elastic fibers.

FIG. 15-49. Syrinx, Chicken. Portion of pessulus and internal tympanic membrane. The latter is lined by both a ciliated, stratified columnar epithelium and by a stratified squamous epithelium.

FIG. 15-50. Tympanic Membrane and Primary Bronchus, Chicken. Three transected bronchial cartilages. Bronchial cartilages are incomplete (C-shaped). They do not extend to the medial side of the bronchus.

FIG. 15-51. Lung, Chicken. Longitudinal section through a secondary bronchus and parabronchi. The presence of numerous cup-shaped atria in the parabronchus distinguish this part of the bronchial tree from the secondary bronchus.

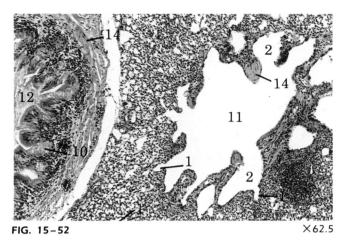

FIG. 15-52   ×62.5

FIG. 15-52. Lung, Chicken. Cross section of a parabronchus and a portion of an adjacent secondary bronchus.

FIG. 15-53. Lung, Chicken. Detail of the wall of a parabronchus. Note the continuity of the air capillaries with the atria. The latter are lined by an epithelium that varies from simple cuboidal to simple squamous.

FIG. 15-54. Abdominal Air Sac, Chicken. The wall of the air sac consists of a connective tissue lamina and an epithelium which may be simple squamous, cuboidal, or ciliated columnar. Air sacs are not well vascularized.

FIG. 15-55. Humerus, x.s., Chicken, Masson's. Many bones of the chicken contain extensions of air sacs.

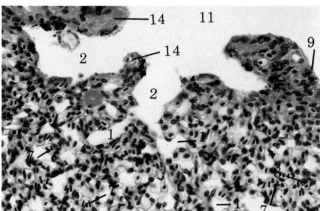

FIG. 15-53   ×250

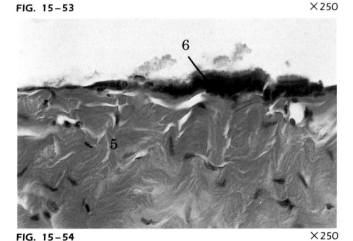

FIG. 15-54   ×250

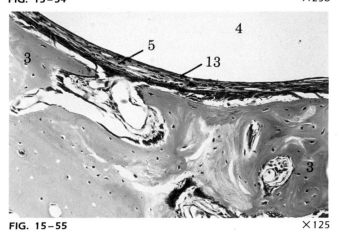

FIG. 15-55   ×125

16

ENDOCRINE SYSTEM

MAMMALS

The pituitary, pineal, thyroid, parathyroid, and adrenal glands possess certain features that distinguish them as organs of the endocrine system. They are very rich in wide, thin-walled vessels called sinusoids. The sinusoids are intimately associated with parenchymal cells, whose secretory products (hormones) pass directly into the circulatory system. Endocrine glands lack ducts. In contrast, exocrine glands convey their secretions (e.g., enzymes, mucus, bile) through ducts to a mucosal or skin surface.

Endocrine cells are not limited to the glands presented in this chapter. For example, hormones are secreted by interstitial cells of the testes, corpora lutea and ovarian follicles, islets of Langerhans, and enterochromaffin cells of the gastrointestinal epithelium.

The **pituitary gland** (hypophysis) is a major endocrine gland that is suspended from the hypothalamus of the brain. It releases several hormones, many of which influence the activity of other endocrine glands. The glandular portion, the **adenohypophysis,** forms from an outpocketing of the ectoderm of the dorsal portion of the oral cavity, called Rathke's pouch. The pars distalis, pars tuberalis, and pars intermedia constitute the adenohypophysis. The neural part of the pituitary gland, the **neurohypophysis,** is derived from a ventral outpocketing of the diencephalon. It is divisible into a median eminence, infundibular stalk, and pars nervosa.

The **pars distalis** is the largest portion of the pituitary gland. The parenchyma consists of irregular cords of cells separated by sinusoids and sparse connective tissue. There are two main types of parenchymal cells: **chromophobes,** characterized by a small amount of cytoplasm that stains poorly, and **chromophils,** with more abundant cytoplasm that is readily stained. The chromophils are classified as **acidophils** (alpha cells) and **basophils** (beta cells). Basophils tend to be larger than acidophils. Chromophobes are smaller than chromophils and are most evident in groups, appearing as clusters of closely packed nuclei.

The **pars intermedia** is situated between the pars distalis and the pars nervosa. In the horse, these regions are closely apposed. In other domestic mammals, the pars intermedia and pars distalis are partially separated by a small cleft, the **hypophyseal cavity,** which is the **vestigial cavity of Rathke's pouch.** The pars intermedia consists predominantly of basophilic cells. Follicles filled with colloid are often present.

The **pars tuberalis** is mainly located around the infundibular stalk. It is composed mainly of cords, clusters, and follicles of small, faintly basophilic cells.

The neurohypophysis contains numerous unmyelinated nerve fibers whose cell bodies are located in the supraoptic and paraventricular nuclei of the hypothalamus. Their axons converge at the **median eminence** (ventral boundary of the third ventricle) and form the hypothalamohypophyseal tract. They pass through the narrow **infundibular stalk** to the **pars nervosa** (infundibular process). The neurosecretions of these cells move along the axons and accumulate at the terminal regions of the nerve fibers as **Herring bodies,** which are best demonstrated with special staining methods. Overall, the pars nervosa has an unorganized, fibrous appearance, and individual axons are indistinct. Numerous **pituicytes** (neuroglial cells) are scattered among the nerve fibers. They possess round to oval nuclei and long cytoplasmic processes. Their cytoplasm cannot be distinguished from nerve fibers in routine histologic preparations.

The **infundibular cavity,** which is continuous with the third ventricle and lined by ependymal cells, extends deep into the pars nervosa in the cat and pig, and to a lesser extent in the dog and horse. In ruminants, the cavity does not reach beyond the infundibular stalk. These relationships are evident in midsagittal sections of the pituitary gland.

The **pineal gland** (pineal body; epiphysis cerebri) is a dorsal evagination of the roof of the diencephalon. It is covered by connective tissue of the pia mater and divided into lobules by connective tissue septa. The parenchyma is composed predominantly of **pinealocytes,** which are arranged as clusters, cords, or follicles. These epithelioid cells have a round nucleus and acidophilic cytoplasm. Neuroglial cells are also present.

Each lobe of the **thyroid gland** is surrounded by a thin capsule of connective tissue and divided into lobules by thin trabeculae. The latter are continuous with sparse intralobular connective tissue that contains numerous sinusoids. In the pig and cow, the connective tissue is abundant. Each lobule consists of numerous **follicles** of various sizes that are frequently filled with colloid. The follicular cells vary in height, depending on the state of activity of the follicle. Their appearance changes from squamous or low cuboidal in the resting stage to cuboidal or columnar in the active stage. In an active follicle, the periphery of the colloid adjacent to the apical surface of the follicular cells is vacuolated. In an inactive follicle, the colloid has a smoother peripheral surface and vacuoles are not present. **Parafollicular (C) cells** occur among the cells that line the thyroid follicles and also between the follicles. They are larger and have a paler cytoplasm than the follicular cells. Their nuclei are relatively large and pale. Parafollicular cells usually occur singly, but may also appear in groups. In the dog, these cells are particularly abundant.

The **parathyroid glands** are classified as internal and external. Those that are adjacent to or embedded in the thyroid gland are the internal parathyroids. The external parathyroids lie a variable distance away from the thyroid gland. The parathyroid glands are surrounded by a thin connective tissue capsule, which may be absent where the glands are deeply embedded within the thyroid gland. A connective tissue stroma is well developed in the pig and cow, but is sparse in other domestic mammals.

The parenchyma of the parathyroid gland consists primarily of clusters and cords of **principal** (chief) **cells.** There are two different functional stages of the principal cell. The **light principal cell** is inactive and has a large, pale nucleus and pale, acidophilic cytoplasm. The **dark principal cell** is a smaller, active cell with a small, dark nucleus and a deeply acidophilic cytoplasm. In the sheep and goat, light cells tend to be located peripheral to the more central, dark cells. In the other domestic mammals, these cells are distributed randomly.

Oxyphilic cells are large cells with an acidophilic cytoplasm and a pyknotic nucleus. They have been reported to occur in small numbers in the parathyroid glands of the horse and cow, particularly older animals.

The paired **adrenal glands** are situated close to the anterior end of the kidneys. The glands are covered by a capsule of dense irregular connective tissue that sometimes contains smooth muscle cells. Clusters of epithelioid cortical cells also occur in the capsule. Thin trabeculae project partially into the parenchyma.

Each adrenal gland is organized into a peripheral cortex and a central medulla. The **adrenal cortex** is divided into four zones. The **zona glomerulosa** (zona multiformis) is the outermost zone. In the carnivore, horse, and pig, the parenchymal cells of this region are columnar and arranged into arcs. In the horse, the columnar cells are especially tall. In ruminants, the zona glomerulosa contains polyhedral cells that form irregular clusters or cords.

The **zona intermedia** lies between the zona glomerulosa and the zona fasciculata. It consists of small, closely packed cells. This zone is seen more often in the horse and carnivore than in the other domestic mammals.

The **zona fasciculata,** the widest zone of the adrenal cortex, is formed by radially arranged cords of cuboidal or polyhedral cells. The cords are one or two cells thick and separated by sinusoids. The cytoplasm of the cells in this zone frequently appears foamy because of the presence of numerous lipid vacuoles.

The **zona reticularis** is the innermost zone of the adrenal cortex. It is arranged as an irregular network of anastomosing cords of cells surrounded by sinusoids.

The **adrenal medulla** is composed mostly of columnar or polyhedral chromaffin cells, which form clusters and anastomosing cords separated by sinusoids. In domestic mammals, an outer and inner zone of the medulla can often be distinguished. The former consists of larger, more darkly stained cells, and the latter contains smaller, more lightly stained cells. Ganglion cells, either individually or in clusters, are scattered through the medulla. Because the cortex and medulla interdigitate at their junction, projections of the zona reticularis may appear within the medulla.

CHICKEN

As in mammals, the **pituitary gland** (hypophysis) of the chicken is attached to the base of the brain below the diencephalon and is encapsulated by the dura mater. The **adenohypophysis** is composed of the pars distalis and pars tuberalis. A pars intermedia is absent. The **pars distalis** is divided into a **cephalic region** and a **caudal region.** Both zones contain cords of acidophils and basophils, and clusters of chromophobes. The acidophils of the cephalic region are pale, and those of the caudal zone are more darkly stained. Thus, the cephalic zone appears more basophilic, and the caudal zone appears more acidophilic. The cords of cells of the former are more closely packed than those of the latter. Some parenchymal cells of the pars distalis may be arranged around a lumen filled with colloid, especially in older birds. Cysts lined by ciliated cells and mucous cells also occur in this part of the pituitary gland.

The **pars tuberalis** surrounds the infundibulum and spreads dorsally over the ventral surface of the brain for a short distance. Ventrally, it extends to the posterior margin of the cephalic zone of the pars distalis. The pars tuberalis contains small, round to elongated, slightly basophilic cells that are arranged in several layers.

The **neurohypophysis** includes the median eminence of the tuber cinereum, the infundibular stalk, and the pars nervosa (infundibular process). The **median eminence** and the **infundibular stalk** consist primarily of nerve fibers, neuroglial cells, and ependymal cells that line the infundibular cavity. The **pars nervosa** has an irregular surface and consists of numerous lobules. Each lobule contains a diverticulum of the infundibular cavity that is lined by ependymal cells. The latter are surrounded by irregular masses of tissue consisting of pituicytes and other neuroglial cells, nerve fibers, and Herring bodies.

The **pineal gland** (epiphysis cerebri) is a small, conical body that is situated between the cerebral hemispheres and the cerebellum. It is surrounded by connective tissue and is composed of a **body** and a narrow, ventral **stalk** that is attached to the roof of the third ventricle. The parenchyma of the gland is arranged into lobules separated by thin connective tissue septa. The lobules contain cells, predominantly pinealocytes, that form rosettes or follicles.

The **thyroid glands** are composed of numerous colloid-filled follicles, as in mammals. Cells that are similar in function to the parafollicular cells of mammals, however, occur in the ultimobranchial bodies, rather than the thyroid glands, of the chicken.

The **parathyroid glands** are each surrounded by a connective tissue capsule. The parenchyma is composed of irregular cords of chief cells, separated by connective tissue and numerous sinusoids.

The **adrenal glands** are enclosed within a capsule of dense connective tissue. Unlike mammals, the parenchyma is not organized into a distinct cortex and medulla. Instead, it is composed of intermingled **cortical (interrenal) tissue** and **medullary** (chromaffin) **tissue.** The cortical cells are arranged as irregular cords. These cells have dark nuclei and appear columnar when the cords are sectioned longitudinally. In a cross section of a cord, the cells appear tall and pyramidal, with several cells arranged radially. Medullary tissue is composed of polygonal cells. They are larger than cortical cells and possess a large, round nucleus and basophilic cytoplasm. Ganglion cells occur among the medullary cells. Two ganglia (the cranial and caudal suprarenal ganglia) are apposed to the surface of the adrenal glands, and are frequently included in histologic sections of this gland.

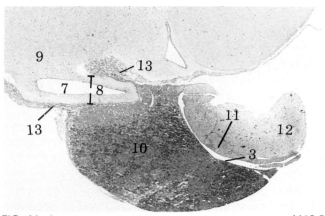

FIG. 16-1   ×12.5

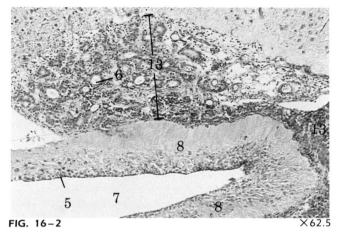

FIG. 16-2   ×62.5

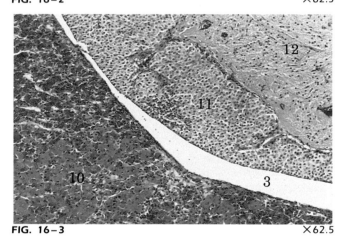

FIG. 16-3   ×62.5

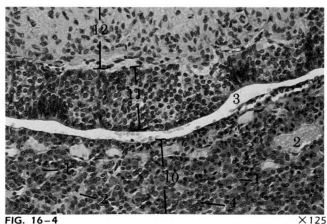

FIG. 16-4   ×125

FIG. 16-5

KEY		
1. Acidophils	**8.**	Infundibular stalk
2. Blood vessel	**9.**	Median eminence
3. Cavity of Rathke's pouch	**10.**	Pars distalis
4. Chromophobes	**11.**	Pars intermedia
5. Ependymal cells	**12.**	Pars nervosa
6. Follicle	**13.**	Pars tuberalis
7. Infundibular cavity		

FIG. 16-1. Pituitary Gland, Cat. Parasagittal section showing all major components. In domestic mammals, except the horse, the cavity of Rathke's pouch persists in the adult. *(Photomicrograph of a histologic section borrowed from the College of Veterinary Medicine, Iowa State University.)*

FIG. 16-2. Pituitary Gland, Cat. Detail of the infundibular stalk and pars tuberalis. Note the presence of small follicles in the pars tuberalis lined by faintly basophilic epithelial cells. *(Photomicrograph of a histologic section borrowed from the College of Veterinary Medicine, Iowa State University.)*

FIG. 16-3. Pituitary Gland, Cat. Pars intermedia, pars distalis, and pars nervosa. *(Photomicrograph of a histologic section borrowed from the College of Veterinary Medicine, Iowa State University.)*

FIG. 16-4. Pituitary Gland, Dog. Detail of the pars distalis, pars intermedia, and pars nervosa.

FIG. 16-5. Pituitary Gland, Parasagittal Section, Horse. Although present in other domestic animals, the cavity of Rathke's pouch is lacking in the horse.

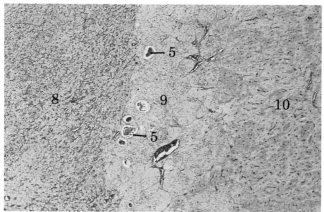

FIG. 16-6   ×12.5

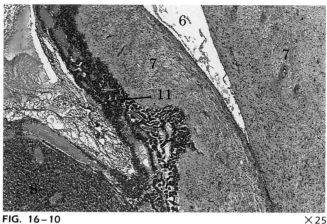

FIG. 16-10   ×25

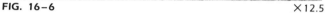
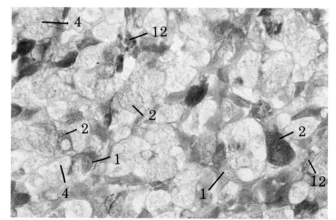

FIG. 16-7   ×125

KEY			
1. Acidophil		**7.** Infundibular stalk	
2. Basophil		**8.** Pars distalis	
3. Blood vessel		**9.** Pars intermedia	
4. Chromophobes		**10.** Pars nervosa	
5. Follicle		**11.** Pars tuberalis	
6. Infundibular cavity		**12.** Sinusoid	

FIG. 16-6. Pituitary Gland, Horse, Alcian Blue, Orange G, Schiff's Reagent. Pars distalis, pars intermedia, and pars nervosa. Note the presence of follicles in the pars intermedia.

FIG. 16-7. Pituitary Gland, Horse, Alcian Blue, Orange G, Schiff's Reagent. Detail of the pars intermedia and pars nervosa. The latter has a distinctive fibrous appearance.

FIG. 16-8. Pituitary Gland, Horse, Alcian Blue, Orange G, Schiff's Reagent. Detail of the pars distalis. In this preparation, acidophils are orange, whereas basophils vary from blue to red. Chromophobes are typically unstained.

FIG. 16-9. Pituitary Gland, Horse. Detail of the pars distalis. Chromophobes appear in clusters and have closely spaced nuclei.

FIG. 16-10. Pituitary Gland, Horse. A portion of the infundibular stalk, pars distalis, and pars tuberalis.

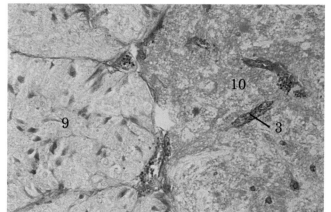

FIG. 16-8   ×250

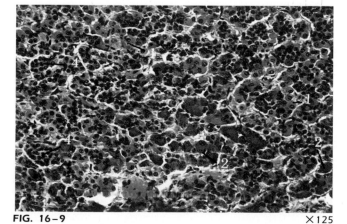

FIG. 16-9   ×125

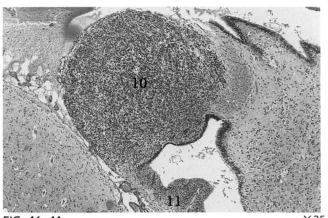

FIG. 16-11 ×25

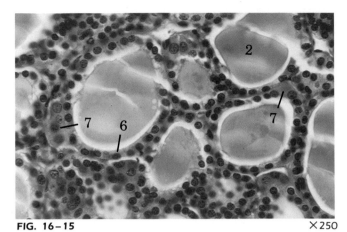

FIG. 16-15 ×250

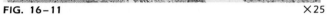

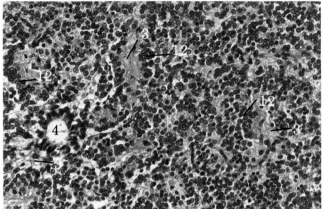

FIG. 16-12 ×125

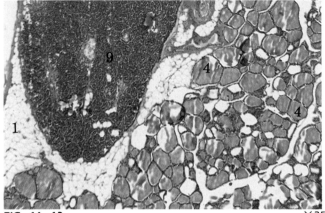

FIG. 16-13 ×25

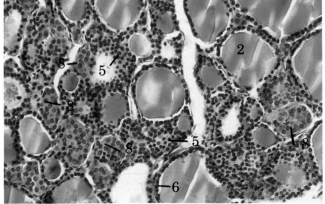

FIG. 16-14 ×125

KEY	
1. Adipose tissue	**7.** Parafollicular cell
2. Colloid	**8.** Parafollicular cells
3. Fibers of neuroglial cells	**9.** Parathyroid gland
4. Follicle	**10.** Pineal gland
5. Follicle, tangential cut	**11.** Pineal stalk
6. Follicular cell	**12.** Pinealocytes

FIG. 16-11. Pineal Gland, Dog. This gland consists primarily of pinealocytes and is located in the midline of the epithalamus.

FIG. 16-12. Pineal Gland, Dog. Detail of the gland.

FIG. 16-13. Thyroid and Parathyroid Glands, Dog. The basophilic, highly cellular parathyroid gland contrasts with the numerous colloid-filled follicles of the thyroid gland.

FIG. 16-14. Thyroid Gland, Inactive, Dog. Parafollicular cells (C-cells) have pale-staining cytoplasm. In the dog, they are particularly numerous and frequently occur in groups.

FIG. 16-15. Thyroid Gland, Inactive, Dog. Large, pale-staining parafollicular cells often form a part of the cellular lining of a thyroid follicle.

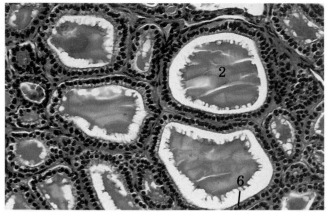

FIG. 16–16   ×125

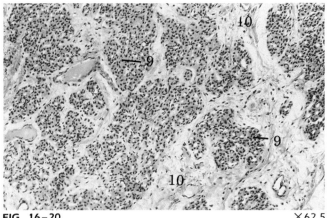

FIG. 16–20   ×62.5

KEY		
1. Cilia	**6.**	Follicular cell
2. Colloid	**7.**	Follicular cell, pigmented
3. Cyst	**8.**	Light cell
4. Dark cell	**9.**	Principal cells
5. Erythrocytes in sinusoid	**10.**	Stroma

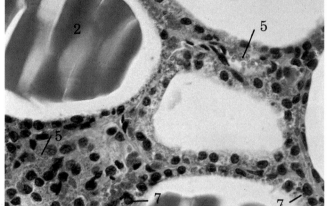

FIG. 16–17   ×250

FIG. 16–16. Thyroid Gland, Active, Horse. Active thyroid follicles are characterized by tall follicular cells and vacuolated colloid. Compare with Figures 16–15 and 16–17.

FIG. 16–17. Thyroid Gland, Inactive, Goat. The high degree of vascularity of the thyroid gland is well illustrated in this micrograph. Pigment granules accumulate in the follicle cells of older animals.

FIG. 16–18. Parathyroid Gland, Dog. Cysts containing colloid frequently occur in the parathyroid gland. Such cysts are lined by a ciliated columnar epithelium.

FIG. 16–19. Parathyroid Gland, Dog. Both light and dark principal cells are visible. The active, dark cells have a nucleus with condensed chromatin and a dark, acidophilic cytoplasm. The inactive, light cells have a larger and paler nucleus and a lighter, acidophilic cytoplasm.

FIG. 16–20. Parathyroid Gland, Cow. The connective tissue stroma of the parathyroid gland of cows and pigs is abundant.

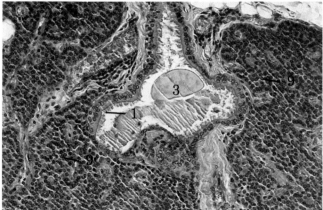

FIG. 16–18   ×125

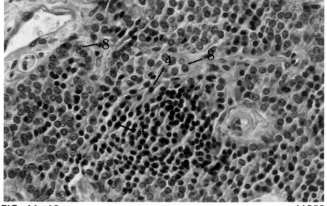

FIG. 16–19   ×250

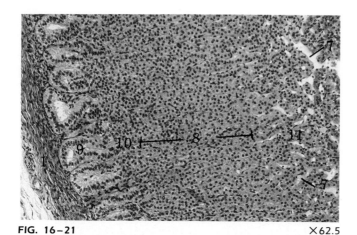

FIG. 16–21   ×62.5

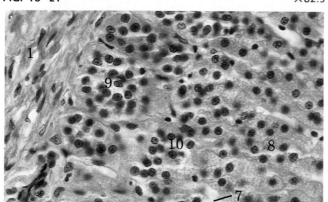

FIG. 16–22   ×250

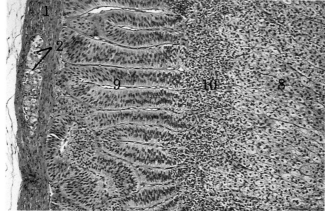

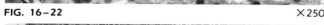

FIG. 16–23   ×62.5

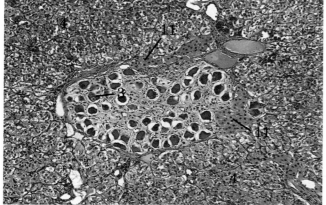

FIG. 16–24   ×62.5

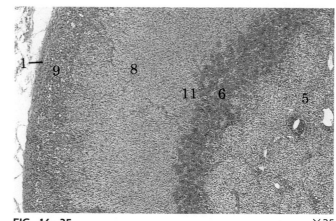

FIG. 16–25   ×25

KEY	
1. Capsule	**7.** Sinusoid
2. Epithelioid cells	**8.** Zona fasciculata
3. Ganglion cell	**9.** Zona glomerulosa
4. Medulla	**10.** Zona intermedia
5. Medulla, inner region	**11.** Zona reticularis
6. Medulla, outer region	

FIG. 16–21. Adrenal Gland, Dog. Adrenal cortex and capsule. The cells of the zona glomerulosa are arranged into arc-like formations in carnivores, horses, and pigs.

FIG. 16–22. Adrenal Gland, Cat. Detail of a portion of the cortex. A zona intermedia occurs between the zona glomerulosa and zona fasciculata. It is especially well developed in carnivores and horses. It consists of small, polyhedral cells. Cells of the zona fasciculata are characteristically highly vacuolated.

FIG. 16–23. Adrenal Gland, Horse. Adrenal cortex and capsule. The zona glomerulosa consists of high arcs composed of especially tall epithelial cells in the horse. Clusters of epithelioid cortical cells frequently occur in the capsule of the adrenal gland. A distinct intermediate zone separates the zona glomerulosa from the zona fasciculata.

FIG. 16–24. Adrenal Gland, Horse. An autonomic ganglion, surrounded by cells of the zona reticularis, is situated in the medulla.

FIG. 16–25. Adrenal Gland, Cow. Portions of the cortex and medulla. The medulla is subdivided into an outer region of darkly stained cells and an inner portion of lightly stained cells.

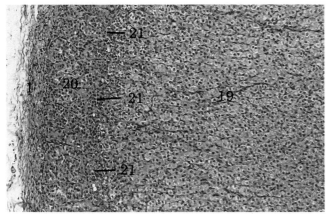

FIG. 16–26   ×62.5

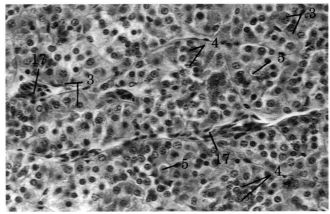

FIG. 16–30   ×250

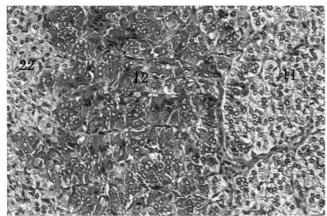

FIG. 16–27   ×125

KEY	
1. Capsule	**12.** Medulla, outer region
2. Chromaffin cells	**13.** Pars distalis, caudal
3. Chromophils	**14.** Pars distalis, cephalic
4. Chromophobes	**15.** Pars nervosa
5. Colloid	**16.** Pars tuberalis
6. Cyst	**17.** Sinusoid
7. Diencephalon	**18.** Skull
8. Ganglion cell	**19.** Zona fasciculata
9. Infundibular cavity	**20.** Zona glomerulosa
10. Infundibular stalk	**21.** Zona intermedia
11. Medulla, inner region	**22.** Zona reticularis

FIG. 16–26. Adrenal Gland, Cow. Portion of the adrenal cortex. The cells of the zona glomerulosa are arranged into irregular groups and cords in ruminants. Compare with Figures 16–21, 16–22, and 16–23.

FIG. 16–27. Adrenal Gland, Cow. The basophilic cells of the outer region of the adrenal medulla contrast with the paler cells of the inner region.

FIG. 16–28. Adrenal Gland, Sheep, Masson's. Adrenal medulla with ganglion cells and cells of the zona reticularis amid the chromaffin cells.

FIG. 16–29. Pituitary Gland, parasagittal section, Chicken. In the chicken, the pars distalis is divisible into a cephalic zone and a caudal zone. The cephalic zone is more basophilic. Ciliated cysts commonly occur within the pars distalis (see Fig. 16–32).

FIG. 16–30. Pituitary Gland, Chicken. The cephalic zone of the pars distalis consists of closely packed cords of chromophils and chromophobes. Some cords have a lumen filled with colloid.

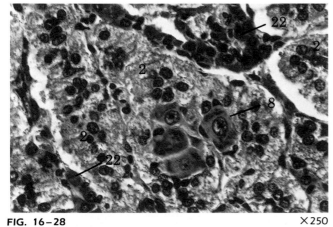

FIG. 16–28   ×250

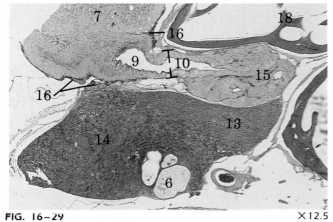

FIG. 16–29   ×12.5

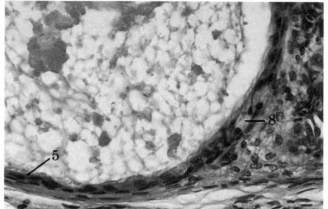

FIG. 16-31 ×250

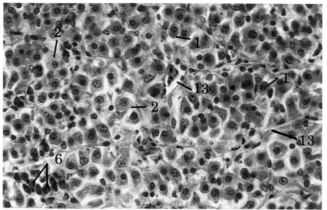

FIG. 16-35 ×25

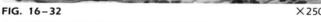

FIG. 16-32 ×250

FIG. 16-31. Pituitary Gland, Chicken. In the caudal zone of the pars distalis, the cells of the cords are more loosely arranged than those of the cephalic zone. Acidophils have a more intensely stained cytoplasm than those of the cephalic zone, and they can be readily distinguished from basophils.

FIG. 16-32. Pituitary Gland, Chicken. Portion of a cyst, in the pars distalis, lined by ciliated cells and mucous cells.

FIG. 16-33. Pituitary Gland, Chicken. Portions of the pars tuberalis and adjacent infundibular stalk. The cells of the pars tuberalis are rounded to elongated with a finely granular, slightly basophilic cytoplasm and a round to oval nucleus.

FIG. 16-34. Pituitary Gland, Chicken. A group of pituicytes within the pars nervosa. Pituicytes have a clear cytoplasm and a large, vesicular nucleus.

FIG. 16-35. Pineal Gland, parasagittal section, Chicken. The body of the pineal gland, portion of the overlying skull, and the cerebellum.

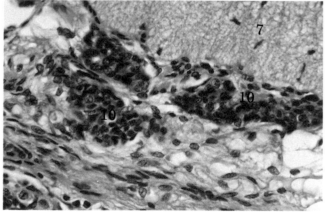

FIG. 16-33 ×250

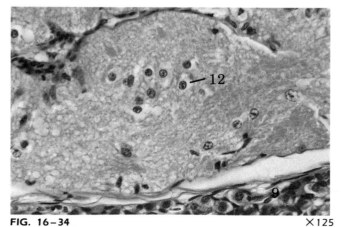

FIG. 16-34 ×125

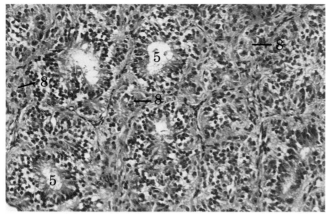

FIG. 16–36   ×125

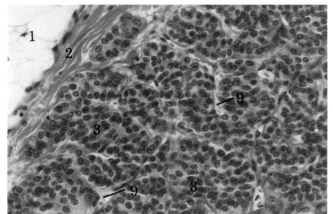

FIG. 16–37   ×250

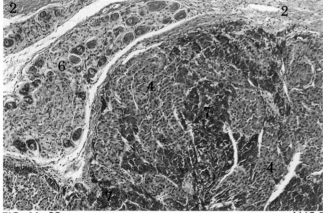

FIG. 16–38   ×62.5

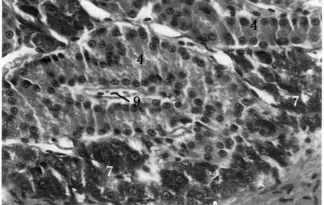

FIG. 16–39   ×250

KEY		
1. Adipose tissue		**6.** Ganglion
2. Capsule		**7.** Medullary cells
3. Chief cells		**8.** Rosette
4. Cortical cells		**9.** Sinusoid
5. Follicle		

FIG. 16–36. Pineal Gland, Chicken. The parenchymal cells of the pineal gland are arranged as compact masses (rosettes) or as round to oval follicles with distinct lumens.

FIG. 16–37. Parathyroid Gland, Chicken. This gland consists of chief cells arranged into a feltwork of anastomosing cords. The cords are surrounded by strands of connective tissue and numerous sinusoids.

FIG. 16–38. Adrenal Gland, Chicken. Cords of cortical cells are interwoven between clumps and irregular masses of medullary cells throughout the gland.

FIG. 16–39. Adrenal Gland, Chicken. Detail of cortical and medullary cells. Cortical cells are columnar. When longitudinal cuts have been made through cords of cortical cells, the cells form a bilayer. When cords are cut transversely, the cells are seen to be arranged radially. Medullary cells are polygonal and larger than cortical cells, and possess basophilic cytoplasm. They are arranged as clumps or irregular masses.

MALE REPRODUCTIVE SYSTEM

MAMMALS

The male reproductive system includes the testes, the system of ducts that leads from them, the penis, and accessory glands.

The **testes** hang in the scrotum and are compound tubular glands that are invested by a thick capsule of dense irregular connective tissue, the **tunica albuginea.** This capsule is rich in smooth muscle in the stallion. The tunica albuginea is covered by a peritoneum, **the visceral layer of the tunica vaginalis.** The latter is composed of a mesothelium and underlying connective tissue that blends with that of the tunica albuginea. Connective tissue **septa** extend from the tunica albuginea into the testis, partially or completely dividing the testis into lobules. These septa are thin in ruminants and thicker in the carnivore, stallion, and boar. Centrally, the septa may merge with the loose connective tissue of the **mediastinum testis.**

Within each lobule of the testis there are convoluted **seminiferous tubules.** They are lined by a stratified epithelium of **spermatogenic cells** and Sertoli cells. The spermatogenic cells give rise to **spermatozoa. Spermatogonia,** the most immature spermatogenic cells, are small round cells with dark, round nuclei that lie adjacent to the basement membrane. These undergo mitotic divisions and produce **primary spermatocytes,** larger cells whose nuclei often show distinct chromatin. Primary spermatocytes undergo the first meiotic division, giving rise to smaller, **secondary spermatocytes.** Secondary spermatocytes are rarely observed because they undergo the second meiotic division shortly after they arise, forming haploid **spermatids.** Early spermatids are round cells with pale nuclei that occur in clusters toward the lumen of the seminiferous tubule. Late spermatids are characterized by small, oval to elongated, dark heads and long, faint tails that project into the lumen. They are released from the seminiferous epithelium as spermatozoa.

The spermatogenic cells of the seminiferous epithelium do not necessarily appear identical from one tubule to the next, or from different locations along the same tubule. There are various combinations of cells in certain stages of development that are always associated with each other. Each particular cell association occurs over a certain distance along the length of a seminiferous tubule. Thus, a cross section of a tubule typically reveals only one of several types of cell associations, while preceding and succeeding segments of the tubule show entirely different associations.

Sertoli cells are fewer in number than the spermatogenic cells. They are distinguished by a pale oval or triangular nucleus that has a prominent nucleolus and occasional cleft-like infoldings. They are tall cells that extend from the basement membrane to the lumen of the tubule, but their boundaries are indistinct in routine histologic preparations. Numerous lateral and apical invaginations of their cell membranes embrace the differentiating spermatogenic cells.

Flattened, contractile **myoid cells** lie just outside the basement membrane of each seminiferous tubule. The connective tissue between adjacent tubules contains polyhedral **interstitial** (Leydig) **cells.** These produce testosterone, and are particularly abundant in the stallion and boar. They are recognized by their small round nucleus and an acidophilic, often foamy cytoplasm.

Near the terminal segment of a seminiferous tubule, the spermatogenic cells decrease in number and the Sertoli cells become more numerous. A **transitional zone,** lined by Sertoli cells, joins a seminiferous tubule to a **straight tubule.** The latter may be lined by simple columnar, cuboidal or squamous cells, and is continuous with a network of anastomosing channels that form the **rete testis.** The rete testis possesses a simple squamous or cuboidal epithelium that may be bistratified cuboidal in the bull. It is surrounded by the loose connective tissue of the **mediastinum testis.**

Efferent ductules, lined by a simple columnar or a pseudostratified epithelium with some ciliated cells, lead from the rete testis and pass through the tunica albuginea to join the **duct of the epididymis** in the head of the **epididymis.** In the stallion, the tubules of the rete testis penetrate the tunica albuginea and form an **extratesticular rete testis,** which is then joined to the duct of the epididymis by efferent ductules. The coiled duct of the epididymis varies in structure from the head to the tail region of the epididymis. Its pseudostratified columnar epithelium, with stereocilia, is thickest in the head region and is encircled by only a few smooth muscle cells. In the body (mid) region, there is less smooth muscle and the epithelium is thinner. In the tail region of the epididymis, the pseudostratified epithelium is thinnest and the surrounding smooth muscle is most abundant. In the stallion, the lining of the duct in the tail region of the epididymis forms short, villus-like projections.

The **vas deferens** (ductus deferens) leads from the duct of the epididymis and joins with the urethra. The vas deferens is lined by a pseudostratified columnar epithelium (some cells with stereocilia) that may become simple columnar distally. The smooth muscle of its thick muscularis presents a variety of arrangements. It may form an inner circular and an outer longitudinal layer, and each of these layers may contain interwoven fibers of smooth muscle. In contrast, the entire muscularis may be interwoven, with no distinct layers of smooth muscle. We have not observed any particular arrangement to be consistent within a species.

The **male accessory glands** include the glands of the ampulla, seminal vesicles, the bulbourethral glands, and the prostate gland. They are composed of branched tubular or tubuloacinar secretory units that often have vesicular dilations. The secretory epithelium of these glands is classified as pseudostratified, because, although consisting primarily of columnar cells (or sometimes cuboidal cells, such as in the prostate) occasional basal cells are present.

Near its junction with the urethra, the vas deferens forms a dilated **ampulla** whose lamina propria and submucosa are filled with glandular secretory units. The ampulla is absent in the tomcat, and the ampullary glands are not well developed in the boar.

The **prostate gland** is a seromucous gland except in the dog, where it is entirely serous. In the boar and ruminants, the prostate gland consists mostly of a **disseminate portion** (pars disseminata), in the form of a glandular layer in the submucosa of the pelvic urethra. In the stallion and carnivores, the disseminate portion is represented only by scattered glands. The **body of the prostate gland** is well developed in the stallion and carnivore, and absent in the ram and billy goat (buck). It is an encapsulated, lobulated gland that partially or completely surrounds a part of the pelvic urethra.

The **seminal vesicles** (vesicular glands) are absent in carnivores. In the stallion, they are true vesicular outpocketings in the form of bladder-like sacs with wide central lumens into which the glands open. In the boar and ruminants, they are compact glands with a lobulated surface.

The mucous-secreting **bulbourethral** (Cowper's)

glands are present in all domestic mammals except the dog. The columnar cells of the pseudostratified epithelium are tall and pale, and possess basally displaced nuclei.

The male **urethra,** which carries both urine and semen, can be divided into a pelvic and a penile portion. The **pelvic urethra** is lined by a transitional epithelium, which may become stratified columnar or cuboidal distally. Along the entire length of the urethra, the connective tissue below the mucosa contains erectile tissue with thin-walled **cavernous spaces** (veins). In the pelvic urethra, this erectile tissue forms the **stratum cavernosum** (vascular stratum). Peripheral to this stratum are the glands of the disseminate portion of the prostate gland. The muscularis of the urethra near the bladder consists of an inner and outer longitudinal layer, and a middle circular layer of smooth muscle. In the vicinity of the prostate gland, most of the smooth muscle is replaced by skeletal urethral muscle. Some longitudinal smooth muscle remains. The muscularis of the pelvic urethra is surrounded by an adventitia.

The **penile urethra,** which courses through the ventral region of the penis, is lined by a mixture of transitional, stratified cuboidal, stratified columnar, or a simple columnar epithelium. The larger, more abundant cavernous spaces of the penile urethra form the **corpus spongiosum** (corpus cavernosum urethra), which is surrounded by a tunica albuginea. Except for a few smooth muscle fibers, the wall of the penile urethra lacks a muscularis.

In the stallion and ruminants, the terminal portion of the urethra extends beyond the penis, forming a **urethral process.** It is covered by a cutaneous membrane and lined by transitional or stratified squamous epithelium. In the stallion, the urethral process contains well developed erectile tissue. In the ram and billy goat, the urethral process contains small cavernous spaces and two cords of fibrocartilage that parallel the urethra.

The **penis** can be divided into the body and glans penis. Both regions contain the penile urethra, with its erectile tissue, the corpus spongiosum. The **body of the penis** (corpus penis) is characterized by two additional masses of erectile tissue called the **corpora cavernosa.** Each corpus cavernosum is enclosed by the dense connective tissue and elastic fibers of the tunica albuginea. The tunic is especially thick in the boar and ruminants, and contains smooth muscle in the stallion. It extends inward to form a network of trabeculae, between which lies the spongy erectile tissue. The latter contains endothelial lined cavernous spaces surrounded by varying proportions of smooth muscle and fibroelastic connective tissue. In the vascular penis of the stallion, the smooth muscle is predominant. In the fibroelastic penis

of the boar and ruminants, the cavernous spaces are surrounded mainly by connective tissue that is rich in elastic fibers and contains only a few or no smooth muscle cells. In the intermediate type of penis of the carnivore, both smooth muscle and connective tissue fill the spaces between the cavernous vessels. The corpus cavernosum of all domestic mammals contains scattered adipose tissue in the connective tissue between the cavernous vessels. This is abundant in the tomcat, especially toward the tip of the corpus cavernosum, where adipose tissue nearly replaces the erectile tissue.

The cavernous spaces receive their blood supply from groups of **helicine arteries.** The walls of these tortuous vessels have cushion-like thickenings formed from longitudinal bundles of smooth muscle and epithelioid cells, and are rich in elastic tissue.

The expanded, distal portion of the penis, called the **glans penis,** is best developed in the stallion and dog. It contains erectile tissue, which is continuous with that of the corpus spongiosum. In carnivores, the glans contains an **os penis.** This bone is small in the tomcat. It is well developed in the dog, and possesses a fibrocartilaginous tip. The surface (visceral prepuce) of the glans penis of the tomcat bears small, keratinized epidermal spines. Small epidermal projections also occur in the stallion and billy goat.

The **prepuce** is a tube-like reflection of skin that covers the distal, free portion of the penis. It is composed of an external, parietal, and visceral layer. The external portion is typical skin that is continuous with the abdominal skin. The external layer turns inward at the preputial opening to form the parietal prepuce (internal layer). This, in turn, reflects at the fornix and continues onto the end of the penis as the visceral prepuce. The stallion has an additional outer fold called the sheath. Hair, sweat glands, and sebaceous glands occur over a variable distance from the external layer to the parietal prepuce. Glands may occur occasionally in the visceral prepuce of the stallion.

CHICKEN

The **testes** are situated in the abdominal cavity of the rooster. They are surrounded by a thin connective tissue capsule, the **tunica albuginea,** which is covered by a **peritoneum.** There are no well developed septa to divide the testes into lobules.

The epithelial cells of the convoluted **seminiferous tubules** are like those of mammals: Sertoli cells; spermatogonia; primary spermatocytes; secondary spermatocytes; spermatids; spermatozoa. Unlike those in mammals, various cell associations do not occur in segments along the length of the seminiferous tubules. Instead, the seminiferous epithelium is arranged into narrow columns of cells that undergo spermatogenesis independently. There is very little connective tissue between adjacent seminiferous tubules, and **interstitial cells** are sparse. They occur singly or in small clusters, primarily in the larger interstitial spaces. They are flattened to polyhedral cells with a relatively large, round nucleus and cytoplasm that is often vacuolated.

The seminiferous tubules are continuous with **straight tubules,** which are lined by Sertoli cells. Straight tubules lead into the anastomosing channels of the **rete testis,** which possess a simple cuboidal to squamous epithelium. The rete testis lies outside the tunica albuginea below the epididymis.

Three types of tubules occur within the **epididymis:** efferent ductules, connecting ducts, and the duct of the epididymis. The numerous, convoluted **efferent ductules** join the rete testis to the connecting ducts. They are lined by a simple epithelium of intermittent groups of tall and low, columnar cells, as well as patches of cells that appear to be pseudostratified. The epithelial cells are arranged into folds, and many of the cells bear tufts of cilia. The **connecting ducts** (excretory canals) are smaller in diameter than the other tubules of the epididymis, and are lined by a pseudostratified columnar epithelium. The epithelial cells are rarely ciliated, and are not arranged into numerous folds as are the cells that line the efferent ductules. Thus, the luminal surface of the connecting ducts has a smooth appearance. The single, convoluted **duct of the epididymis** is similar in structure to the connecting ducts, except that it is much larger in diameter. All of the tubules of the epididymis are surrounded and bound by connective tissue.

At the terminal portion of the epididymis, the duct of the epididymis joins the **vas deferens.** The latter is a convoluted duct, with a pseudostratified columnar epithelium, underlying smooth muscle, and a more peripheral layer of dense connective tissue. Each vas deferens merges with a small, conical **ejaculatory duct,** whose submucosa contains erectile tissue. The ejaculatory duct protrudes and opens into the urodeum of the **cloaca,** marking the termination of the duct system of the male.

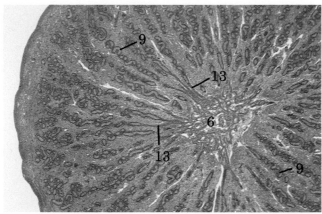

FIG. 17-1 ×12.5

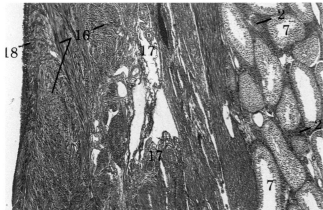

FIG. 17-2 ×62.5

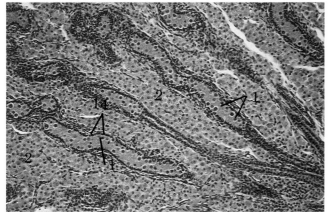

FIG. 17-3 ×25

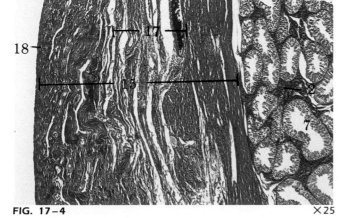

FIG. 17-4 ×25

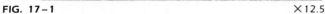

FIG. 17-5 ×250

KEY	
1. Gonocyte	**11.** Spermatid, late
2. Interstitial cells	**12.** Spermatogonia
3. Lumen	**13.** Straight tubule
4. Myoid cell, nucleus	**14.** Supporting cells
5. Primary spermatocyte	**15.** Tunica albuginea
6. Rete testis	**16.** Tunica albuginea, smooth muscle
7. Seminiferous tubule	
8. Sertoli cell, nucleus	**17.** Tunica albuginea, vascular layer
9. Sex cord	
10. Spermatid, early	**18.** Tunica vaginalis

FIG. 17-1. Testis, x.s., Baby Boar. Developing sex cords in the testis of a two-day-old boar.

FIG. 17-2. Testis, x.s., Baby Boar. Detail of developing sex cords and interstitial cells. Two types of cells can be distinguished in the sex cord. Supporting cells (small with dark nuclei) are positioned along the edges of the cords. They will develop into Sertoli cells. Gonocytes, precursors of spermatogonia, are located in the interior of the cords. They have large, pale nuclei.

FIG. 17-3. Testis, Stallion, Mallory's. The tunica albuginea of the stallion is characterized by the presence of smooth muscle.

FIG. 17-4. Testis, Boar, Mallory's. The tunica albuginea consists of dense irregular connective tissue. It lacks smooth muscle in domestic mammals, except the stallion.

FIG. 17-5. Seminiferous Tubules, Testis, Dog. A portion of each of three adjacent seminiferous tubules is shown.

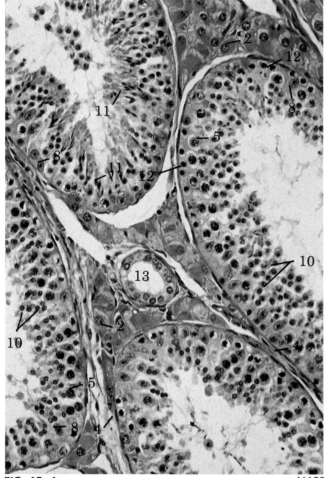

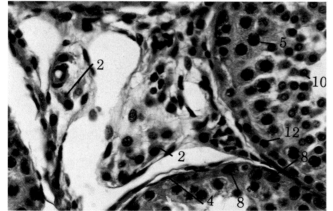

FIG. 17-6 ×180

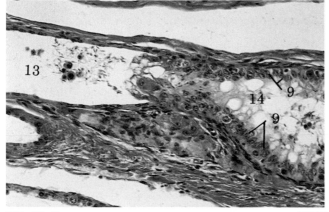

FIG. 17-7 ×250

FIG. 17-8 ×125

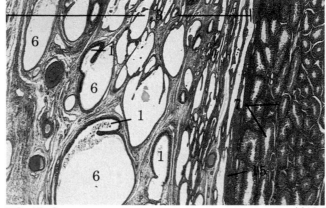

FIG. 17-9 ×12.5

KEY	
1. Efferent ductule	**9.** Sertoli cells
2. Interstitial cell	**10.** Spermatid, early
3. Mediastinum testis	**11.** Spermatid, late
4. Myoid cell, nucleus	**12.** Spermatogonium
5. Primary spermatocyte	**13.** Straight tubule
6. Rete testis, channel	**14.** Transitional zone
7. Seminiferous tubules	**15.** Tunica albuginea
8. Sertoli cell, nucleus	

FIG. 17-6. Seminiferous Tubules, Testis, Stallion. Four portions of seminiferous tubules are visible. Note the numerous interstitial cells (abundant in the boar and stallion) and the section through a straight tubule.

FIG. 17-7. Interstitial Tissue, Testis, Ram. Interstitial tissue and three portions of seminiferous tubules are shown. Interstitial cells are relatively sparse in carnivores and ruminants.

FIG. 17-8. Transitional Zone and Straight Tubule, Testis, Stallion. A transitional zone joins a seminiferous tubule to a straight tubule. Sertoli cells line this zone and protrude into the lumen of the straight tubule.

FIG. 17-9. Rete Testis, Stallion. Anastomosing channels form the rete testis, which is surrounded by the loose connective tissue of the mediastinum testis. In the stallion, the rete testis extends through the tunica albuginea and becomes extratesticular, as it is in this micrograph. Junctions of rete tubules and efferent ductules are shown (see Fig. 17-10).

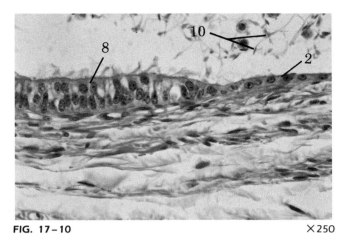

FIG. 17-10   ×250

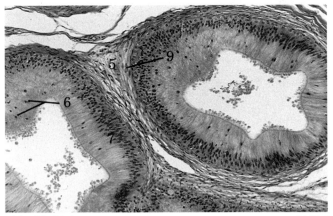

FIG. 17-14   ×62.5

KEY	
1. Columnar epithelium	8. Pseudostratified
2. Cuboidal epithelium, rete	epithelium, efferent ductule
testis	9. Smooth muscle
3. Duct of the epididymis	10. Spermatozoa
4. Efferent ductule	11. Tunica albuginea, smooth
5. Loose connective tissue	muscle
6. Lymphocyte, migrating	12. Tunica vaginalis,
7. Pseudostratified epithelium	mesothelium

FIG. 17-10. Junction of Rete Testis and Efferent Ductule, Stallion. The rete testis is lined by cuboidal cells, whereas the efferent ductule is lined by a ciliated, pseudostratified columnar epithelium.

FIG. 17-11. Efferent Ductules, Stallion. Various cuts through the tortuous efferent ductules are surrounded by loose connective tissue.

FIG. 17-12. Efferent Ductules, Stallion. Efferent ductules are lined by a ciliated, pseudostratified columnar epithelium. The epithelium may be simple columnar in some regions.

FIG. 17-13. Head of Epididymis, Stallion, Masson's. The epididymis is surrounded by a tunica albuginea of dense irregular connective tissue, which contains smooth muscle in the stallion. Portions of the coiled duct of the epididymis are shown.

FIG. 17-14. Head of Epididymis, Stallion. In this region, the pseudostratified columnar epithelium of the duct of the epididymis is thickest. Smooth muscle fibers surrounding the duct are scarce (compare with Figs. 17-15 and 17-16).

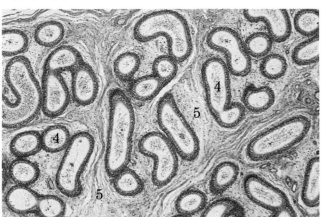

FIG. 17-11   ×25

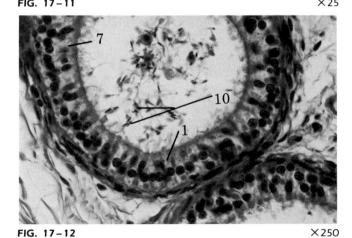

FIG. 17-12   ×250

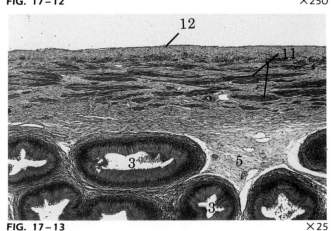

FIG. 17-13   ×25

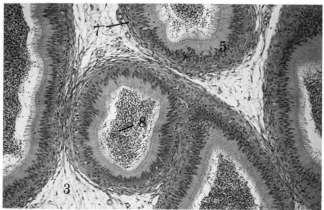

FIG. 17-15 ×62.5

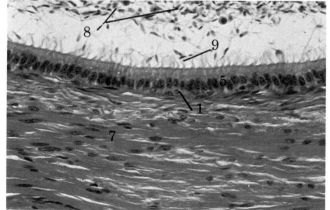

FIG. 17-16 ×62.5

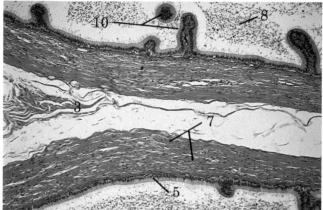

FIG. 17-17 ×250

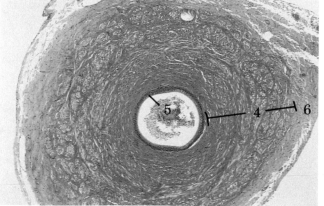

FIG. 17-18 ×25

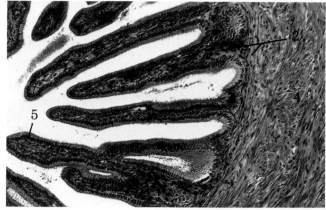

FIG. 17-19 ×62.5

KEY	
1. Basal cell	**6.** Serosa
2. Lamina propria	**7.** Smooth muscle
3. Loose connective tissue	**8.** Spermatozoa
4. Muscularis	**9.** Stereocilia
5. Pseudostratified epithelium	**10.** Villus-like projection

FIG. 17-15. Body of Epididymis, Stallion. The duct of the epididymis in this region is surrounded by more smooth muscle than in the head of the epididymis, and the pseudostratified columnar epithelium is not as thick.

FIG. 17-16. Tail of Epididymis, Stallion. A low, pseudostratified columnar epithelium and abundant circular smooth muscle characterize the duct of the epididymis in this region. In the stallion, the caudal segment of the duct of the epididymis has villus-like projections.

FIG. 17-17. Tail of Epididymis, Stallion. Detail of the duct of the epididymis lined by low, pseudostratified columnar epithelium and surrounded by abundant circular smooth muscle.

FIG. 17-18. Vas Deferens, x.s., Dog. The bulk of the wall consists of smooth muscle cells, which form an inner circular and an outer predominantly longitudinal layer with some randomly arranged cells.

FIG. 17-19. Vas Deferens, x.s., Stallion, Masson's. This section of the vas deferens, taken from near the epididymis, has long mucosal folds. The inner layer of the muscularis contains interwoven bundles of smooth muscle. Although out of the field of view in this micrograph, the smooth muscle of the outer layer of the muscularis is mostly arranged longitudinally.

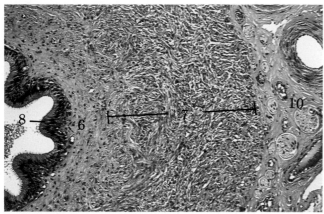

FIG. 17-20   ×62.5

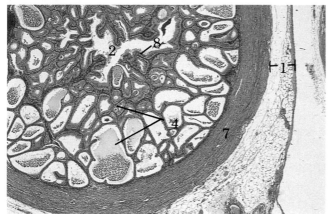

FIG. 17-21   ×12.5

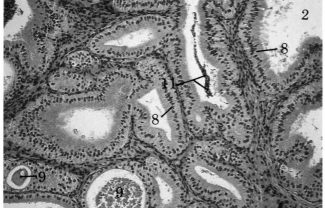

FIG. 17-22   ×62.5

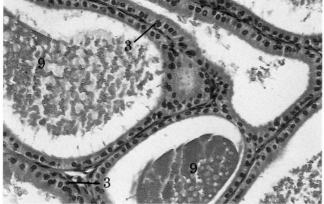

FIG. 17-23   ×125

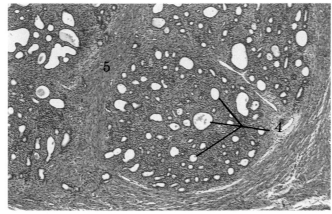

FIG. 17-24   ×25

KEY	
1. Adventitia	**7.** Muscularis
2. Ampulla, lumen	**8.** Pseudostratified epithelium
3. Basal cell, nucleus	**9.** Secretion
4. Gland	**10.** Serosa
5. Interlobular septum	**11.** Spermatozoa
6. Lamina propria	

FIG. 17-20. Vas Deferens, x.s., Boar, Masson's. The muscularis consists of an admixture of longitudinally and randomly arranged smooth muscle. The epithelium is pseudostratified columnar with stereocilia present intermittently.

FIG. 17-21. Ampulla, x.s., Ram. The terminal segment of the vas deferens, the ampulla, contains branched tubuloalveolar glands in the dog, stallion, and ruminants. The glands are poorly developed in the boar. The ampulla is absent in the tomcat.

FIG. 17-22. Ampulla, Ram. Detail of the mucosa. Spermatozoa are stored in the glands close to their openings into the lumen of the ampulla.

FIG. 17-23. Ampulla, Ram. The secretory alveoli are lined by a pseudostratified epithelium composed of cuboidal to columnar cells and occasional basal cells.

FIG. 17-24. Seminal Vesicle, Castrated Billy Goat. In the castrated male, the glandular tissue of the accessory glands is greatly reduced (compare with Fig. 17-25).

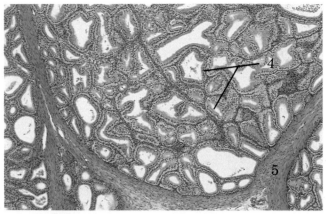

FIG. 17-25 ×25

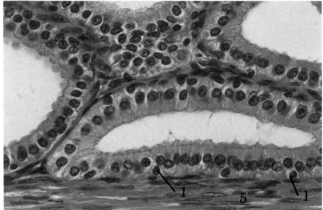

FIG. 17-26 ×250

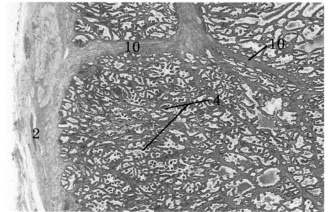

FIG. 17-27 ×12.5

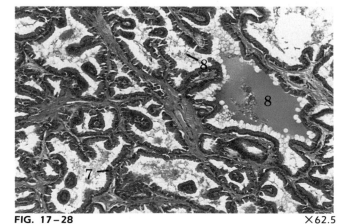

FIG. 17-28 ×62.5

FIG. 17-29 ×12.5

KEY	
1. Basal cell	**7.** Pseudostratified epithelium
2. Capsule	**8.** Secretion
3. Duct	**9.** Stratum cavernosum
4. Gland	**10.** Trabecula
5. Interlobular septum	**11.** Transitional epithelium
6. Prostate gland	**12.** Urethra, lumen

FIG. 17-25. Seminal Vesicle, Ram. Lobules of tubuloalveolar glands are divided by interlobular septa, which contain an abundance of smooth muscle in ruminants. In the stallion and boar, the septa consist predominantly of connective tissue, with some smooth muscle. Seminal vesicles are absent in carnivores.

FIG. 17-26. Seminal Vesicle, Ram. The pseudostratified glandular epithelium is characterized by sparse basal cells. Note the muscular septum.

FIG. 17-27. Body of the Prostate, Dog. The body of the prostate, which is well developed in carnivores and the stallion, is surrounded by a capsule of dense connective tissue and smooth muscle. Trabeculae from the capsule divide the gland into lobules.

FIG. 17-28. Body of the Prostate, Dog. In the dog, this is a serous gland. (Compare with Fig. 17-31.)

FIG. 17-29. Disseminate Portion of the Prostate, x.s., Ram, Masson's. This portion of the prostate is well developed in the boar and ruminants. The glands are located within the submucosa of the pelvic urethra. The stratum cavernosum of the pelvic urethra contains cavernous spaces that are smaller and less numerous than those of the corpus spongiosum of the penile urethra.

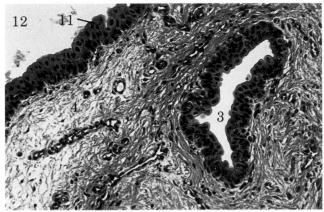

FIG. 17–30   ×125

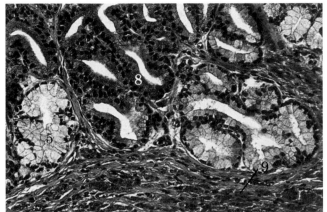

FIG. 17–31   ×125

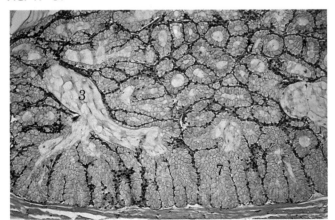

FIG. 17–32   ×25

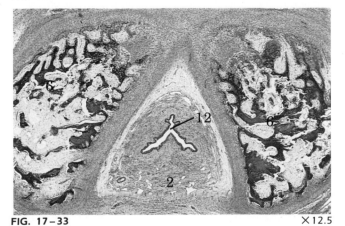

FIG. 17–33   ×12.5

FIG. 17–34   ×62.5

KEY	
1. Cavernous space	**7.** Secretory cells
2. Corpus spongiosum	**8.** Serous cells
3. Duct	**9.** Smooth muscle
4. Lamina propria	**10.** Spongy bone
5. Mucous cells	**11.** Transitional epithelium
6. Os penis	**12.** Urethra, lumen

FIG. 17–30. Disseminate Portion of the Prostate, x.s., Ram, Masson's. The transitional epithelium of both the pelvic urethra and a duct of the prostate gland is shown.

FIG. 17–31. Disseminate Portion of the Prostate, x.s., Ram, Masson's. The prostate is a mixed gland except in the dog, where there are no mucous secretory units.

FIG. 17–32. Bulbourethral Gland, Boar. This gland is a compound tubular gland in the boar, tomcat, and billy goat and a tubuloalveolar gland in the stallion, bull, and ram. It is absent in the dog. The pale-staining secretory cells are columnar or pyramidal, with basally displaced nuclei.

FIG. 17–33. Penis, x.s., Puppy. Section is through the developing os penis, which is present in carnivores.

FIG. 17–34. Penis, x.s., Puppy. Detail of the urethra and portion of the os penis.

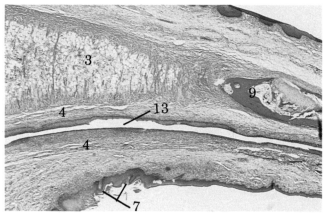

FIG. 17–35   ×12.5

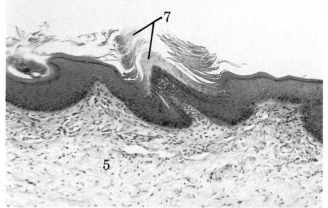

FIG. 17–36   ×62.5

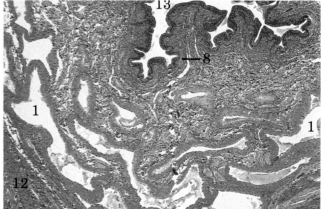

FIG. 17–37   ×12.5

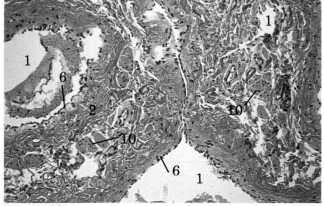

FIG. 17–38   ×62.5

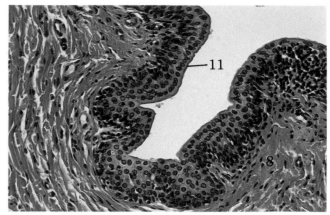

FIG. 17–39   ×125

KEY	
1. Cavernous space	**8.** Lamina propria
2. Connective tissue	**9.** Os penis
3. Corpus cavernosum	**10.** Smooth muscle
4. Corpus spongiosum	**11.** Stratified columnar
5. Dermis	epithelium
6. Endothelium	**12.** Tunica albuginea
7. Epidermal spine	**13.** Urethra, lumen

FIG. 17–35. Penis, l.s., Tomcat. In the tomcat, the distal portion of the corpus cavernosum consists largely of nonerectile, adipose tissue. A small os penis is present in the glans, and small spines are present on the surface of the glans of the tomcat. *(Photomicrograph of a histologic section borrowed from the College of Veterinary Medicine, Iowa State University.)*

FIG. 17–36. Glans Penis, l.s., Tomcat. Detail of a keratinized epidermal spine. *(Photomicrograph of a histologic section borrowed from the College of Veterinary Medicine, Iowa State University.)*

FIG. 17–37. Penile Urethra, x.s., Stallion. Portion of the penile urethra with abundant cavernous spaces of the corpus spongiosum.

FIG. 17–38. Corpus Spongiosum, Body of Penis, Stallion. The cavernous spaces of the stallion and carnivore are surrounded by connective tissue rich in elastic fibers and by many bundles of smooth muscle.

FIG. 17–39. Penile Urethra, x.s., Stallion. The epithelial lining of the urethra in this section is stratified columnar. The epithelium, however, is variable in the penile urethra, and in places may also be simple columnar, transitional, or stratified cuboidal.

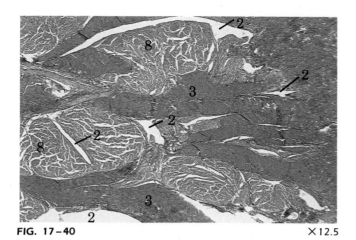

FIG. 17–40 ×12.5

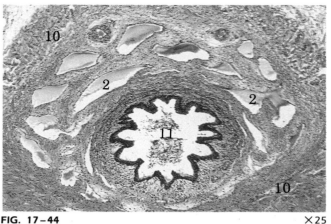

FIG. 17–44 ×25

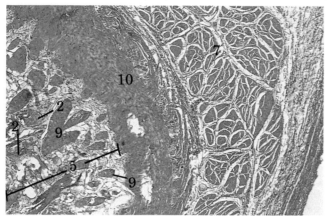

FIG. 17–41 ×12.5

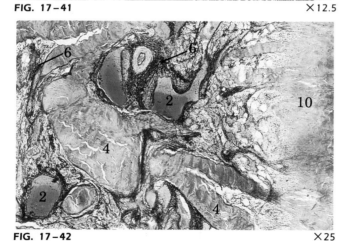

FIG. 17–42 ×25

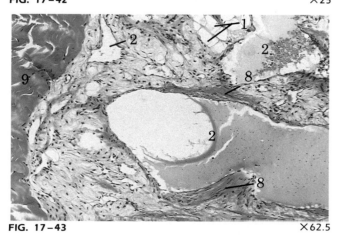

FIG. 17–43 ×62.5

KEY		
1. Adipose tissue	**7.**	Retractor penis muscle
2. Cavernous space	**8.**	Smooth muscle
3. Connective tissue	**9.**	Trabecula
4. Connective tissue trabecula	**10.**	Tunica albuginea
5. Corpus cavernosum	**11.**	Urethra, lumen
6. Elastic fibers		

FIG. 17–40. Body of Penis, Stallion. Large masses of smooth muscle surround the cavernous spaces of the corpus cavernosum of the stallion.

FIG. 17–41. Body of Penis, x.s., Boar. A portion of the sigmoid flexure including the retractor penis muscle.

FIG. 17–42. Body of Penis, x.s., Boar, Orcein. The connective tissue surrounding the cavernous spaces of the corpus cavernosum is rich in elastic fibers in the boar and ruminants.

FIG. 17–43. Body of Penis, Boar. In the boar and ruminant, the cavernous spaces of the corpus cavernosum are invested largely by connective tissue and only a smattering of smooth muscle.

FIG. 17–44. Penile Urethra, x.s., Ram. The distribution of the cavernous spaces of the corpus spongiosum of the penile urethra is especially well represented in this section.

MALE REPRODUCTIVE SYSTEM **201**

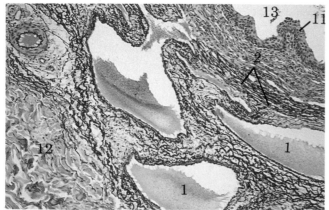

FIG. 17–45 X62.5

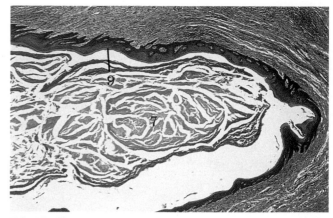

FIG. 17–49 X12.5

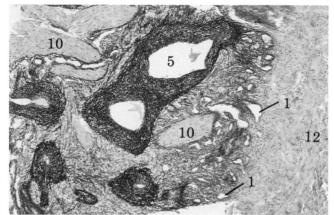

FIG. 17–46 X25

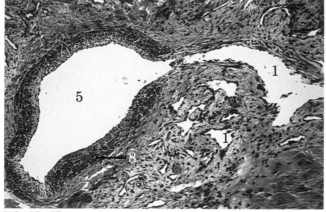

FIG. 17–47 X62.5

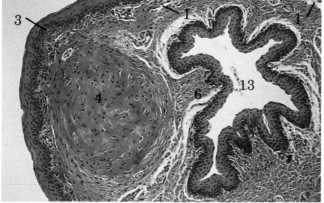

FIG. 17–48 X62.5

KEY	
1. Cavernous space	**8.** Smooth muscle
2. Elastic fibers	**9.** Stratified squamous
3. Epidermis	epithelium
4. Fibrocartilaginous cord	**10.** Trabecula
5. Helicine artery	**11.** Transitional epithelium
6. Lamina propria	**12.** Tunica albuginea
7. Smegma	**13.** Urethra, lumen

FIG. 17–45. Body of Penis, x.s., Ram, Orcein. The cavernous spaces of the corpus spongiosum are surrounded by connective tissue rich in elastic fibers in boars and ruminants.

FIG. 17–46. Helicine Artery, Body of Penis, Ram, Orcein. The corpus cavernosum contains helicine arteries, which are tortuous vessels with an abundance of elastic fibers throughout their walls.

FIG. 17–47. Helicine Artery, Body of Penis, Ram, Masson's. Junction of a helicine artery with a cavernous space in the corpus cavernosum.

FIG. 17–48. Urethral Process, x.s., Ram. The urethral process is a tortuous, worm-like extension of the urethra in the ram and billy goat. One of the two fibrocartilaginous cords that parallel the urethra is shown.

FIG. 17–49. Urethral Pouch, Stallion. The urethral pouch, found only in the stallion, is filled with smegma, which is composed of desquamated epithelial cells and the secretion of the preputial glands.

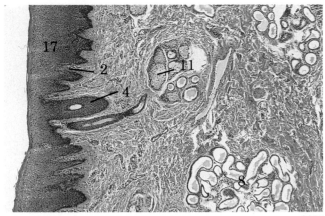

FIG. 17-50 ×25

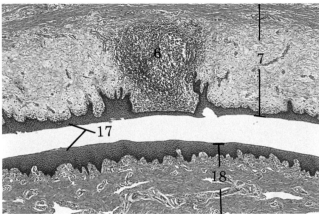

FIG. 17-51 ×25

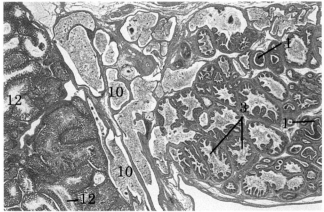

FIG. 17-52 ×12.5

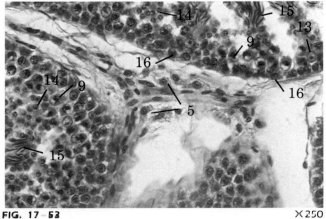

FIG. 17-53 ×250

KEY		
1. Connecting duct	**11.** Sebaceous gland	
2. Dermal papilla	**12.** Seminiferous tubule	
3. Efferent ductule	**13.** Sertoli cell, nucleus	
4. Hair follicle	**14.** Spermatid, early	
5. Interstitial cell	**15.** Spermatid, late	
6. Lymphatic nodule	**16.** Spermatogonium	
7. Parietal prepuce	**17.** Stratified squamous	
8. Preputial gland	epithelium	
9. Primary spermatocyte	**18.** Visceral prepuce	
10. Rete testis		

FIG. 17-50. Parietal Prepuce, Stallion. The dermis contains sebaceous glands and tubular preputial (sweat) glands.

FIG. 17-51. Prepuce, Boar. The parietal and visceral prepuce are shown.

FIG. 17-52. Testis and Epididymis, x.s., Rooster. Seminiferous tubules, the rete testis, and portions (efferent ductules and connecting ducts) of the epididymis.

FIG. 17-53. Interstitial Tissue, Testis, Rooster. Interstitial (Leydig) cells are found principally in the larger intertubular spaces. These cells are either polyhedral or elongated, and may contain vacuoles.

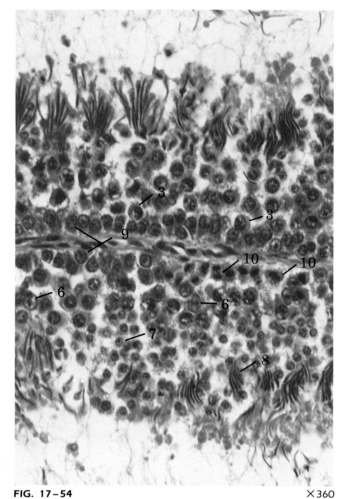

FIG. 17-54   ×360

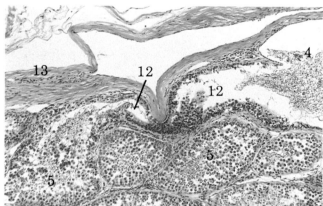

FIG. 17-55   ×62.5

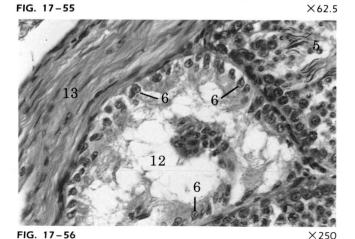

FIG. 17-56   ×250

FIG. 17-57   ×250

KEY	
1. Cilia	**8.** Spermatid, late
2. Efferent ductule	**9.** Spermatogonium
3. Primary spermatocyte	**10.** Spermatogonium, dividing
4. Rete testis	**11.** Spermatozoa
5. Seminiferous tubule	**12.** Straight tubule
6. Sertoli cell, nucleus	**13.** Tunica albuginea
7. Spermatid, early	

FIG. 17-54. Seminiferous Tubules, Testis, Rooster. Detail of portions of adjacent seminiferous tubules. Note that the seminiferous epithelial cells are organized into narrow columns.

FIG. 17-55. Testis, Rooster. A straight tubule, lined by Sertoli cells, connects a seminiferous tubule with the rete testis.

FIG. 17-56. Straight Tubule, Testis, Rooster. Sertoli cells form the epithelium of straight tubules.

FIG. 17-57. Junction of Rete Testis and Efferent Ductule, Rooster. The epithelial cells lining efferent ductules vary in shape and many possess cilia. The rete testis is lined by squamous epithelial cells.

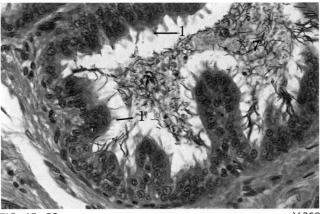

FIG. 17-58   ×250

KEY	
1. Cilia	**5.** Pseudostratified epithelium
2. Connecting duct	**6.** Smooth muscle
3. Duct of the epididymis	**7.** Spermatozoa
4. Efferent ductule	

FIG. 17–58. Efferent Ductule, x.s., Rooster. Detail of an efferent ductule. The epithelial cells vary in shape, and many bear cilia. The epithelium is folded and is surrounded by loose connective tissue. Occasionally, smooth muscle cells may be present.

FIG. 17–59. Connecting Duct and Efferent Ductule, Rooster. Connecting ducts present a smooth inner surface and are lined by a pseudostratified columnar epithelium with occasional basal cells. The epithelial cells are generally without cilia. In contrast, the efferent ductule has a folded lining, and its epithelial cells are mostly ciliated.

FIG. 17–60. Duct of the Epididymis, Rooster. The duct of the epididymis has a larger diameter than a connecting duct, but otherwise is comparable in structure to the latter.

FIG. 17–61. Vas Deferens, Distal, Rooster. The lining epithelium is similar to that of the epididymis. A layer of smooth muscle separates the epithelium from the surrounding connective tissue.

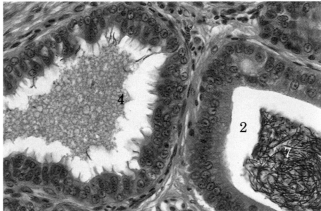

FIG. 17–59   ×250

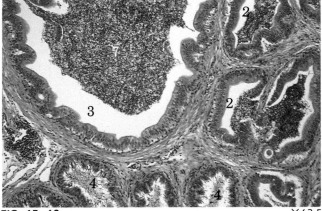

FIG. 17–60   ×62.5

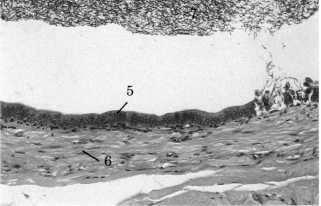

FIG. 17–61   ×125

FEMALE REPRODUCTIVE SYSTEM

MAMMALS

The ovaries, oviducts, uterus, vagina, and vulva are the major components of the mammalian female reproductive system. A simple squamous or cuboidal epithelium, **germinal epithelium,** often missing from histologic preparations, covers the **cortex** of the **ovary.** Beneath the epithelium is a layer of dense connective tissue, the **tunica albuginea.** A **cortical stroma,** containing ovarian **follicles** in various stages of development, lies internal to the tunica albuginea. In bitches and queens, but ordinarily not in other domestic mammals, cords of epithelioid cells called **interstitial gland cells** occur throughout the stroma. The epithelioid cells are derived from the theca interna of atretic, antral follicles or from the granulosa cells of atretic, preantral follicles.

A **medulla** consisting of richly vascularized loose connective tissue lies internal to the ovarian cortex. In the mare, the medullary tissue is located external to the cortex. Channels, lined by a cuboidal epithelium and called the **rete ovarii,** are conspicuous components of the medulla in carnivores and ruminants. **Hilus cells** (groups of epithelioid cells) may be found close to the rete ovarii in the region of the hilus in some mammals.

Primordial follicles are the least developed and most numerous follicles of the ovary. They lie just below the tunica albuginea. Each consists of a **primary oocyte** surrounded by a layer of simple squamous **follicle cells.** In response to periodic hormonal stimulation, growth is initiated in some of the primordial follicles. The earliest growing follicle, the **primary follicle,** consists of an enlarging oocyte surrounded by a layer of cuboidal cells. Proliferation of the follicle cells results in the formation of a **multilaminar** (late primary) **follicle.** Fluid-filled spaces appearing between the follicle cells gradually coalesce, forming an antrum. Concomitantly, an acidophilic, translucent membrane, the **zona pellucida,** appears around the oocyte. Further growth results in the formation of a **secondary follicle** with a C-shaped **antrum.** Its follicle cells are now called the **membrana granulosa.** A sheath of stromal cells, the **theca folliculi,** forms around the follicle. The theca differentiates into a cellular, vascular inner layer, the **theca interna,** and an outer, connective tissue layer, the **theca externa.** The boundary between the stroma and the theca externa and that between the theca externa and theca interna is often indistinct. Continued growth results in the formation of a large **tertiary** (Graafian) **follicle** whose oocyte is surrounded by a multilayer of membrana granulosa cells, the **cumulus oophorus.** The columnar cells of the innermost portion of the latter constitute the **corona radiata,** which is separated from the oocyte by the zona pellucida.

Ordinarily, each mature tertiary follicle contains a single oocyte. The follicles of certain animals (carnivores, sows, and ewes) may, however, contain as many as six oocytes.

Mature follicles vary widely in size. They are about 2 mm in diameter in the bitch and queen, 15 mm in the cow, and as large as 70 mm in the mare. Maximum size is reached just prior to ovulation. Following ovulation, granulosa cells, and cells of the theca interna of most species, multiply, hypertrophy, and differentiate into granulosa lutein cells and smaller, more peripheral theca lutein cells respectively of the **corpus luteum.** A yellow pigment (lutein) is formed by the luteal cells of the cow, mare, and carnivores, but is lacking in ewes, nanny goats (does), and sows. Luteal cells produce progesterone. Regression of the corpus luteum occurs during late diestrus, leaving scar tissue, the **corpus albicans.**

Although many primordial follicles begin the process of growth and differentiation, few become mature. The majority undergo a degenerative regression, called **atresia.** The oocyte and membrana granulosa degenerate first. Cells of the theca interna hypertrophy and the zona pellucida becomes swollen. Eventually, the entire follicle is resorbed.

The **oviduct** is a muscular tube consisting of an **isthmus,** which arises from the uterus, a middle segment, the **ampulla,** and a funnel-shaped **infundibulum,** which lies next to the ovary. From the outside inward, the wall of the oviduct is comprised of a serosa, muscularis, lamina propria, and epithelium. The muscularis, which is thickest in the isthmus, is formed mainly from circular smooth muscle with a modicum of longitudinally arranged smooth muscle external to it. Many of the cells of the simple columnar epithelium are ciliated. In part, the epithelium of ruminants and sows is pseudostratified. The mucosa is thrown into longitudinal folds, with less folding occurring in the isthmus than in the ampulla.

The wall of the bicornuate **uterus** of domestic mammals has three layers: the outer **perimetrium** (serosa), middle **myometrium,** and inner **endometrium** (mucosa). The myometrium is divisible into a thick, inner circular layer and a thin, outer longitudinal layer. A richly vascularized and well innervated **stratum vasculare** usually separates the muscle layers. The stratum vasculare, however, is indistinct in the sow and may be located in the outer half of the circular layer in the cow.

The epithelium of the endometrium is simple cuboidal or columnar in the bitch, queen, and mare, but may be stratified or pseudostratified in ruminants and sows. Simple, branched **uterine** (endometrial) **glands** extend into the lamina propria. These may be considerably coiled in the mare, sow, and ruminants. Nonglandular regions of the endometrium, called **caruncles,** occur in ruminants.

The mucosa of the uterine **cervix** is elevated into longitudinal folds, which may become subdivided into secondary and tertiary folds. The epithelium is simple columnar with goblet cells. In the bitch, however, it is stratified squamous. Glandular tissue fades in the cervix, extending to the cervical os only in carnivores. An inner circular and an outer longitudinal layer of smooth muscle form the muscularis.

The **estrous cycle** consists of a succession of stages. The first stage, **proestrus,** is characterized by endometrial growth. It is followed by **estrus,** or period when the female is receptive to the male. In most species, ovulation occurs during estrus. The development of the corpus luteum occurs during the next stage, **metestrus. Diestrus** follows metestrus and coincides with the presence of a fully functional corpus luteum. During this time, the development and secretory activity of the endometrial glands peak. **Anestrus,** a period of sexual inactivity, follows diestrus.

The **placenta** is derived from the endometrium and the chorioallantoic membrane (CAM). The degree of intimacy between these two components varies and is a basis for classifying placentas. A placenta is **indeciduate** when these two membranes are in contact but are not intimately fused. The placenta is **deciduate** when the membranes have become fused. Little or no endometrium is lost during the birth process in animals having an indeciduate placenta (mare, ruminants, and sow).

Conversely, considerable mucosa is lost at parturition in animals with deciduate placentas (carnivores).

The extent to which the CAM contributes to the placenta is variable. If most of the CAM contributes, as in the mare and sow, the placenta is **diffuse;** if numerous but isolated areas contribute, as in ruminants, the placenta is **cotyledonary;** when a belt-like portion of the CAM contributes, as in carnivores, the placenta is **zonary.**

The surfaces of the chorioallantoic membrane and the endometrium may contact one another in three different ways. These types of contact are designated as **folded, villous,** and **labyrinthine.** In the sow, both surfaces are folded and are closely applied to each other. In the mare and ruminants, chorioallantoic villi insert into pockets (crypts) in the endometrium. In carnivores, the apposed surfaces form a complex, interlinked, fused labyrinth.

Classification of the placenta can also be based on the number of tissue layers separating the fetal and maternal blood. In the mare and sow, six layers intervene: the endothelium, connective tissue, and epithelium of the CAM; and the epithelium, connective tissue, and endothelium of the endometrium. This configuration characterizes the **epitheliochorial placenta.** In ewes and nanny goats (does), the epithelium of the **caruncles** (endometrial elevations where functional contact with the CAM is made) is lost, thereby reducing the number of tissue layers to five **(syndesmochorial placenta).** In the cow, the epithelium of the caruncle remains intact (epitheliochorial), but portions of the intercaruncular epithelium degenerate. In carnivores, both the endometrial epithelium and the endometrial connective tissue are lost, bringing the epithelium of the CAM and the endothelium of the endometrium into contact. Only four tissue layers separate the fetal and maternal blood in this type, the **endotheliochorial placenta.**

A mucosa, muscularis, and adventitia or serosa (cranial region only) form the wall of the **vagina.** The mucosa is lined, throughout, by a stratified squamous epithelium in all species except the cow. In the anterior portion of the vagina of the cow, the epithelium is stratified columnar with goblet cells. In carnivores, the epithelial cells become keratinized during estrus. A lamina propria and submucosa are present. Usually, the inner layer of the muscularis is thick and consists of circularly arranged smooth muscle, while the outer layer is thin and consists of longitudinally organized smooth muscle. In some animals (bitch, queen, and sow) a thin layer of longitudinal muscle occurs internal to the circular layer. An adventitia or serosa is present.

Vaginal cytology provides a way of determining stages of the estrous cycle of the bitch or queen and therefore can be helpful to the practitioner who is trying to determine the best time to breed an animal. In the bitch, for example, **proestrus, estrus, diestrus,** and **anestrus** are stages of the estrous cycle. The formation of the corpus luteum occurs during late estrus in the bitch. Therefore there is no **metestrus.** Proestrus lasts an average of 9 days and is characterized by a watery, bloody discharge and swollen vulva. Estrus is evidenced when a bitch is willing to stand for mating, and ordinarily lasts about 9 days. A clear or bloody discharge is present. Diestrus lasts for about 2 months and begins on the day when the bitch no longer tolerates a male's advances. Anestrus follows diestrus and may last from two to ten months.

Various types of epithelial cells are found in vaginal smears taken during the estrous cycle. **Parabasal cells** are the smallest. They are round cells with round nuclei, and have the highest nucleocytoplasmic ratio of any of the sloughed cells. **Intermediate cells** are larger than parabasal cells. Their nuclei are similar in size and shape to those of the latter. The corners of intermediate cells are rounded. **Superficial intermediate cells** (transitional cells) are bigger than intermediate cells and have angular edges. Their nuclei resemble those of parabasal and intermediate cells. **Superficial cells** are similar in size to superficial intermediate cells. Their edges are angular and may be folded. Their nuclei are pyknotic, faded, or lacking.

Smears taken during proestrus (early to mid) may contain erythrocytes and neutrophils as well as parabasal, intermediate, superficial intermediate, and superficial cells. During late proestrus, superficial intermediate and superficial cells are the most numerous, and neutrophils decline.

The vast majority (90% or more) of cells found in smears taken during estrus are superficial cells. During late proestrus, similar smears may be obtained. Ordinarily, during estrus, neutrophils are not observed. Erythrocytes show a reduction in number, but in many bitches they can be found throughout estrus and into early diestrus. Bacteria may be found in estrous smears.

During diestrus, superficial cells decrease by a minimum of twenty percent. Parabasal and intermediate cells, which may have been absent or very sparse, increase to more than 10% and frequently rise to more than 50%. Although neutrophils reappear during diestrus, smears from some bitches contain few or none. Because erythrocytes may be present in smears from early diestrus, it is not possible to distinguish proestrus from diestrus without taking more than one smear.

During anestrus, parabasal and intermediate cells predominate in smears. Bacteria may be found, but will be less abundant than in proestrus or estrus. Neutrophils may occur, but are ordinarily less abundant than in early diestrus.

In domestic mammals, the **vulva** includes the **vesti-**

bule, **labia,** and **clitoris.** The mucosal epithelium is stratified squamous. The major vestibular glands are bilateral, mucus-secreting, tubuloacinar glands in the submucosa, found in ruminants and the queen. Minor vestibular glands occur in the mucosa of most domestic animals. They are small, branched, tubular, mucous glands distributed through the vestibular mucosa.

The integument of the labia (lips of the vulva) has a structure like that of the external skin. It is well endowed with both sebaceous and tubular apocrine glands.

The clitoris consists of **erectile tissue** (corpus cavernosum clitoridis), a **glans,** and a **prepuce.** The amount of erectile tissue varies. The prepuce has parietal and visceral components as in males.

CHICKEN

The left **ovary** and oviduct represent the reproductive organs of the hen. The ovary consists of an outer **cortex,** which envelops a vascular **medulla.** Ovarian follicles of various sizes occur within the cortex. A layer (germinal epithelium) of cuboidal or flattened cells covers the cortex. The **tunica albuginea,** composed of dense connective tissue, lies below the epithelium. A **stroma** of loose connective tissue occurs below the tunica albuginea.

Developing follicles occur throughout the stroma of the cortex. Large follicles are suspended from the surface of the ovary by stalks of cortical tissue. Each follicle consists of a growing, yolk-laden oocyte with a rounded nucleus **(germinal vesicle).** The oocyte is surrounded by several layers. These are, from the outside inward, the **theca externa, theca interna, membrana granulosa,** and **perivitelline membrane.** The latter abuts the surface membrane of the oocyte.

The theca externa is formed from a compact connective tissue, which contains groups of pale **interstitial (luteal) cells.** The latter may also be found, in groups, in the cortical stroma and medulla. The theca interna is only about one quarter as thick as the externa. It is formed from a compact layer of spindle-shaped cells. The membrana granulosa consists of a single layer of cuboidal cells in the smallest and largest follicles, but in those of intermediate size, the epithelium is pseudostratified columnar.

The cortex of the mature ovary also contains concentrations of fat-filled **vacuolar cells.** Numerous fat vacuoles occur throughout the cytoplasm of these cells, and their nuclei are pyknotic. Collections of these cells are believed to represent regressing postovulatory follicles.

Atretic follicles are commonly found in normal active ovaries. In the most common type of atretic follicle, cells of the membrana granulosa proliferate, forming a number of irregular layers around the oocyte. The oocyte becomes smaller and is eventually replaced by granulosa cells. Ultimately, scar tissue replaces the granulosa cells. In older birds, the oocyte becomes surrounded by hyperplastic and hypertrophied interstitial (luteal) cells during atresia. Both the oocyte and the cells of the membrana granulosa eventually degenerate.

The **oviduct** of the chicken is tortuous and muscular. It consists, in anterioposterior sequence, of the following five regions: **infundibulum, magnum, isthmus, shell gland** (uterus), and **vagina.** From the outside inward, the wall of the oviduct consists of a serosa, muscularis (outer longitudinal and inner circular smooth muscle), lamina propria, and epithelium. In most regions, the lamina propria contains glands.

The infundibulum is composed of a thin-walled funnel and a neck region. Scattered bundles of smooth muscle lie within the connective tissue between the serosa and ciliated, simple columnar epithelium. Longitudinal folds are present in the mucosa within the interior of the funnel near the neck. The folds increase in depth within the neck, and secondary folds appear. The muscularis becomes sorted out into circular and longitudinal layers in the neck.

The magnum is the longest part of the oviduct. Its well developed tubular glands produce albumin. Its mucosal folds are more numerous and taller than those of the infundibulum. Tertiary folds are present. The muscularis is better developed than in the infundibulum. The pseudostratified epithelium is composed of ciliated columnar cells and secretory (goblet) cells.

The isthmus is a relatively short region with a diameter less than that of the magnum. Its longitudinal mucosal folds possess numerous secondary folds. The muscularis is better developed than the magnum's. The epithelium is ciliated, pseudostratified columnar with secretory cells. Its numerous tubular glands secrete the shell membranes.

The uterus is an expanded portion of the oviduct. Its walls are not as thick as those of the preceding segments. The muscularis is well developed, especially the longitudinal layer. The mucosa is thrown into longitudinal, leaf-shaped folds, which are covered by a ciliated, pseudostratified, columnar epithelium. The shell of the egg is produced from secretions of its tubular glands.

The vagina is a short, narrow duct. Its muscularis is well developed, especially the circular layer. Its mucosa is thrown into numerous tall, narrow folds bearing many small secondary folds. The surface is covered by a ciliated, pseudostratified columnar epithelium with mucous cells. Sperm storage occurs in the **sperm-host glands.** These tubular glands occur within the connective tissue of the mucosa of the vagina near the junction between the uterus and vagina. After insemination, sperm appear in compact masses within the glands. The vagina of the oviduct opens into the urodeum of the cloaca.

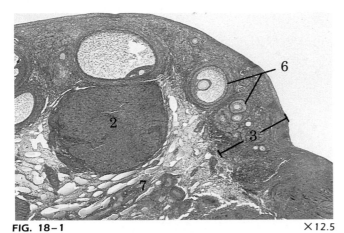

FIG. 18-1   ×12.5

FIG. 18–1. Ovary, Queen. Follicles of various ages and a corpus luteum can be seen in the cortex. A portion of the vascular medulla is present.

FIG. 18–2. Ovary, Queen. Early follicles in the outer region of the cortex.

FIG. 18–3. Ovary, Bitch. A multilaminar, primary follicle.

FIG. 18–4. Ovary, Queen. A young, tertiary follicle.

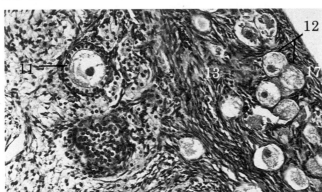

FIG. 18–2   ×125

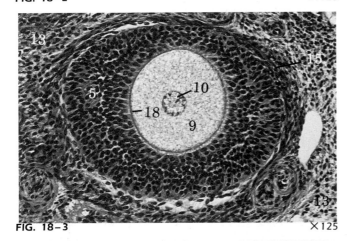

FIG. 18–3   ×125

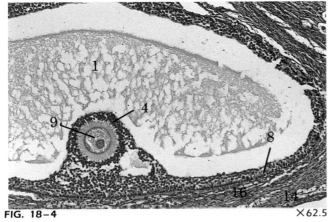

FIG. 18–4   ×62.5

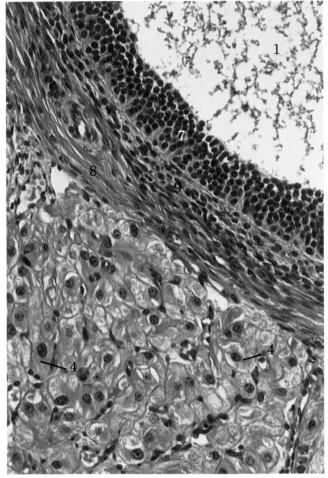

FIG. 18–5 ×180

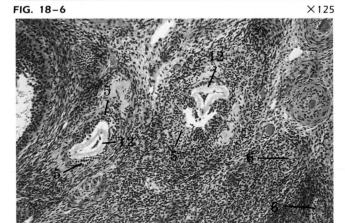

FIG. 18–6 ×125

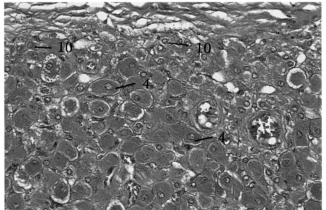

FIG. 18–7 ×62.5

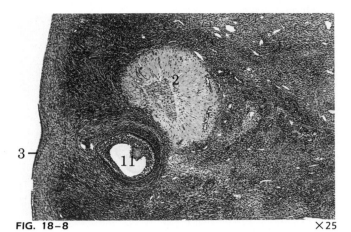

FIG. 18–8 ×25

KEY	
1. Antrum	**7.** Membrana granulosa
2. Corpus albicans	**8.** Theca externa
3. Germinal epithelium	**9.** Theca interna
4. Granulosa lutein cell	**10.** Theca lutein cell
5. Hypertrophied theca cells	**11.** Young tertiary follicle
6. Interstitial gland	**12.** Zona pellucida

FIG. 18–5. Ovary, Bitch. Portion of the wall of a tertiary follicle, and part of an adjacent corpus luteum.

FIG. 18–6. Corpus Luteum, Ovary, Sow. Peripheral region of a corpus luteum showing theca lutein cells (small) and granulosa lutein cells (large).

FIG. 18–7. Ovary, Bitch. Atretic follicles, each with a swollen zona pellucida.

FIG. 18–8. Corpus Albicans, Ovary, Cow, Masson's. The scar tissue of the corpus albicans is stained bright blue-green in this preparation.

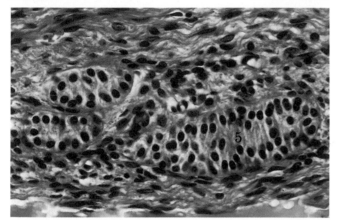

FIG. 18-9   ×62.5

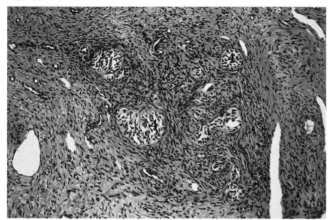

FIG. 18-10   ×250

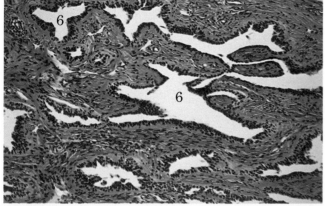

FIG. 18-11   ×62.5

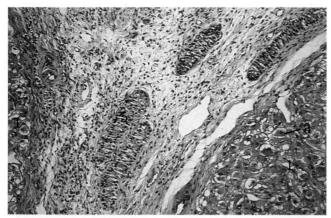

FIG. 18-12   ×62.5

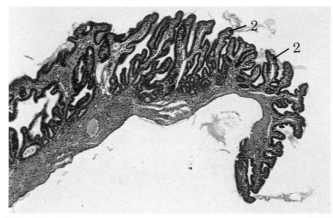

FIG. 18-13   ×25

KEY		
1. Corpus luteum	**4.** Hilus cells	
2. Folds	**5.** Interstitial gland	
3. Granulosa lutein cell	**6.** Rete ovarii	

FIG. 18-9. Ovary, Bitch. Several interstitial glands within the stroma between two corpora lutea.

FIG. 18-10. Interstitial Glands, Ovary, Bitch. Cords of epithelioid cells form the parenchyma of interstitial glands. These glands are well developed in queens and bitches.

FIG. 18-11. Hilus Cells, Ovary, Cow. Clusters of epithelioid cells, located in the vicinity of the hilus, are called hilus cells. They resemble the epithelioid cells of the interstitial glands. See Figure 18-10.

FIG. 18-12. Rete Ovarii, Ovary, Cow. Cords of cells, or channels lined by cuboidal epithelial cells, located in the medulla of the ovary are called the rete ovarii. They are considered to be homologous to the rete testis.

FIG. 18-13. Fimbria of Infundibulum, Oviduct, Mare. The mucosa of the fimbria is highly folded.

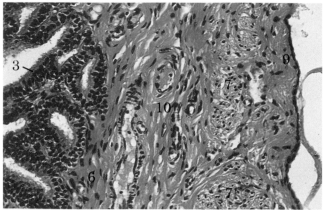

FIG. 18–14 ×125

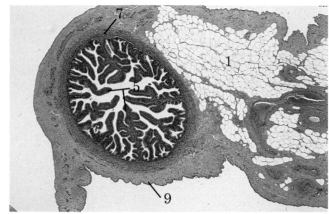

FIG. 18–18 ×12.5

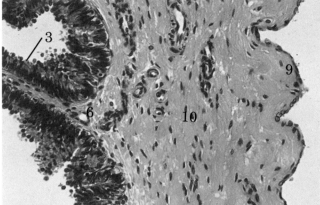

FIG. 18–15 ×125

FIG. 18–14. Fimbria of Infundibulum, Oviduct, Mare. Detail of the wall. Note the smooth muscle of the thin muscularis.

FIG. 18–15. Fimbria of Infundibulum, Oviduct, Cow. Portions of the fimbria may lack smooth muscle, as in this example.

FIG. 18–16. Infundibulum, Oviduct, Cow, Masson's. The epithelium consists of ciliated, columnar epithelial cells and nonciliated, secretory cells. Extruded nuclei, which appear to arise from epithelial cells, are common.

FIG. 18–17. Infundibulum, Neck, Oviduct, x.s., Cow. The mucosa is highly folded, and the muscularis is thin.

FIG. 18–18. Ampulla, Oviduct, x.s., Cow. The mucosa is highly folded. The muscularis is relatively thick. Compare to Figure 18–17.

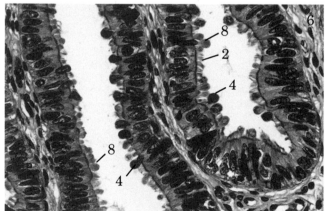

FIG. 18–16 ×250

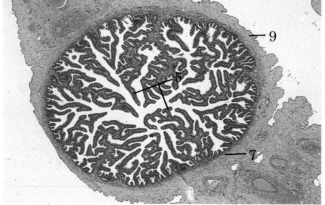

FIG. 18–17 ×12.5

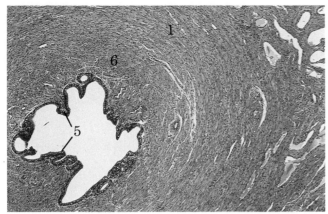

FIG. 18–19 ×25

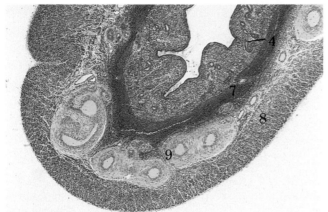

FIG. 18–20 ×25

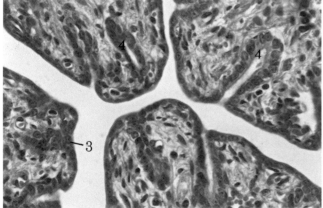

FIG. 18–21 ×250

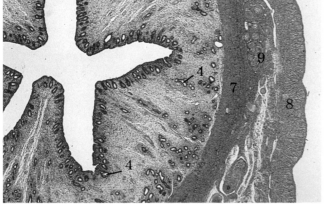

FIG. 18–22 ×12.5

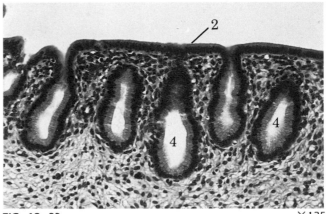

FIG. 18–23 ×125

KEY	
1. Circular muscle	**6.** Longitudinal muscle
2. Columnar epithelium	**7.** Myometrium, circular
3. Cuboidal epithelium	**8.** Myometrium, longitudinal
4. Endometrial gland	**9.** Stratum vasculare
5. Folds	

FIG. 18–19. Isthmus, Oviduct, x.s., Mare. The mucosa of the isthmus has fewer folds than any other part of the oviduct. The muscularis is thickest in this part of the oviduct.

FIG. 18–20. Uterine Horn, x.s., Anestrus, Bitch. The endometrium is thin and the glands are sparse in anestrus.

FIG. 18–21. Uterine Horn, x.s., Anestrus, Queen. The lumen of the anestrus uterus is lined by a simple cuboidal epithelium.

FIG. 18–22. Uterine Horn, x.s., Proestrus, Bitch. In proestrus, the endometrium becomes thicker and the glands enlarge.

FIG. 18–23. Uterine Horn, x.s., Proestrus, Bitch. Luminal epithelial cells become columnar during proestrus and estrus.

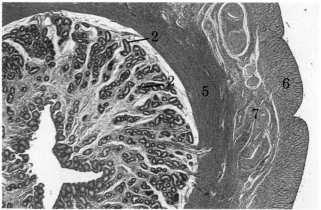

FIG. 18-24 ×12.5

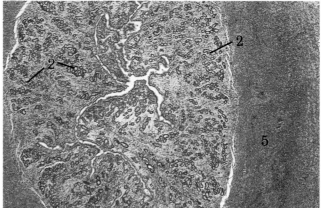

FIG. 18-25 ×12.5

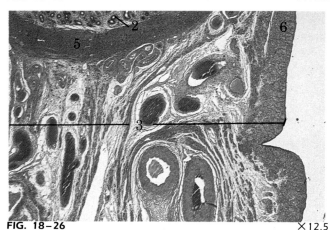

FIG. 18-26 ×12.5

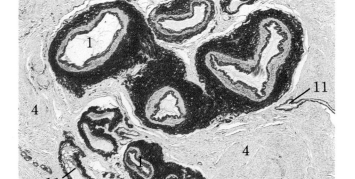

FIG. 18-27 ×25

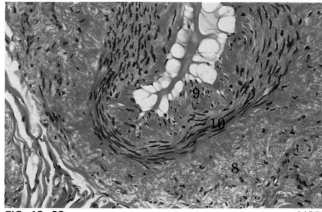

FIG. 18-28 ×250

KEY	
1. Artery	**7.** Stratum vasculare
2. Endometrial gland	**8.** Tunica adventitia
3. Mesometrium	**9.** Tunica intima
4. Myometrium	**10.** Tunica media
5. Myometrium, circular	**11.** Vein
6. Myometrium, longitudinal	

FIG. 18-24. Uterine Horn, x.s., Estrus, Bitch. A thick endometrium and highly developed glands are characteristic of the estrous uterus.

FIG. 18-25. Uterine Horn, x.s., Diestrus, Bitch. The endometrium and its glands become fully developed during diestrus.

FIG. 18-26. Mesometrium, Bitch. The mesometrium contains an abundance of smooth muscle and numerous blood vessels. Smooth muscle of the mesometrium is continuous with the outer, longitudinal layer of the myometrium.

FIG. 18-27. Uterine Horn, Brood Mare, Orcein. There is an abundance of elastic fibers (red-brown in this micrograph) in the intima and adventitia of blood vessels of the uterus of animals that have been through a pregnancy. The section is from the midregion of the myometrium.

FIG. 18-28. Uterine Horn, Brood Mare. Detail of a portion of an artery in the myometrium. The intima becomes thickened with elastic fibers and smooth muscle in animals who have experienced a pregnancy. The adventitia also becomes heavily infiltrated with elastic fibers.

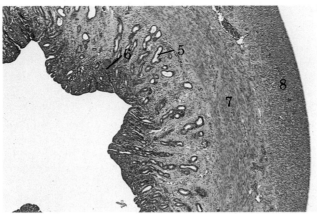

FIG. 18-29   ×25

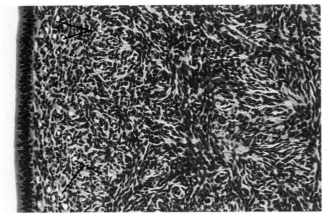

FIG. 18-33   ×125

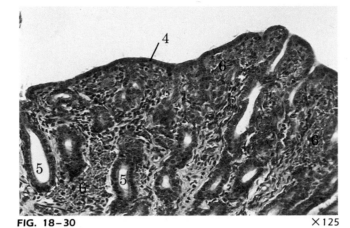

FIG. 18-30   ×125

KEY	
1. Blood vessels	**6.** Hemorrhagic region
2. Caruncle	**7.** Myometrium, circular
3. Cilia	**8.** Myometrium, longitudinal
4. Cuboidal epithelium	**9.** Pseudostratified epithelium
5. Endometrial gland	

FIG. 18-29. Uterine Horn, x.s., Metestrus, Cow. Metestrous bleeding occurs in the cow. Numerous erythrocytes of hemorrhagic regions can be seen beneath the surface epithelium. See Figure 18-30.

FIG. 18-30. Uterus, Metestrus, Cow. Detail of Figure 18-29. Hemorrhagic regions are evident in the endometrium beneath the surface epithelium. The epithelial cells are cuboidal during metestrus in the cow.

FIG. 18-31. Uterine Horn, Cow, Masson's. The epithelial cells lining the uterine glands are sometimes ciliated, as in this section.

FIG. 18-32. Caruncle, Uterus, x.s., Cow. The endometrium of the uterus of ruminants contains nonglandular, highly cellular prominences called caruncles. Uterine glands that lie deep to the caruncle open near its base.

FIG. 18-33. Caruncle, Uterus, Cow. The caruncle consists of highly cellular (mostly fibroblasts) connective tissue, and numerous blood vessels located beneath the epithelium.

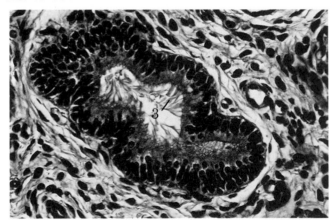

FIG. 18-31   ×250

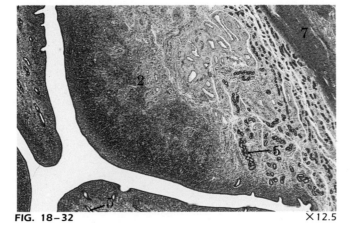

FIG. 18-32   ×12.5

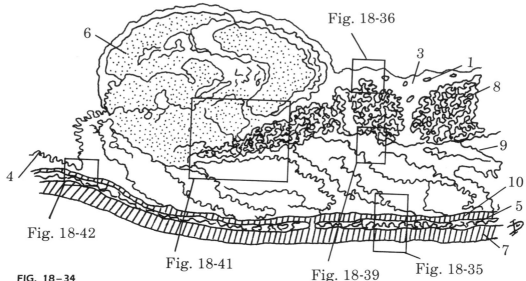

FIG. 18-34

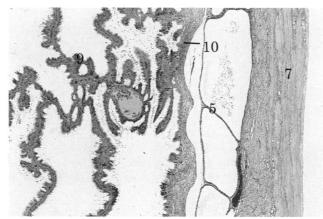

FIG. 18-35   ×25

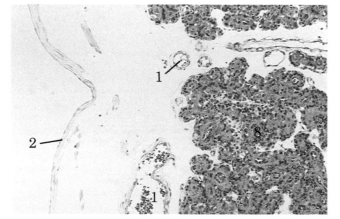

FIG. 18-36   ×62.5

FIG. 18-34. Placenta, Bitch. The placenta of carnivores is of the zonary type. A section through a portion of one of the edges of this belt-like structure is shown in this drawing. The regions enclosed by rectangles refer to subsequent micrographs found in this chapter.

FIG. 18-35. Zonary Placenta, Bitch, Trichrome. Section through the deepest layers of the placenta (see Fig. 18-34 for location). The spongy zone is formed by the occluded uterine glands in the midregion of the endometrium. The deep glandular layer consists of the bases of the uterine glands. The supraglandular layer is a sheet of connective tissue between the deep glandular and spongy layers. *(Photomicrograph of a histologic section borrowed from the College of Veterinary Medicine, Iowa State University.)*

FIG. 18-36. Zonary Placenta, Bitch, Trichrome. Portion of the chorioallantoic membrane and the placental labyrinth. The chorioallantoic membrane in this micrograph appears thicker than normal because of the presence of extensive space artifact. Note the presence of fetal blood vessels in the chorioallantoic membrane. *(Photomicrograph of a histologic section borrowed from the College of Veterinary Medicine, Iowa State University.)*

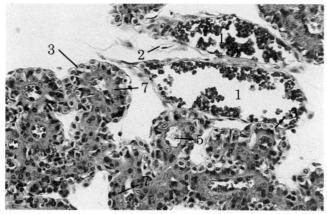

FIG. 18–37   ×125

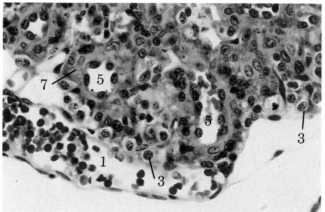

FIG. 18–38   ×250

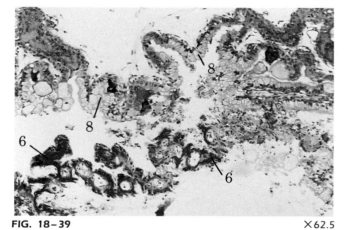

FIG. 18–39   ×62.5

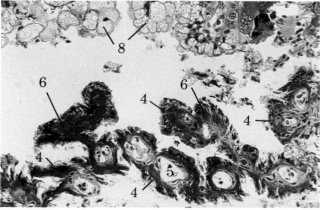

FIG. 18–40   ×125

FIG. 18–37. Zonary Placenta, Bitch, Trichrome. Section is through the placental labyrinth. Both maternal and fetal components of this endotheliochorial placenta can be seen. *(Photomicrograph of a histologic section borrowed from the College of Veterinary Medicine, Iowa State University.)*

FIG. 18–38. Zonary Placenta, Bitch, Trichrome. Detail of the placental labyrinth. The maternal blood vessels are lined by endothelial cells with bulging nuclei. *(Photomicrograph of a histologic section borrowed from the College of Veterinary Medicine, Iowa State University.)*

FIG. 18–39. Zonary Placenta, Bitch, Trichrome. Trophoblastic projections, lined by large, pale, vacuolated cells, protrude into spaces (areolae) in the region where the placental labyrinth is forming. A portion of the maternal tissue, which has been partially destroyed by the invading trophoblast, is represented by the red-stained, necrotic tissue seen in the lower left quadrant of the micrograph. *(Photomicrograph of a histologic section borrowed from the College of Veterinary Medicine, Iowa State University.)*

FIG. 18–40. Zonary Placenta, Bitch, Trichrome. Detail of Fig. 18–39. *(Photomicrograph of a histologic section borrowed from the College of Veterinary Medicine, Iowa State University.)*

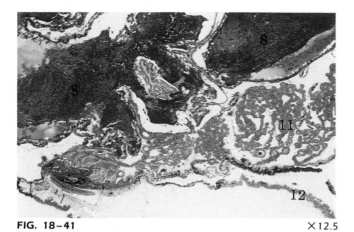

FIG. 18-41   ×12.5

KEY	
1. Allantoic blood vessel	**8.** Marginal hematoma
2. Chorioallantoic membrane	**9.** Maternal blood vessel
3. Chorioallantoic villus	**10.** Microplacentome
4. Chorioallantoic villus, epithelium	**11.** Placental labyrinth
5. Chorion laeve, epithelium	**12.** Spongy zone
6. Crypt	**13.** Uterine gland
7. Crypt, epithelium	**14.** Uterus, epithelium

FIG. 18-41. Zonary Placenta, Bitch, Trichrome. A portion of a marginal hematoma, consisting of large compartments filled with blood derived from hemorrhaging uterine blood vessels, is shown. See Figure 18-34 for location. *(Photomicrograph of a histologic section borrowed from the College of Veterinary Medicine, Iowa State University.)*

FIG. 18-42. Chorion Laeve, Bitch, Trichrome. The chorion laeve is the part of the chorioallantoic sac that is not involved in the formation of the placenta. Its surface is smooth and is apposed to the uterine epithelium. This section is from the region adjacent to the hematoma of the placenta. *(Photomicrograph of a histologic section borrowed from the College of Veterinary Medicine, Iowa State University.)*

FIG. 18-43. Diffuse Placenta, Mare. In the horse, small tufts of branched chorioallantoic villi interdigitate with crypts of the endometrium. Together, the tufts and the crypts form structures called microplacentomes. *(Photomicrograph of a histologic section borrowed from the College of Veterinary Medicine, Iowa State University.)*

FIG. 18-44. Diffuse Placenta, Mare. Detail of a microplacentome. Longitudinal and cross sections of chorioallantoic villi are surrounded by endometrial crypts. The epithelium of the crypts, which may vary in height, is flattened in this region. The villi contain blood vessels and connective tissue and are covered by pink-stained trophoblast cells. *(Photomicrograph of a histologic section borrowed from the College of Veterinary Medicine, Iowa State University.)*

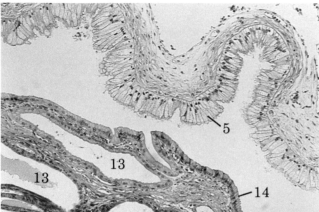

FIG. 18-42   ×62.5

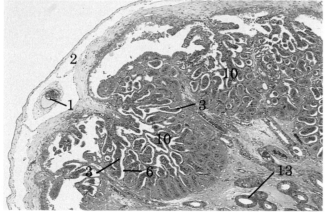

FIG. 18-43   ×25

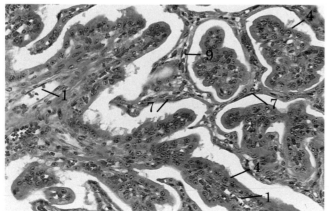

FIG. 18-44   ×125

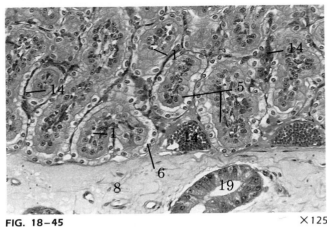

FIG. 18–45   ×125

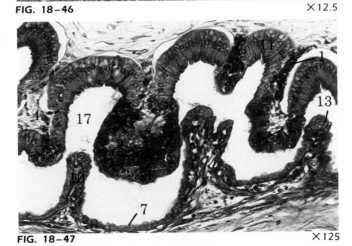

FIG. 18–46   ×12.5

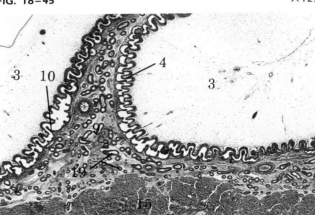

FIG. 18–47   ×125

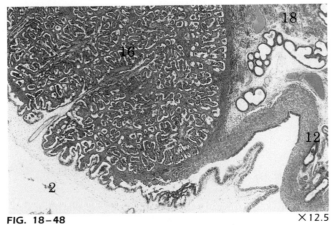

FIG. 18–48   ×12.5

KEY	
1. Allantoic blood vessel	**10.** Endometrium, secondary fold
2. Chorioallantoic membrane	**11.** High columnar cells
3. Chorioallantoic membrane, primary fold	**12.** Intercotyledonary endometrium
4. Chorioallantoic membrane, secondary fold	**13.** Low columnar cells
5. Chorioallantoic villus, epithelium	**14.** Maternal blood vessel
6. Crypt, epithelium	**15.** Myometrium
7. Cuboidal cells	**16.** Placentome
8. Endometrium, connective tissue	**17.** Space artifact
9. Endometrium, primary fold	**18.** Stalk of placentome
	19. Uterine gland

FIG. 18–45. Diffuse Placenta, Mare. Detail of a placentome adjacent to the endometrium. The epithelium of the endometrial crypt consists of pale, cuboidal cells. The epithelium of the chorioallantoic villi is formed from pink-stained cuboidal and low columnar cells. *(Photomicrograph of a histologic section borrowed from the College of Veterinary Medicine, Iowa State University.)*

FIG. 18–46. Diffuse Placenta, Sow, Trichrome. The placenta of the sow is folded, diffuse, and epitheliochorial. Folds of the chorioallantoic membrane interdigitate with folds of the uterus. *(Photomicrograph of a histologic section borrowed from the College of Veterinary Medicine, Iowa State University.)*

FIG. 18–47. Diffuse Placenta, Sow, Trichrome. Interdigitating secondary folds of the chorioallantoic membrane and endometrium. The bases of the folds of the chorioallantoic membrane are lined by high columnar epithelial cells, whereas the crests of the maternal folds are covered by shorter columnar cells. The remainder of both epithelial surfaces is lined by cuboidal or flattened cells. Note that the chorioallantoic epithelial surface is invaded by capillaries. *(Photomicrograph of a histologic section borrowed from the College of Veterinary Medicine, Iowa State University.)*

FIG. 18–48. Cotyledonary Placenta, Cow. A section through a placentome formed from the association of a cotyledon (clumps of chorioallantoic villi) with a uterine caruncle (endometrial elevation). Note that the endometrium of the intercotyledonary region is discontinuous.

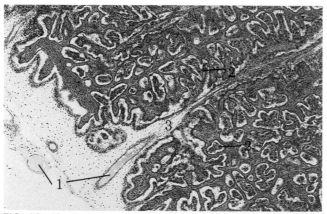

FIG. 18–49 ×25

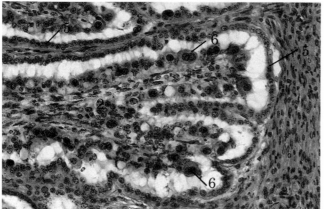

FIG. 18–50 ×125

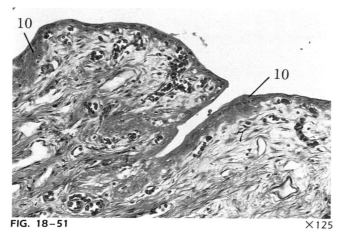

FIG. 18–51 ×125

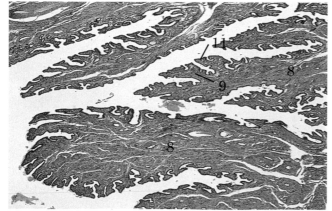

FIG. 18–53 ×250

KEY	
1. Allantoic blood vessel	**6.** Diplokaryocyte
2. Chorioallantoic villus, branch	**7.** Lamina propria
	8. Primary fold
3. Chorioallantoic villus, main stem	**9.** Secondary fold
	10. Stratified squamous epithelium
4. Cilia	
5. Cryptal epithelium	**11.** Tertiary fold

FIG. 18–49. Cotyledonary Placenta, Cow. Detail of Figure 18–48. Highly branched chorioallantoic villi interdigitate with uterine crypts.

FIG. 18–50. Cotyledonary Placenta, Cow. Detail of a portion of a placentome adjacent to the stalk. Note that the cryptal epithelium is cuboidal or flattened. The epithelium of the chorioallantoic villus consists of irregularly shaped cells and binucleate giant cells (diplokaryocytes).

FIG. 18–51. Cervix of Uterus, Bitch. The mucosa of the cervix is thrown into folds. The epithelium of the bitch's cervix is stratified squamous. *(Photomicrograph of a histologic section borrowed from the College of Veterinary Medicine, Iowa State University.)*

FIG. 18–52. Cervix of Uterus, Mare. Cervical folds are evident.

FIG. 18–53. Cervix of Uterus, Mare, Masson's. The cervical epithelium is simple columnar, except in the bitch (see Fig. 18–51). Epithelial cells may be ciliated.

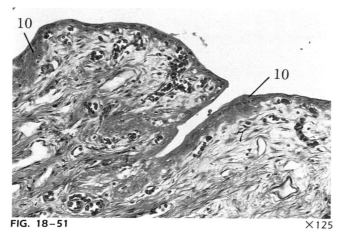

FIG. 18–52 ×12.5

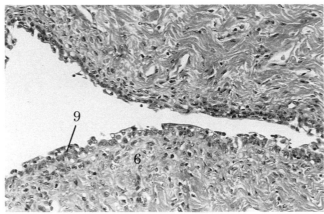

FIG. 18–54   ×125

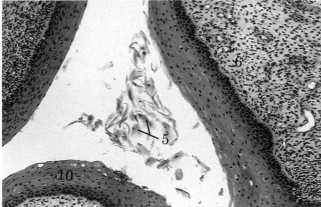

FIG. 18–55   ×62.5

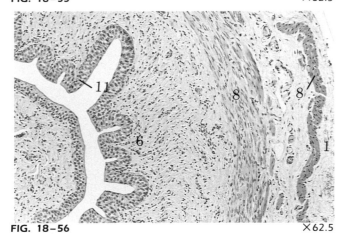

FIG. 18–56   ×62.5

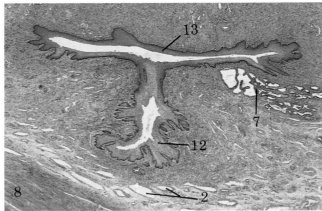

FIG. 18–57   ×12.5

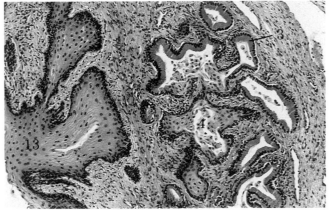

FIG. 18–58   ×62.5

KEY	
1. Adventitia	**8.** Muscularis
2. Cavernous spaces	**9.** Stratified epithelium
3. Columnar cells	**10.** Stratified squamous
4. Duct	epithelium
5. Keratinized cells	**11.** Transitional epithelium
6. Lamina propria	**12.** Urethral epithelium
7. Minor vestibular gland	**13.** Vestibular epithelium

FIG. 18–54. Vagina, Anestrus, Bitch. The epithelium of the carnivore's anestrous vagina is stratified squamous to stratified cuboidal. *(Photomicrograph of a histologic section borrowed from the College of Veterinary Medicine, Iowa State University.)*

FIG. 18–55. Vagina, Estrus, Queen. In carnivores, the vagina is lined by a thickened, keratinized, stratified squamous epithelium during estrus. Exfoliated keratinized cells are visible in the vaginal lumen in this micrograph.

FIG. 18–56. Urethra, x.s., Queen. Section was taken from the region close to the bladder. This portion of the urethra is lined by a transitional epithelium. *(Photomicrograph of a histologic section borrowed from the College of Veterinary Medicine, Iowa State University.)*

FIG. 18–57. Junction of Vestibule and Urethra, x.s., Queen. Near the vestibule, the urethra is lined by a stratified squamous epithelium. Note the presence of cavernous spaces in the connective tissue adjacent to the muscularis. Such spaces occur only in the distal two thirds of the urethra in the doe, ewe, and queen. In all other domestic mammals, cavernous spaces occur throughout the entire length of the urethra.

FIG. 18–58. Vestibule, Queen. Detail of a minor vestibular gland. The secretory tubules of these branched, tubular glands are lined by columnar cells. Their ducts are lined by stratified squamous epithelium.

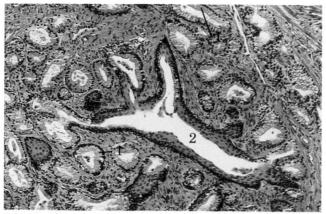

FIG. 18-59 ×62.5

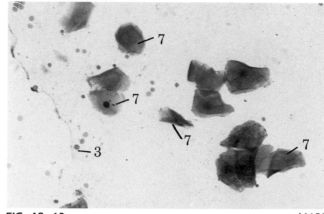

FIG. 18-63 ×125

KEY	
1. Columnar cells	**5.** Neutrophil
2. Duct	**6.** Parabasal cell
3. Erythrocyte	**7.** Superficial cell
4. Intermediate cell	**8.** Superficial intermediate cell

FIG. 18-59. Vestibule, Queen. Detail of a major vestibular gland. These glands are found in queens and ruminants. They are compound tubular glands with secretory units like those of the minor vestibular glands (see Fig. 18-58).

FIG. 18-60. Vaginal Smear, Anestrus, Bitch, Hema-3. During anestrus, parabasal and intermediate cells are the predominant epithelial cells present (see introduction for description of cell types). Neutrophils and bacteria may be present in limited numbers.

FIG. 18-61. Vaginal Smear, Early Proestrus, Bitch, Hema-3. During early to mid proestrus, smears may contain neutrophils, erythrocytes, and various epithelial cell types (parabasal, intermediate, superficial intermediate, and superficial cells).

FIG. 18-62. Vaginal Smear, Mid to Late Proestrus, Bitch, Diff-Quik. In late proestrus, superficial intermediate and superficial cells are predominant. Neutrophils decrease in number at this time.

FIG. 18-63. Vaginal Smear, Estrus, Bitch, Diff-Quik. Most (90% or more) of the epithelial cells from a bitch in estrus are superficial cells. Erythrocytes may be present in small numbers. Some estrous smears may contain large numbers of bacteria. Neutrophils are not normally present.

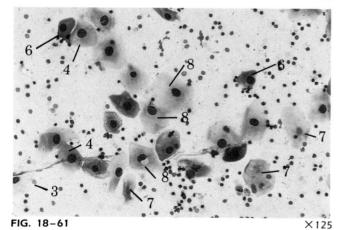

FIG. 18-60 ×125

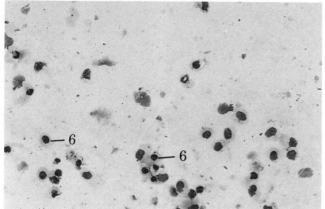

FIG. 18-61 ×125

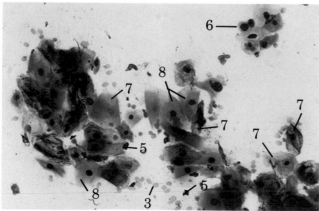

FIG. 18-62 ×125

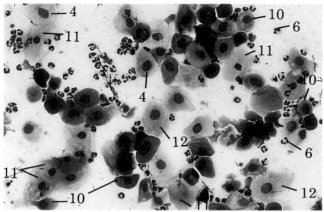

FIG. 18-64 ×125

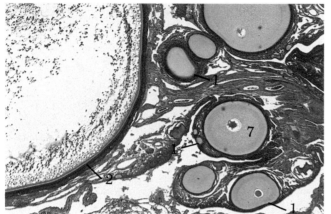

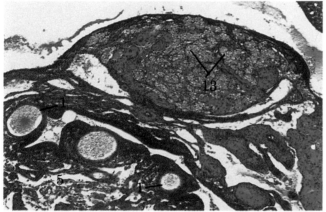

FIG. 18-65 ×12.5

FIG. 18-66 ×62.5

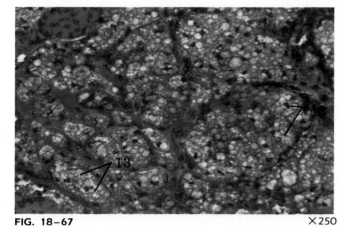

FIG. 18-67 ×250

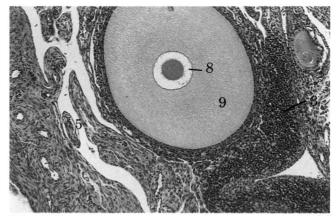

FIG. 18-68 ×62.5

KEY	
1. Follicle, early	**8.** Oocyte, nucleus
2. Follicle, late	**9.** Oocyte, yolk-laden
3. Granulocytes	cytoplasm
4. Intermediate cell	**10.** Parabasal cell
5. Medulla	**11.** Superficial cell
6. Neutrophil	**12.** Superficial intermediate cell
7. Oocyte	**13.** Vacuolar cells

FIG. 18-64. Vaginal Smear, Diestrus, Bitch, Diff-Quik. There is a significant change in the numbers of epithelial cell types during diestrus. Superficial cells decrease, and parabasal and intermediate cells increase. Neutrophils usually reappear during diestrus. Because erythrocytes may be present in smears from bitches in early diestrus, it is not possible to distinguish proestrus from diestrus on the basis of a single smear.

FIG. 18-65. Ovary, Hen. A portion of the ovarian cortex with developing follicles.

FIG. 18-66. Ovary, Vacuolar Cells, Hen. A portion of the cortex with a mass of fat-laden vacuolar cells. The latter may represent regressing postovulatory follicles.

FIG. 18-67. Ovary, Vacuolar Cells, Hen. Detail of Figure 18-66. Vacuolar cells have pyknotic nuclei and contain numerous fat vacuoles. Cell boundaries are often indistinct.

FIG. 18-68. Ovary, Granulocytes, Hen. Granulocytes are often found in the cortex of mature ovaries. The acidophilic granules of these cells impart a red tinge to a large area of the cortex in this micrograph.

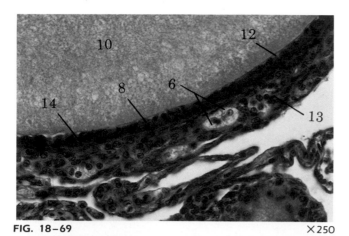

FIG. 18-69   ×250

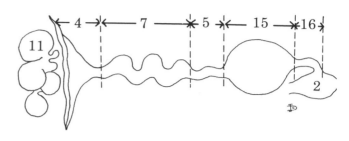

FIG. 18-73

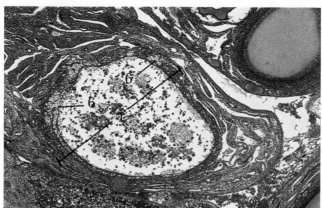

FIG. 18-70   ×25

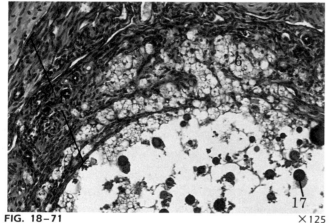

FIG. 18-71   ×125

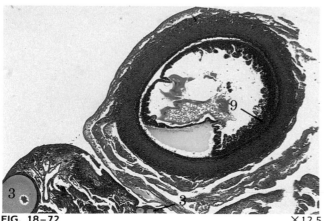

FIG. 18-72   ×12.5

KEY	
1. Atretic follicle	**10.** Oocyte, yolk-laden
2. Cloaca	cytoplasm
3. Developing follicle	**11.** Ovary
4. Infundibulum	**12.** Perivitelline membrane
5. Isthmus	**13.** Theca externa
6. Interstitial cells	**14.** Theca interna
7. Magnum	**15.** Uterus
8. Membrana granulosa	**16.** Vagina
9. Membrana granulosa,	**17.** Yolk sphere
thickened	

FIG. 18-69. Ovary, Developing Follicle, Hen. A portion of the wall of a developing follicle. Note the flattened cells of the theca interna and the presence of interstitial cells in the theca externa.

FIG. 18-70. Ovary, Atretic Follicle, Hen. In some atretic follicles, interstitial (luteal) cells proliferate, hypertrophy, and migrate inward (see Fig. 18-71).

FIG. 18-71. Ovary, Atretic Follicle, Hen. Detail of Figure 18-70.

FIG. 18-72. Ovary, Atretic Follicle, Hen. Cells of the membrana granulosa have proliferated, forming a thick layer characteristic of many atretic follicles.

FIG. 18-73. Oviduct, Diagrammatic, Hen.. The oviduct of the hen is divisible into an infundibulum, magnum, isthmus, uterus, and vagina.

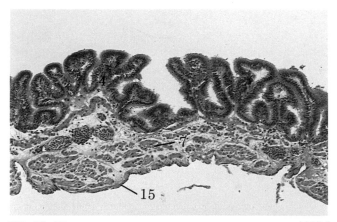

FIG. 18-74   ×62.5

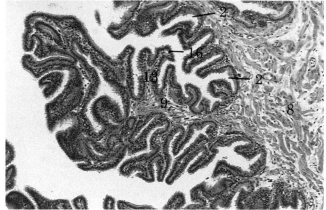

FIG. 18-75   ×62.5

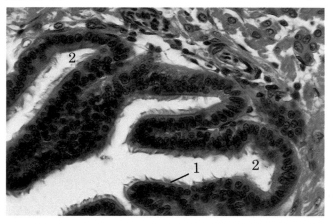

FIG. 18-76   ×250

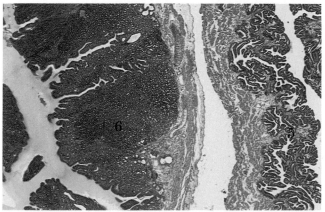

FIG. 18-77   ×12.5

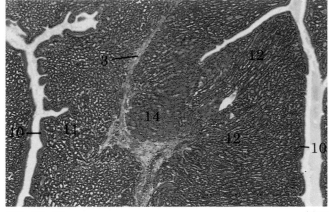

FIG. 18-78   ×25

KEY	
1. Ciliated epithelium	**10.** Pseudostratified columnar epithelium
2. Glandular groove	**11.** Regenerating gland
3. Lamina propria	**12.** Resting gland
4. Mucosa	**13.** Secondary fold
5. Mucosal fold, infundibulum	**14.** Secretory gland
6. Mucosal fold, magnum	**15.** Serosa
7. Muscularis	**16.** Tertiary fold
8. Muscularis, circular	
9. Primary fold	

FIG. 18-74. Funnel of Infundibulum, Oviduct, x.s., Hen. The mucosa is thrown into shallow ridges, which increase in height as the funnel narrows toward the neck region. The epithelium is ciliated, simple columnar. Scattered bundles of smooth muscle form the muscularis. A serosa covers the funnel externally.

FIG. 18-75. Neck of Infundibulum, x.s., Oviduct, Hen. Tall primary mucosal folds bear secondary and tertiary folds.

FIG. 18-76. Neck of Infundibulum, x.s., Oviduct, Hen. Detail of mucosa showing folds lined by ciliated columnar cells. The bases of the grooves between the folds are lined by nonciliated secretory cells, which collectively line the glandular grooves.

FIG. 18-77. Neck of Infundibulum and Magnum, x.s., Oviduct, Hen. The primary mucosal folds of the magnum are taller and broader vis-à-vis the infundibulum, because of the presence of numerous tubular glands.

FIG. 18-78. Magnum, x.s., Oviduct, Hen. Portion of a fold. Depending upon their activity, the tubular glands of the magnum exhibit distinctive features. Three morphologic phases of activity can be recognized (regenerating, secretory, resting). See Figures 18-80 and 18-81 for details.

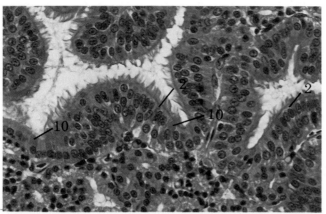

FIG. 18–79   ×250

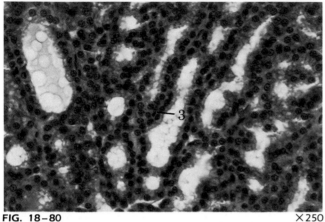

FIG. 18–80   ×250

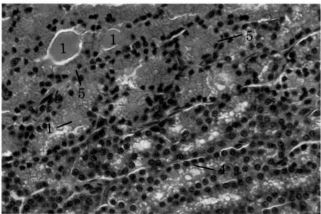

FIG. 18–81   ×250

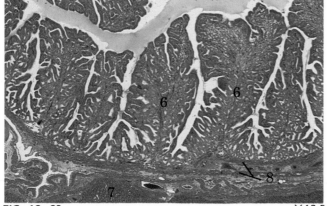

FIG. 18–82   ×12.5

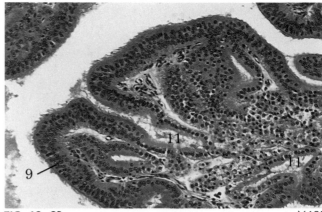

FIG. 18–83   ×125

KEY	
1. Albumen	**6.** Isthmus, primary fold
2. Ciliated cell	**7.** Magnum
3. Epithelium, regenerating gland	**8.** Muscularis
	9. Pseudostratified epithelium
4. Epithelium, resting gland	**10.** Secretory cell
5. Epithelium, secretory gland	**11.** Tubular gland

FIG. 18–79. Magnum, Oviduct, Hen. Detail of the epithelium. Ciliated columnar and secretory (goblet) cells comprise the epithelium of the magnum. The nuclei of the secretory cells are round and are located close to the base of the cell, whereas the nuclei of the ciliated cells are oval and occupy the central to apical region of the cell. Accordingly, the epithelium is pseudostratified columnar.

FIG. 18–80. Magnum, Oviduct, Hen. Detail of regenerating tubular glands. These glands have clearly defined lumens. The secretory cells are cuboidal.

FIG. 18–81. Magnum, Oviduct, Hen. Detail of secretory tubular glands and resting tubular glands. The cells of the secretory stage are characterized by pyknotic, basal nuclei. The entire cytoplasm is filled with strongly acidophilic granules. The glandular lumens may be dilated by secreted albumen. The cytoplasm of the cells in the resting stage has a frothy appearance, and the lumens of the glands are obscure.

FIG. 18–82. Isthmus, x.s., Oviduct, Hen. The primary folds of the isthmus are not as broad as those of the magnum (compare with Fig. 18–77). They are somewhat angular in appearance. A portion of an adjacent region of the magnum is present in this micrograph.

FIG. 18–83. Isthmus, Oviduct, Hen. A portion of the epithelium and underlying tubular glands. The epithelium is ciliated and pseudostratified columnar. A tubular gland can be seen opening to the surface. The glandular cells do not undergo obvious cyclic changes as in the magnum.

FIG. 18-84   ×12.5

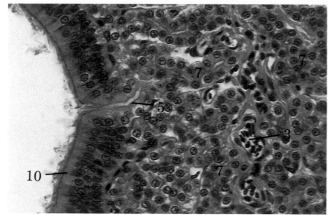

FIG. 18-85   ×250

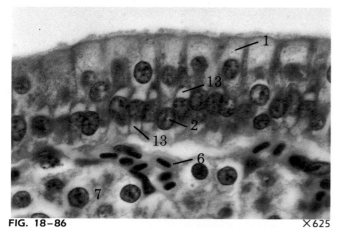

FIG. 18-86   ×625

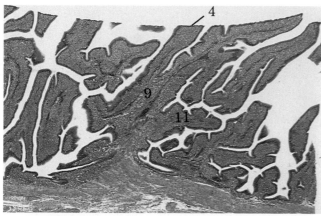

FIG. 18-87   ×25

FIG. 18-88   ×125

KEY	
1. Apical cell	**8.** Muscularis
2. Basal cell, nucleus	**9.** Primary fold
3. Blood vessel	**10.** Pseudostratified epithelium
4. Concave surface	**11.** Secondary fold
5. Duct	**12.** Sperm-host gland
6. Erythrocyte in capillary	**13.** Vacuole
7. Glandular epithelium	

FIG. 18-84. Uterus (Shell Gland), Oviduct, Hen. The folds of the uterus are not as broad as those of the magnum, and there is less glandular tissue. This section was taken from a uterus that had been fixed while containing an egg. Accordingly, the luminal surface is somewhat concave.

FIG. 18-85. Uterus (Shell Gland), Oviduct, Hen. Ducts of complex, branched, tubular glands pierce the pseudostratified columnar epithelium at intervals. Ducts are formed from polygonal gland cells.

FIG. 18-86. Uterus (Shell Gland), Oviduct, Hen. Basal cells (nuclei close to the basement membrane) of the pseudostratified epithelium may contain vacuoles above and below their nuclei. Apical cells (nuclei centrally located) contain numerous granules before releasing their secretion.

FIG. 18-87. Vagina, x.s., Oviduct, Hen. The mucosa of the vagina is characterized by long, slender, primary folds bearing numerous small secondary folds. The muscularis is highly developed.

FIG. 18-88. Vagina, Proximal, Oviduct, Hen. Sperm-host glands are tubular glands, lined by tall columnar cells, and are located within the mucosa of the vagina near the uterovaginal junction. Sperm are stored in these glands, remaining functional for up to 21 days.

19

THE EYE

MAMMALS

The eye is a sensory organ designed for vision. Basically, it is composed of a **lens** and a wall that is divided into three layers: an outer **fibrous tunic** (corneoscleral layer), a middle **vascular tunic** (uvea), and an inner **retinal tunic.** The fibrous tunic is divided into the posterior, opaque sclera and the anterior, transparent cornea. The vascular tunic includes the choroid, ciliary body, and iris. The retinal tunic consists of a ten-layered, photosensitive retina and a bilayered, nonphotosensitive portion that covers the ciliary body and the posterior surface of the iris.

The eye contains three fluid-filled regions. The **anterior chamber** is bordered by the cornea, iris, and lens. The **posterior chamber** is located between the iris, lens, zonular fibers, and ciliary processes. Both of these chambers contain aqueous humor. The most posterior compartment, the **cavity of the vitreous humor,** lies behind the lens.

The transparent, biconvex **lens** is avascular. It is composed entirely of epithelial cells enclosed within a homogeneous capsule. The cells on the anterior surface of the lens just below the capsule are simple cuboidal and form the **lens epithelium.** Toward the equator of the lens, the cells become long, prismatic, and arranged in meridional rows, forming **lens fibers.** As new lens fibers develop from the lens epithelium at the germinal zone of the equator, older lens fibers are displaced centrally and lose their nuclei. The lens is suspended by **zonular fibers** that attach to the lens capsule from the ciliary processes.

The **sclera** consists of densely interwoven bundles of collagenous fibers arranged parallel to the surface of the wall of the eye. There are also fibroblasts, some fine elastic fibers, and scattered melanocytes, especially in the innermost region of the sclera.

The **cornea** is avascular. Its anterior (outer) surface is covered by the nonkeratinized, stratified squamous **anterior epithelium.** Below this layer is **Bowman's membrane,** which is not distinct in domestic mammals. The underlying **stroma** (substantia propria) is composed of thin lamellae of collagenous fibers oriented parallel to the corneal surface. Fibroblasts occur between the layers of fibers. **Descemet's membrane** is a relatively thick membrane that separates the stroma from the **posterior epithelium.** The latter consists of a single layer of squamous to low cuboidal cells that covers the posterior surface of the cornea.

The corneoscleral junction is called the **limbus.** Here, the regular collagenous lamellae of the corneal stroma merge with the interwoven fibers of the sclera. The appearance of the stratified squamous epithelium of the cornea differs from that of the bulbar conjunctiva, which overlies the sclera near the limbus. The deepest cells in the epithelium of the bulbar conjunctiva are smaller and more closely packed than those of the anterior epithelium of the cornea. In addition, the basal border of the conjunctival epithelium is uneven with the presence of an underlying, papillated layer of loose connective tissue. The boundary between the corneal epithelium and the underlying stroma, however, is smooth.

The **choroid** is the portion of the vascular tunic of the eye that lies between the sclera and the photosensitive retina. It contains numerous melanocytes. The fine network of connective tissue of the **suprachoroid layer** joins the sclera to the **vascular layer** of the choroid. The latter is composed of a profusion of blood vessels surrounded by loose connective tissue. The **choriocapillary layer** contains a thin network of capillaries that are distributed in a single plane. **Bruch's membrane,** a refractile membrane that lies between the choriocapillary layer and the pigment epithelium of the retina, is difficult to resolve.

A reflective **tapetum lucidum** is located between the choriocapillary and vascular layers of the choroid in the dorsal portion of the eye. It is present in all domestic mammals except the pig. The horse and ruminants have a **fibrous tapetum** composed of layers of collagenous fibers and fibroblasts. The cat and dog have a **cellular tapetum** formed by flattened, pentagonal or hexagonal cells that appear brick-like in profile. The tapetal cells are filled with numerous rod-shaped granules. The flat surfaces of the cells and the long axes of their rod-shaped granules lie parallel to the surface of the retina.

The **ciliary body** is an anterior continuation of the choroid that extends to the base of the iris. The loose connective tissue of the stroma contains smooth muscle, the **ciliary muscle,** that lies peripheral to an inner, vascular region. The epithelium of the ciliary body, which is formed by cells of the nonphotosensitive portion of the retina, is called the **pars ciliaris retinae.** It is a bilayer of cells consisting of a basal layer of pigmented cells and a surface layer of nonpigmented columnar cells. Short folds of the posterior surface of the ciliary body become longer toward the iris and form **ciliary processes** that project toward the lens. Zonular fibers extend from the processes to the lens capsule near the equator of the lens.

The **iris** is the most anterior part of the uveal tract. It forms a thin, contractile diaphragm with a central aperture, the **pupil.** The base of the iris is attached to the anterior portion of the ciliary body. The connective tissue **stroma** of the iris contains many melanocytes and blood vessels. The stroma contains circumferentially arranged bundles of smooth muscle that form the **sphincter** (constrictor) **muscle.** The anterior surface of the iris is not covered by an epithelium, but rather by a discontinuous layer of stromal cells (fibroblasts and melanocytes). The posterior surface is covered by a bilayer of epithelial cells, the **pars iridica retinae,** which represents the most anterior continuation of the nonphotosensitive portion of the retina. It consists of a superficial layer of **pigmented columnar cells** and a basal layer of partially **pigmented myoepithelial cells.** The latter are elongated, radially arranged, contractile cells that form the dilator "muscle" of the iris. They have an apical, pigmented portion containing the nucleus and a nonpigmented basal portion. The nonpigmented regions of these cells border the stroma and appear as an acidophilic band. The pigmented portion of each myoepithelial cell lies just below the layer of pigmented columnar cells. In the horse, pig, and ruminant, a number of **corpora nigra** (iris granules) project from the pupillary margin of the iris. They are highly vascularized proliferations of the stroma and the pigmented epithelial cells of the iris.

At the peripheral margin of the anterior chamber is the **filtration angle,** the area between the limbus, the base of the iris, and the ciliary body. This triangular region is spanned by a latticework of trabeculae and intertrabecular, fluid-filled spaces. The trabeculae are composed of connective tissue and pigment cells, and are covered by a single layer of squamous cells. They form the **pectinate ligament,** the **uveal trabecular meshwork,** and the **corneoscleral trabecular meshwork.** At the peripheral margin of the anterior chamber, excess aqueous humor passes through the openings between the pectinate ligament into the **spaces of Fontana** within the uveal trabecular meshwork. These spaces communicate with those of the corneoscleral trabecular meshwork, which drain into the **scleral venous plexus.** In the horse, the limbus does not overlap the pectinate ligament of the filtration angle, so that the pectinate ligament is apparent by direct examination of the eye. In the other domestic mammals, the limbus covers the pectinate ligament, which is, therefore, obscured from view by the opaque sclera.

The **retina** is the innermost layer of the wall of the eye. The photosensitive portion lines the inner surface of the eye (adjacent to the cavity of the vitreous humor) posteriorly from the **ora ciliaris retinae.** The latter is the point of transition from the photosensitive retina to the nonphotosensitive retina. From the ora ciliaris retinae, the nonphotosensitive portion continues anteriorly as a bilayer of cells, forming the pars ciliaris retinae and the pars iridica retinae, which cover the ciliary body and the posterior surface of the iris, respectively.

From the choroid to the cavity of the vitreous humor, the 10 layers of the photosensitive retina are: **pigment epithelium, layer of rods and cones, outer limiting membrane** (usually not apparent), **outer nuclear layer, outer plexiform layer, inner nuclear layer, inner plexiform layer, ganglion cell layer, nerve fiber layer,** and **inner limiting membrane.** In the region of the eye where the tapetum is present in the choroid, the cuboidal cells of the pigment epithelium of the retina contain few or no pigment granules. Pigment granules are numerous where a tapetum is absent.

The nerve fiber layer consists of axonal processes of the ganglion cells that converge at the **optic disc** and form the optic nerve. Because photoreceptor cells are not present here, this region is also referred to as the blind spot. Bundles of fibers of the optic nerve pass through perforations of the sclera. This sievelike part of the sclera is the **lamina cribrosa.**

The **conjunctiva** is a thin transparent mucous membrane. The **bulbar conjunctiva** is continuous with the anterior surface of the cornea at the limbus and covers the sclera for a short distance. The **palpebral conjunctiva** lines the internal surface of the eyelids. The **fornix of the conjunctiva** is the point of reflexion of the bulbar and palpebral conjunctiva. The epithelium of the conjunctiva varies from stratified squamous to stratified columnar, and may even appear transitional. Goblet cells are often present. The underlying layer of loose connective tissue may contain diffuse or nodular lymphatic tissue.

The **eyelids** are covered internally by the palpebral conjunctiva and externally by thin skin. The skin contains hair follicles, **sweat glands** (glands of Moll), and sebaceous glands (glands of Zeiss). In the pig, the glands are particularly well developed. Between the dermis of the skin and the lamina propria of the palpebral conjunctiva is a plate of dense connective tissue, the **tarsus** (tarsal plate). Large, multilobular sebaceous glands, called **tarsal** (Meibomian) **glands,** are embedded in the tarsus. Their central ducts open onto the palpebral surface near its junction with the skin.

The **nictitating membrane** (third eyelid) is a ventromedial fold of conjunctiva. It is supported by hyaline cartilage in the dog and ruminants, and by elastic cartilage in the cat, horse, and pig. The **superficial gland of the nictitating membrane** surrounds the base of the cartilage. It is a serous gland in the horse and cat, mixed in the dog and ruminants, and mucous in the pig. The pig also has a **Harderian gland** (deep gland of the nictitating membrane) that produces a fatty secretion.

The **lacrimal gland** is a tubuloacinar gland, serous in the cat and mixed in the horse, ruminant, dog, and pig. It is predominantly a mucous gland in the pig and mostly serous in the horse and ruminant. There are also accessory lacrimal glands, such as Krause's gland, which may be serous or mixed.

CHICKEN

The eye of the chicken is quite different from that of mammals. Within the **capsule,** the **lens** is divided into the **annular pad** and the **lens body.** The annular pad forms an outer ring around the equator of the lens body. It consists of radially arranged lens fibers with peripheral nuclei. In the lens body, the lens fibers are oriented parallel to the optical axis of the eye, and some nuclei are present, primarily near the annular pad.

A remarkable feature of the avian **sclera** is the presence of a ring of overlapping **scleral ossicles** anteriorly, and a cup-shaped layer of hyaline cartilage, the **scleral cartilage,** posteriorly. The latter terminates internal to the scleral ossicles. Dense connective tissue encloses the scleral ossicles and extends posteriorly, peripheral to the cartilage layer.

The layers of the **cornea** of the chicken are similar to those of mammals. Bowman's membrane, however, is thicker and therefore more apparent in histologic preparations. Decemet's membrane is relatively thin and less distinct.

The **choroid** is a thick vascularized coat with numerous pigment cells. The suprachoroid abuts the thin perichondrium of the scleral cartilage. The vascular layer of the choroid contains blood vessels and large spaces embedded in loose connective tissue. The choriocapillary layer is separated from the pigment epithelium of the retina by an indistinct Bruch's membrane. No tapetum lucidum is present.

The **ciliary body** is a thin layer of loose connective tissue with a thick outer region of numerous elastic fibers. It is covered by a bilayer of more or less cuboidal pigmented basal cells and cuboidal to columnar, nonpigmented surface cells. Folds of the lining of the ciliary body form ciliary processes that fuse to the lens capsule in the region of the equator of the lens. More posteriorly, zonular fibers extend from the ciliary body to the lens capsule. The ciliary muscles (Crampton's and Brücke's) are skeletal muscles that lie across from the ciliary body, just inside the main portion of the sclera.

The **iris** is thickest just above its narrow base, then tapers toward the pupillary margin. The stroma contains a sphincter and dilator muscle. Both of these are formed from small skeletal muscle cells that contain lipid vacuoles. The dilator muscle is sparse and posterior to the thicker sphincter muscle. The anterior (corneal) surface of the iris is covered by a simple layer of nonpigmented, flattened epithelial cells. The posterior (lens) surface is covered by a stratified layer of pigmented epithelial cells, three to five cells thick.

The photosensitive **retina** of the chicken is composed of 10 layers, as in mammals, but unlike in mammals is avascular. The cells of the pigment epithelium are considerably different in the chicken. They are tall and narrow rather than cuboidal. The nucleus occupies the smaller, basal region of each cell, which contains few or no pigment granules. The apical portion is filled with rod-shaped pigment granules that are oriented parallel to the long axis of the cell. The apical cytoplasm often appears to be separated into tufts or strands of pigment granules.

The **pecten** is a thin, highly vascular, pleated membrane that protrudes into the cavity of the vitreous humor from the ventral surface of the eye. Its base is secured intermittently to the linear, optic disc. The apical surface is attached to a thickened mass of pectineal tissue called the **bridge.** The pecten is characterized by an extensive network of capillaries lined by thick endothelial cells with plump nuclei. Polymorphic pigment cells fill the spaces between the capillaries and larger vessels. The pecten is draped by a **covering membrane,** which is thought to be continuous with the inner limiting membrane of the retina.

The **filtration angle** of the chicken is somewhat different from that of mammals. It is filled by a trabecular meshwork formed by the **pectinate ligament** (uveal meshwork) and the **scleral trabecular meshwork.** The pectinate ligament is a loose network of elastic fibers covered by simple squamous cells. It spans the filtration angle from the scleral trabecular meshwork to the iris and the elastic tissue of the ciliary body. The trabecular meshwork of the pectinate ligament encloses the **spaces of Fontana.** The latter communicate with the spaces of the scleral trabecular meshwork, which is formed by collagenous and elastic fibers. These spaces communicate with the **canal of Schlemm** within the sclera.

The chicken has a thin, well developed **nictitating membrane.** A supportive cartilage is absent. The inner surface of the **eyelids** is lined by the palpebral conjunctiva. The external surface is covered by thin skin with sparse feathers. No glands are present.

The **lacrimal gland** is a small, tubular gland that produces a mucous secretion. It lies medial to the caudal part of the lower eyelid. The **Harderian gland** is a larger gland that lies on the dorsal posterior surface of the eye. It is characterized by numerous plasma cells that surround the tubular secretory units.

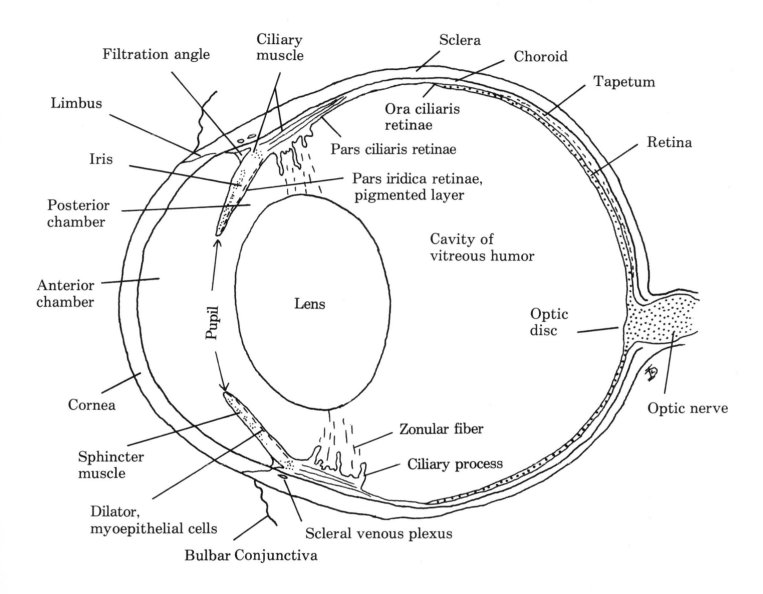

FIG. 19–1. Eye, sagittal section, Dog.

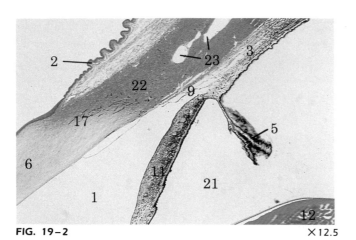

FIG. 19-2 ×12.5

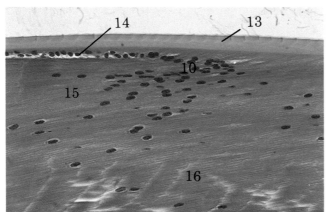

FIG. 19-3 ×125

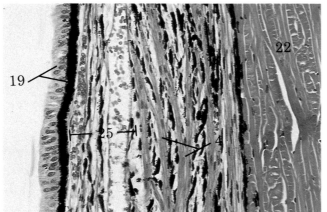

FIG. 19-4 ×125

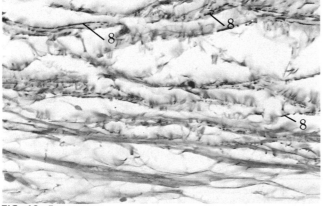

FIG. 19-5 ×250

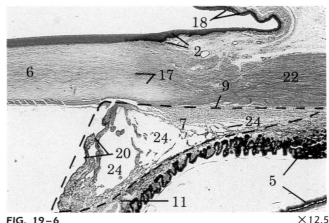

FIG. 19-6 ×12.5

KEY	
1. Anterior chamber	**13.** Lens capsule
2. Bulbar conjunctiva	**14.** Lens epithelium
3. Ciliary body	**15.** Lens fibers, new
4. Ciliary muscle	**16.** Lens fibers, old
5. Ciliary process	**17.** Limbus
6. Cornea	**18.** Palpebral conjunctiva
7. Corneoscleral trabecular meshwork	**19.** Pars ciliaris retinae
8. Elastic fiber	**20.** Pectinate ligament
9. Filtration angle	**21.** Posterior chamber
10. Germinal zone	**22.** Sclera
11. Iris	**23.** Scleral venous plexus
12. Lens	**24.** Spaces of Fontana
	25. Vascular layer, choroid

FIG. 19-2. Eye, Dog. Anterior, peripheral portion of the eye.

FIG. 19-3. Lens, Equator, Horse. Newly formed and older lens fibers are visible in this section through the germinal zone. The latter is the marginal band of lens epithelium that lies around the equator. Its cells are capable of dividing throughout adult life.

FIG. 19-4. Ciliary Body, Dog. The epithelium of the ciliary body is called the pars ciliaris retinae. This portion of the nonphotosensitive retina consists of an inner (closer to the cavity of the vitreous humor) nonpigmented layer, and an outer heavily pigmented layer of cells.

FIG. 19-5. Ciliary Body, Cat, Orcein. In addition to smooth muscle (see Fig. 19-4), the ciliary body contains an abundance of elastic fibers.

FIG. 19-6. Eye, Horse. In a section through a horse's eye, the limbus does not overlap the pectinate ligament. Compare with Fig. 19-7. The filtration angle is indicated by the triangular-shaped area marked by the dashed line.

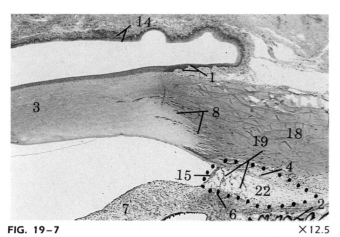

FIG. 19–7   ×12.5

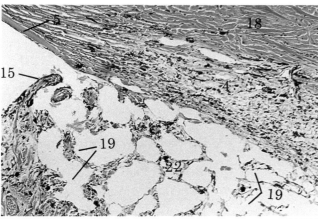

FIG. 19–8   ×62.5

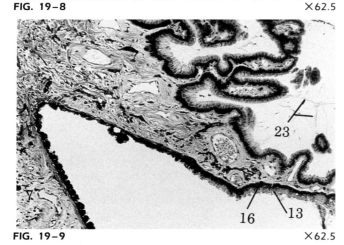

FIG. 19–9   ×62.5

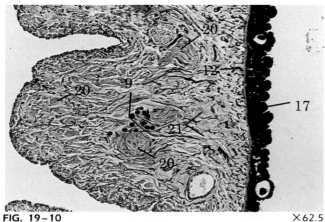

FIG. 19–10   ×62.5

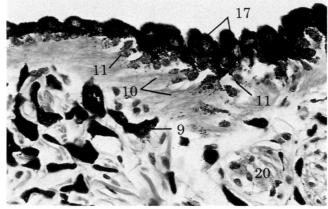

FIG. 19–11   ×250

KEY	
1. Bulbar conjunctiva	**12.** Myoepithelial cells
2. Ciliary process	**13.** Nonpigmented cells
3. Cornea	**14.** Palpebral conjunctiva
4. Corneoscleral trabecular meshwork	**15.** Pectinate ligament
5. Decemet's membrane	**16.** Pigmented cells
6. Filtration angle	**17.** Pigmented surface cells
7. Iris	**18.** Sclera
8. Limbus	**19.** Spaces of Fontana
9. Melanocyte	**20.** Sphincter muscle
10. Myoepithelial cell, cytoplasm	**21.** Stroma
11. Myoepithelial cell, nucleus	**22.** Uveal trabecular meshwork
	23. Zonular fibers

FIG. 19–7. Eye, Pig. In a section through the eye of a domestic mammal other than the horse, the limbus overlaps the pectinate ligament. The area of the filtration angle is outlined by dots.

FIG. 19–8. Filtration Angle, Pig. Collagenous fibers, elastic fibers, fibroblasts, and pigment cells form the pectinate ligament and the uveal trabecular meshwork. The corneoscleral trabecular meshwork is a three-dimensional latticework of fine connective tissue fibers and fibroblasts lying adjacent to the sclera.

FIG. 19–9. Ciliary Processes, Pig. The nonpigmented cells of the epithelium of the ciliary processes cover the pigmented cells. Together these two layers of cells comprise the pars ciliaris retinae, which extends from the ora ciliaris retinae to the iris. The nonpigmented cells give rise to the zonular fibers.

FIG. 19–10. Iris, Horse. The back surface of the iris is covered by a continuation of the pars ciliaris retinae and is called the pars iridica retinae. The surface layer of the pars iridica retinae consists of heavily pigmented cells, and its inner layer is formed by the contractile, pigmented myoepithelial cells that dilate the iris. Anteriorly, the iris is covered by a discontinuous layer of stromal cells.

FIG. 19–11. Iris, Dog. The heavily pigmented cells of the pars iridica retinae cover the posterior surface of the iris. The myoepithelial cells of the pars iridica retinae are partially pigmented in the region of their nuclei.

FIG. 19-12   ×625

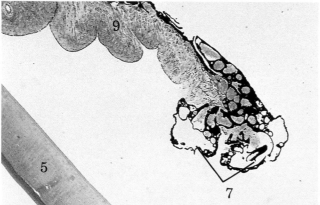

FIG. 19-13   ×12.5

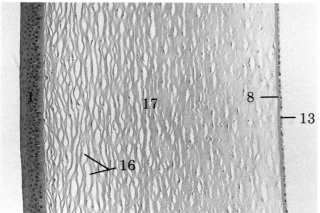

FIG. 19-14   ×62.5

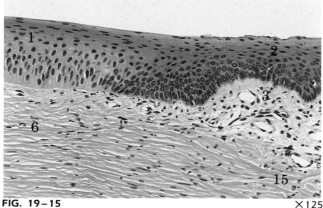

FIG. 19-15   ×125

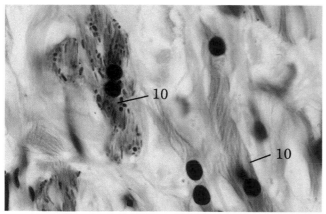

FIG. 19-16   ×62.5

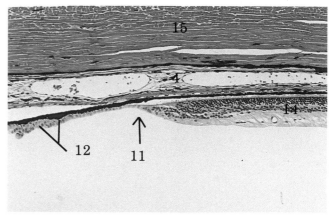

KEY	
1. Anterior epithelium	**9.** Iris
2. Bulbar conjunctiva, epithelium	**10.** Melanocyte
	11. Ora ciliaris retinae
3. Bulbar conjunctiva, lamina propria	**12.** Pars ciliaris retinae
	13. Posterior epithelium
4. Choroid	**14.** Retina, photosensitive
5. Cornea	**15.** Sclera
6. Corneal stroma	**16.** Space artifacts
7. Corpus nigrum	**17.** Stroma
8. Descemet's membrane	

FIG. 19-12. Iris, Cat. In the cat, melanocytes of the iris are binucleate and contain rod-shaped melanosomes.

FIG. 19-13. Corpus Nigrum, Goat. In ungulates, the pupillary border of the iris is differentiated into corpora nigra, which are vascularized outgrowths of the stroma and pigmented epithelium of the iris.

FIG. 19-14. Cornea, Dog. The anterior surface is covered by a nonkeratinized stratified squamous epithelium. The posterior surface is covered by squamous or low cuboidal cells.

FIG. 19-15. Junction of Cornea and Bulbar Conjunctiva, Pig. Both the cornea and bulbar conjunctiva are covered by a nonkeratinized stratified squamous epithelium at their junction. The basal border of the conjunctiva is irregular and the cells of its deepest layers are smaller than those of the anterior epithelium of the cornea.

FIG. 19-16. Ora Ciliaris Retinae, Dog. The transition zone between the photosensitive and the nonphotosensitive (pars ciliaris retinae) regions of the retina.

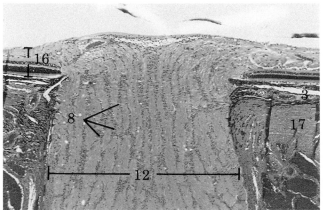

FIG. 19–17   ×25

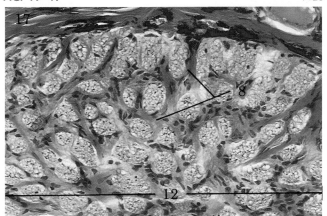

FIG. 19–18   ×125

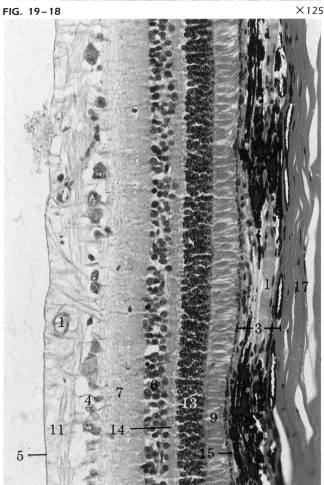

FIG. 19–19   ×180

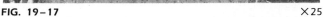

FIG. 19–20   ×250

KEY	
1. Blood vessel	**11.** Nerve fiber layer
2. Choriocapillary layer	**12.** Optic nerve
3. Choroid	**13.** Outer nuclear layer
4. Ganglion cell layer	**14.** Outer plexiform layer
5. Inner limiting membrane	**15.** Pigment epithelium
6. Inner nuclear layer	**16.** Retina
7. Inner plexiform layer	**17.** Sclera
8. Lamina cribrosa	**18.** Tapetum
9. Layer of rods and cones	**19.** Vascular layer, choroid
10. Melanocytes	

FIG. 19–17. Optic Nerve, sagittal section, Dog. Nerve fibers of the retina converge to form the optic nerve at the optic disc (blind spot).

FIG. 19–18. Lamina Cribrosa, x.s., Dog. At the lamina cribrosa the connective tissue of the sclera forms a sievelike framework, which subdivides the optic nerve into bundles of fibers.

FIG. 19–19. Retina, Choroid, and Part of the Sclera, Pig. Note that the dendrites (cones) of cone cells of the pig are particularly plump and easily recognized.

FIG. 19–20. Fibrous Tapetum, Sheep. The tapetum of ruminants and horses is a compact connective tissue membrane sandwiched between the choriocapillary and vascular layers of the choroid. The cells of the pigment epithelium of the retina contain few or no pigment granules where a tapetum is present.

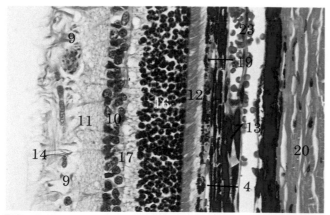

FIG. 19–21   ×250

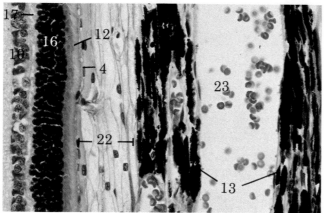

FIG. 19–22   ×250

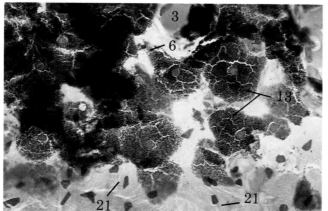

FIG. 19–23   ×250

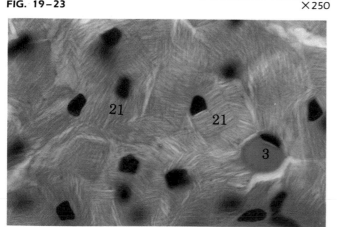

FIG. 19–24   ×625

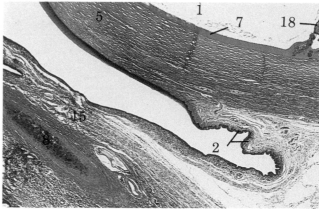

FIG. 19–25   ×12.5

KEY	
1. Anterior chamber	**13.** Melanocytes
2. Bulbar conjunctiva	**14.** Nerve fiber layer
3. Capillary, x.s.	**15.** Nictitating membrane,
4. Choriocapillary layer	bulbar surface
5. Cornea	**16.** Outer nuclear layer
6. Cytoplasmic process	**17.** Outer plexiform layer
7. Descemet's membrane	**18.** Pectinate ligament
8. Elastic cartilage	**19.** Pigment epithelium
9. Ganglion cell layer	**20.** Sclera
10. Inner nuclear layer	**21.** Tapetal cell
11. Inner plexiform layer	**22.** Tapetum lucidum
12. Layer of rods and cones	**23.** Vascular layer, choroid

FIG. 19–21. Retina, Choroid, and Part of the Sclera, Dog. Where the tapetum lucidum is lacking from the choroid layer, the cells of the pigment epithelium of the retina contain numerous melanosomes.

FIG. 19–22. Cellular Tapetum, Dog. In profile, the cells of the tapetum lucidum of carnivores are brick-like. Note that in this section the cells of the pigment epithelium of the retina are indistinct (compare with Fig. 19–21).

FIG. 19–23. Melanocytes of Choroid Layer, Dog. Melanocytes of the choroid layer are flat polygonal cells with cytoplasmic processes. Their polygonal shape is evident in this tangential cut through the choroid layer.

FIG. 19–24. Tapetum Lucidum, Dog. Tapetal cells are flattened and have a pentagonal or hexagonal outline, which is apparent in this tangential section through the choroid layer. The cells are filled with numerous small rods, whose long axes parallel the flat surfaces of the cells.

FIG. 19–25. Nictitating Membrane and Cornea, Horse. A portion of the bulbar surface of the nictitating membrane and its supportive cartilage are shown. The nictitating membrane is a fold of the ventromedial portion of the conjunctiva. It contains elastic cartilage in the horse, pig, and cat, and hyaline cartilage in the dog and ruminants.

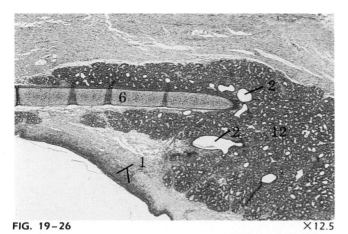

FIG. 19–26 ×12.5

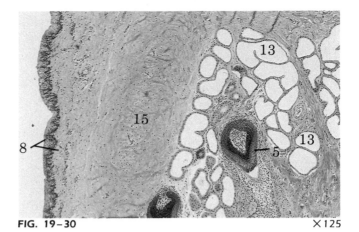

FIG. 19–30 ×125

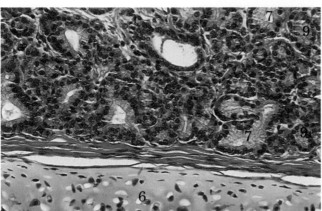

FIG. 19–27 ×125

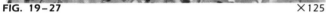
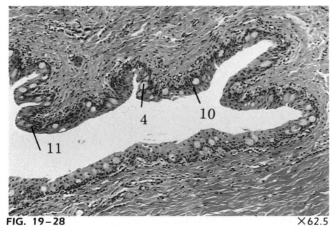

FIG. 19–28 ×62.5

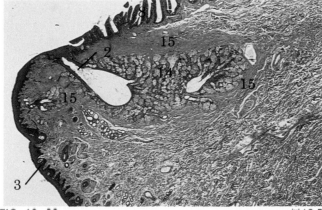

FIG. 19–29 ×12.5

KEY	
1. Diffuse lymphatic tissue	**10.** Stratified columnar
2. Duct	epithelium
3. Epidermis	**11.** Stratified squamous
4. Goblet cell	epithelium
5. Hair follicle	**12.** Superficial gland
6. Hyaline cartilage	**13.** Sweat gland
7. Mucous acinus	**14.** Tarsal gland
8. Palpebral conjunctiva	**15.** Tarsus
9. Serous acinus	

FIG. 19–26. Superficial Gland of the Nictitating Membrane, Dog. The base of the cartilage of the nictitating membrane is surrounded by the superficial gland.

FIG. 19–27. Superficial Gland of the Nictitating Membrane, Dog. This gland is mixed in the dog and ruminants. It is serous in the horse and cat, and mucous in the pig.

FIG. 19–28. Palpebral Conjunctiva, Pig. The palpebral conjunctiva is a mucous membrane that lines the inner surface of the eyelid. Its stratified epithelium varies from squamous through columnar, and may even appear transitional. Goblet cells may be present.

FIG. 19–29. Eyelid, Lower, Horse. The outer surface of the eyelid is covered by thin skin, while the inner surface is lined by the palpebral conjunctiva. The tarsal gland is a multilobulated gland whose duct opens onto the palpebral surface near the margin of the eyelid. The tarsal gland is surrounded by a condensed layer of connective tissue, the tarsus.

FIG. 19–30. Eyelid, Upper, Pig. Numerous tubular sweat glands (and sebaceous glands, not shown) occur in the skin surface of the eyelid of the pig.

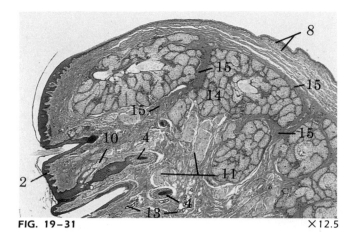

FIG. 19-31   ×12.5

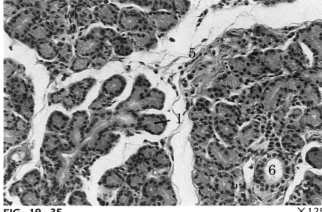

FIG. 19-35   ×125

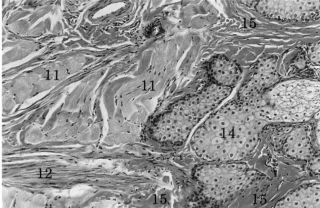

FIG. 19-32   ×62.5

FIG. 19-31. Eyelid, Lower, Goat. The skin surface of the eyelid contains hair follicles, sweat glands, and sebaceous glands.

FIG. 19-32. Eyelid, Lower, Goat. Bundles of smooth and skeletal muscle fibers are scattered in the connective tissue between the tarsus and the skin surface of the eyelid.

FIG. 19-33. Krause's Gland, Pig. Krause's gland is a small accessory lacrimal gland (serous in this preparation) located near the fornix of the conjunctiva.

FIG. 19-34. Harderian Gland, Pig. Among domestic mammals, this gland is present only in the pig. It secretes a fatty product.

FIG. 19-35. Lacrimal Gland, Cow. A compound tubular acinar gland. The lacrimal gland is predominantly a serous gland in ruminants and horses.

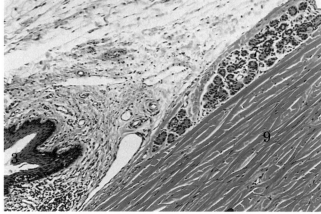

FIG. 19-33   ×62.5

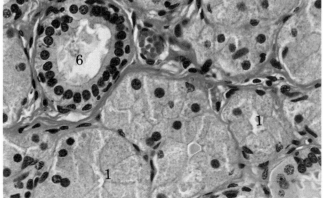

FIG. 19-34   ×250

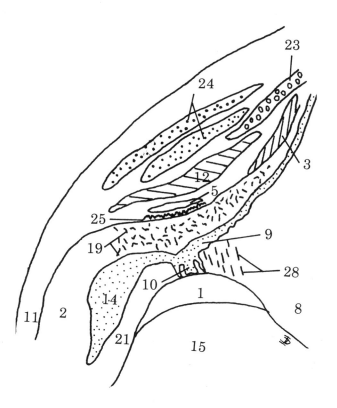

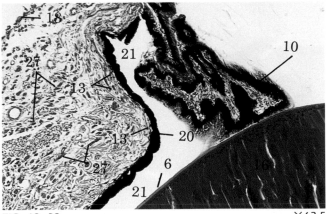

FIG. 19–39 ×62.5

KEY	
1. Annular pad	**16.** Lens fibers, annular pad
2. Anterior chamber	**17.** Lens fibers, lens body
3. Brücke's muscle	**18.** Nonpigmented epithelium, iris
4. Bulbar conjunctiva	
5. Canal of Schlemm	**19.** Pectinate ligament
6. Capsule	**20.** Pigmented epithelium, iris
7. Cavity of the lens	**21.** Posterior chamber
8. Cavity of vitreous humor	**22.** Sclera
9. Ciliary body	**23.** Scleral cartilage
10. Ciliary process	**24.** Scleral ossicle
11. Cornea	**25.** Scleral trabecular meshwork
12. Crampton's muscle	
13. Dilator muscle	**26.** Spaces of Fontana
14. Iris	**27.** Sphincter muscle
15. Lens body	**28.** Zonular fibers

FIG. 19–36. Eye, Anterolateral Segment, Chicken.

FIG. 19–37. Lens, Chicken. A portion of the annular pad and lens body.

FIG. 19–38. Filtration Angle, Chicken. The filtration angle is bordered by the cornea, iris, ciliary body, and sclera in the chicken. It is bridged by a trabecular meshwork of the pectinate ligament, which encloses the spaces of Fontana.

FIG. 19–39. Ciliary Process, Chicken, Masson's. Ciliary processes occur below the base of the iris and fuse with the lens capsule of the annular pad. The ciliary epithelium also attaches to the capsule by zonular fibers.

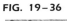
FIG. 19–36

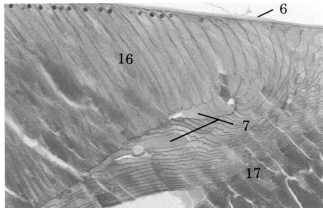

FIG. 19–37 ×125

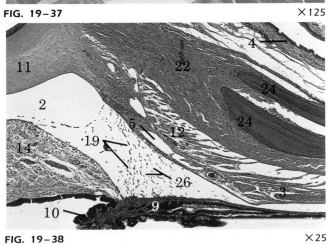

FIG. 19–38 ×25

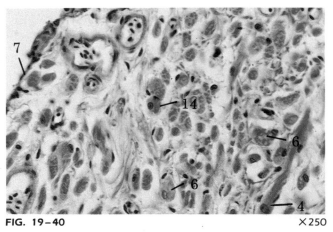

FIG. 19-40 ×250

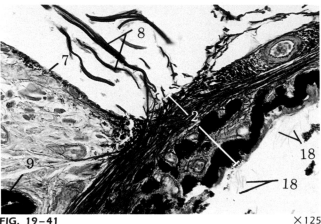

FIG. 19-41 ×125

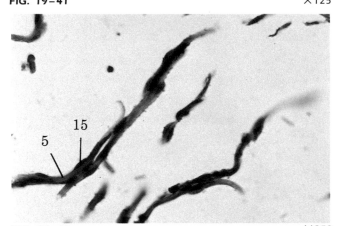

FIG. 19-42 ×250

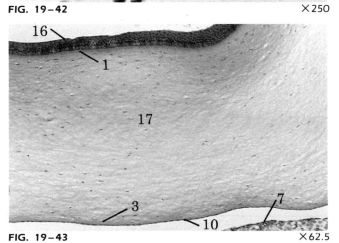

FIG. 19-43 ×62.5

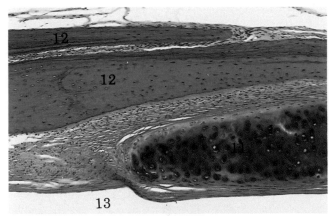

FIG. 19-44 ×62.5

KEY	
1. Bowman's membrane	**10.** Posterior epithelium
2. Ciliary body	**11.** Scleral cartilage
3. Decemet's membrane	**12.** Scleral ossicle
4. Dilator muscle cell	**13.** Space artifact
5. Elastic fiber	**14.** Sphincter muscle cell
6. Lipid vacuole	**15.** Squamous cell, nucleus
7. Nonpigmented epithelium, iris	**16.** Stratified squamous epithelium
8. Pectinate ligament	**17.** Stroma
9. Pigmented epithelium, iris	**18.** Zonular fibers

FIG. 19-40. Iris, Chicken. The iridial musculature of the chicken is composed of skeletal muscle cells, which are characterized by the presence of numerous lipid vacuoles. Unlike mammals, the corneal surface of the iris is covered by a layer of flattened, nonpigmented epithelial cells. The lens surface of the iris (see Fig. 13-39) is covered by a stratified pigmented epithelium that is three to five cells thick.

FIG. 19-41. Junction of Ciliary Body and Iris, Chicken, Orcein. The elastic fibers of the pectinate ligament insert into an elastic meshwork of the ciliary body.

FIG. 19-42. Pectinate Ligament, Chicken. The elastic fibers of the pectinate ligament are covered by a simple squamous epithelium.

FIG. 19-43. Cornea, Chicken. A well developed Bowman's membrane separates the anterior, stratified squamous epithelium of the cornea from the underlying stroma.

FIG. 19-44. Sclera, Chicken. The sclera is strengthened anteriorly by overlapping bony plates (scleral ossicles). Posteriorly, it consists of a thin layer of cartilage. The region of overlap of these skeletal elements is shown here. In this section, the ciliary body has separated from the sclera, creating a space artifact.

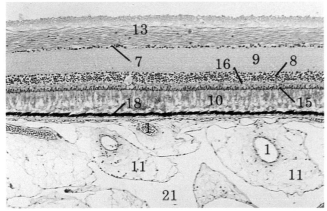

FIG. 19-45   ×62.5

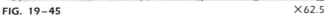

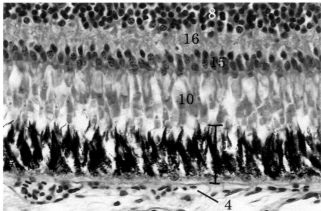

FIG. 19-46   ×250

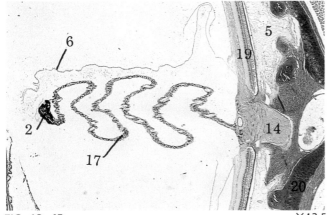

FIG. 19-47   ×12.5

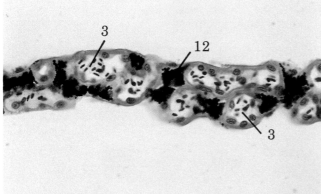

FIG. 19-48   ×250

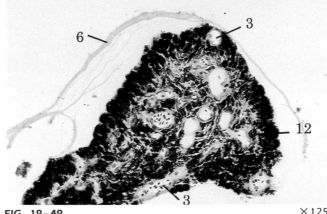

FIG. 19-49   ×125

KEY	
1. Blood vessels	**12.** Melanocyte
2. Bridge	**13.** Nerve fiber layer
3. Capillary	**14.** Optic nerve
4. Choriocapillary layer	**15.** Outer nuclear layer
5. Choroid	**16.** Outer plexiform layer
6. Covering membrane	**17.** Pecten
7. Ganglion cell layer	**18.** Pigment epithelium
8. Inner nuclear layer	**19.** Retina
9. Inner plexiform layer	**20.** Scleral cartilage
10. Layer of rods and cones	**21.** Space
11. Loose connective tissue	

FIG. 19-45. Retina and Choroid, Chicken. The bulk of the choroid is composed of blood vessels and large spaces supported by a loose connective tissue. The layers of the retina are comparable to those of mammals.

FIG. 19-46. Retina and Choroid, Chicken. Cells of the pigment epithelium of the retina are tall and contain rod-shaped pigment granules. The basal region of each cell contains the nucleus and a few pigment granules.

FIG. 19-47. Pecten, Chicken. The pecten is a thin, folded, and heavily pigmented membrane that projects into the vitreous humor from the posteroventral surface of the eye.

FIG. 19-48. Pecten, Chicken. Numerous, polymorphic melanocytes are interspersed through this highly vascularized, nutritive membrane. The large capillaries are lined by thick endothelial cells with plump nuclei.

FIG. 19-49. Bridge of Pecten, Chicken. This thickened, highly pigmented mass of pectineal tissue is located along the free edge of the pecten.

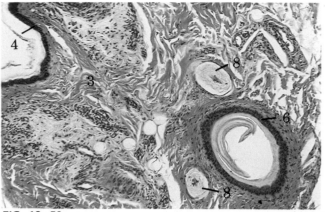

FIG. 19–50   ×62.5

FIG. 19–50. Eyelid, Chicken. A thin epidermis covers the eyelid. Herbst corpuscles are associated with a feather follicle.

FIG. 19–51. Lacrimal Gland, Chicken. This compound tubular gland produces a mucoid secretion and is organized into lobules.

FIG. 19–52. Harderian Gland, Chicken. This accessory immunologic gland contains a multitude of plasma cells. It is located on the dorsal posterior surface of the eye.

FIG. 19–53. Harderian Gland, Chicken. Detail of the Harderian gland showing numerous plasma cells surrounding the vacuolated cells of the tubular secretory units.

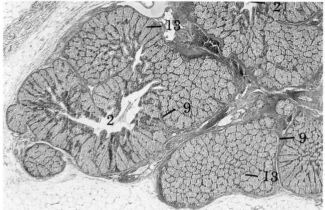

FIG. 19–51   ×25

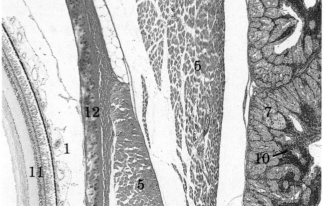

FIG. 19–52   ×25

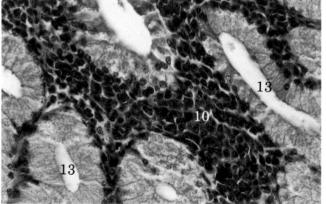

FIG. 19–53   ×250

THE EAR

Sensations of sound and balance are received by separate and specialized areas of the ear before being transmitted to the brain, where they are interpreted. Based on anatomy, location, and function, the ear is divisible into external, middle, and internal components. The **external ear** collects sound waves, which it channels to the tympanic membrane. Vibrations produced in the latter are transmitted by the ossicles of the **middle ear** to fluids of the **internal ear,** where they generate movements of the delicate basilar membrane. Such movements stimulate sensory hair cells from which impulses are relayed by sensory nerves to the brain, where the sound is identified.

MAMMALS

The external ear of domestic mammals is comprised of the **pinna** (auricle), which collects sound, and an **external auditory meatus,** which conveys the sound waves to the **tympanic membrane.**

The external auditory meatus is lined by a continuation of the surface skin. Hair, sebaceous glands, and tubular ceruminous glands are present. The combined secretions of these glands, plus sloughed epithelial cells, form cerumen (ear wax). The initial portion of the meatus is supported by cartilage, the remainder by bone.

Middle ear ossicles **(malleus, incus,** and **stapes)** are located in the **tympanic cavity.** They bridge the cavity from the tympanic membrane to the oval window located within the petrous part of the temporal bone.

The tympanic cavity is surrounded by bone. The tympanic membrane forms the lateral wall of the cavity. It is composed of a thin outer layer of epithelium that is continuous with the skin of the external auditory meatus, a thin connective tissue layer, and an inner layer of simple squamous or cuboidal epithelium. The remainder of the cavity is lined by ciliated columnar and simple squamous cells. The latter cover the ossicles as well as portions of the wall of the cavity.

The **membranous labyrinth** of the inner ear consists of the **cochlear duct, sacculus, utriculus,** and **semicircular ducts.** Cavities within the petrous segment of the temporal bone, lined by periosteum and containing **perilymph** (a fluid similar to cerebrospinal fluid), house the membranous labyrinth. Those cavities containing the semicircular ducts are called the **semicircular canals;** the one containing the sacculus and utriculus is called the **vestibule;** and the one containing the **cochlear duct** (membranous cochlea) is named the **cochlear canal** (bony cochlea, scala media). The cochlear canal spirals like a snail shell around a central pillar of bone, the **modiolus.** A thin shelf of bone, the **osseous spiral lamina,** travels up the modiolus like the thread of a screw. The number of turns in the cochlear canal varies. There are two and one half in the horse, three in the cat, and four in the pig, for example.

Each semicircular duct is lined by a mesothelium, is filled with **endolymph,** and bears an expansion, the **ampulla.** A sensory structure, the **crista ampullaris,** is located in each ampulla. The **sensory hair cells** and **supporting cells** of each crista are covered by a **gelatinous cupula.** When the latter is deflected during rotational movements of the head, the sensory cells are stimulated and impulses are sent to the brain, where the signals are interpreted.

Both the sacculus and utriculus are filled with endolymph and are lined, in part, by **maculae,** which are patch-like collections of sensory hair cells and supporting cells. The remainder of these structures is lined by mesothelium. Embedded in the outer surface of the gelatinous otolithic membrane covering the maculae are numerous crystalline particles of calcium carbonate called **otoliths** (otoconia or statoconia). As the membrane shifts in response to gravity acting upon the otoliths, sensory cells of the maculae are stimulated. Impulses sent to the brain in response to the stimulus make the animal aware of the position of its head in space. The maculae also detect linear acceleration or deceleration of the head because of the inertia provided to their otolithic membranes by the weight of the otoliths.

The spirally organized cochlear duct is filled with endolymph and is roughly triangular in cross section. One side of the duct is attached to the **spiral ligament,** a thickening of the periosteal lining of the cochlear canal.

This side consists of a stratified cuboidal epithelium, the **stria vascularis.** Capillaries occur among the superficial cuboidal cells of the stria. The side of the duct opposite the stria is pointed. The floor of the duct is formed from the fibrous **basilar membrane,** which extends from the spiral ligament to the osseous spiral lamina. The roof is formed from the **vestibular** (Reissner's) **membrane.** This consists of two adjacent layers of simple squamous epithelium. Above the roof is a large chamber, the **scala vestibuli,** which is filled with perilymph. Below the floor of the cochlear duct is another large chamber filled with perilymph, the **scala tympani.** All three scalas follow a spiral path to the top of the cochlear canal. At the apex, the scala vestibuli communicates with the scala tympani through a tiny opening called the **helicotrema.**

The upper surface of the basilar membrane supports the acoustically sensitive **organ of Corti,** which is bathed by the endolymph within the cochlear duct. The lower surface of the basilar membrane is lined by a simple squamous epithelium which faces the scala tympani. The organ of Corti is comprised of sensory hair cells and various different supporting cells. Overlying the organ of Corti and extending from the **spiral limbus** (an elevation of connective tissue above the osseous spiral lamina) is the proteinaceous, **tectorial membrane.** Stereocilia of the sensory cells contact the tectorial membrane. The stereocilia are displaced when the basilar membrane vibrates in response to sound waves passing through the fluid-filled scalas. The sensory cells respond to this perturbation by initiating impulses in the cochlear nerve, which are transmitted to the brain for interpretation. The stimulatory sound waves are dissipated through the secondary tympanic membrane of the round window located in the lower part of the medial wall of the tympanic cavity.

CHICKEN

The ear of the chicken consists of the same basic components as that of the mammal, but there are some differences.

Although an external auditory meatus is present in the chicken, it is relatively short, and there is no pinna.

The middle ear is lined by a cuboidal epithelium that also covers the columella, a single partially ossified rod, which extends from the tympanic membrane to the oval window. The columella transmits vibrations from the tympanic membrane to the internal ear, taking the place of the malleus, incus, and stapes of mammals.

Unlike that of mammals, the sacculus of the internal ear contains two maculae. The cochlear duct is a short, narrow, slightly curved tube. It possesses a terminal expansion, the **lagena,** a structure peculiar to birds. The lagena contains a macula that is similar in structure and function to other maculae (see under Mammals). The cochlear duct is separated from the overlying scala vestibuli by the **tegmentum vasculosum.** The latter is composed of a thin connective tissue membrane integrated with a highly folded epithelium containing numerous blood vessels. The epithelium faces the cavity of the cochlear duct. The tegmentum occupies the same position as the vestibular membrane in mammals. The common wall separating the cochlear duct from the scala tympani below is formed from the basilar membrane, a platform that supports the organ of Corti (papilla acustica or basilaris). As in mammals, the organ of Corti is composed of sensory and supporting cells, and is overlain by a tectorial membrane that is in contact with the sensory hairs (stereocilia) of the sensory cells.

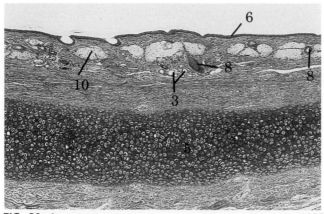

FIG. 20–1 ×25

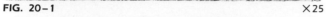

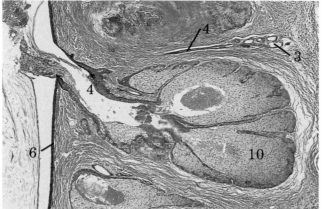

FIG. 20–2 ×25

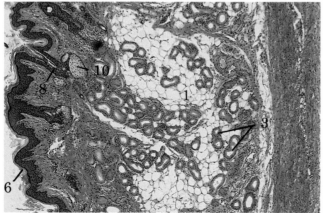

FIG. 20–3 ×25

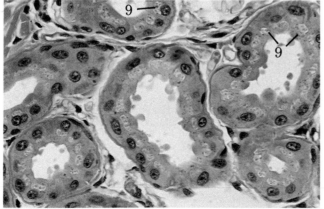

FIG. 20–4 ×250

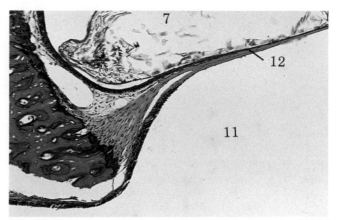

FIG. 20–5 ×62.5

KEY	
1. Adipose tissue	**7.** External auditory meatus
2. Bone	**8.** Hair follicle
3. Ceruminous gland	**9.** Pigment granules
4. Duct	**10.** Sebaceous gland
5. Elastic cartilage	**11.** Tympanic cavity
6. Epidermis	**12.** Tympanic membrane

FIG. 20–1. External Auditory Meatus, Puppy. The outer portion of the meatus is supported by elastic cartilage. The thin epidermis is underlain by numerous sebaceous glands and a few ceruminous glands. Small hair follicles are present.

FIG. 20–2. External Auditory Meatus, Puppy. The external auditory meatus, near the tympanic membrane, contains large sebaceous glands.

FIG. 20–3. External Auditory Meatus, Goat. Outer portion of the meatus with numerous ceruminous glands. Hair follicles and portions of sebaceous glands are also present.

FIG. 20–4. Ceruminous Gland, Goat. The secretory epithelium of these apocrine glands varies from cuboidal to columnar. The cells contain brown pigment granules.

FIG. 20–5. Tympanic Membrane, Periphery, Puppy. The tympanic membrane has a core of collagenous fibers. Its outer (external auditory meatus) surface is covered by a stratified squamous epithelium; its inner (tympanic cavity) surface is covered by a simple squamous or cuboidal epithelium.

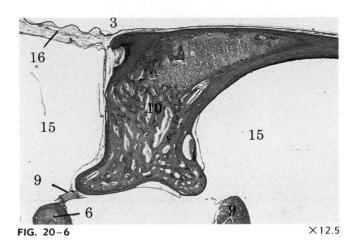

FIG. 20–6 ×12.5

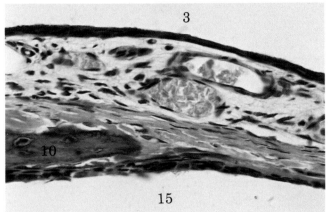

FIG. 20–7 ×250

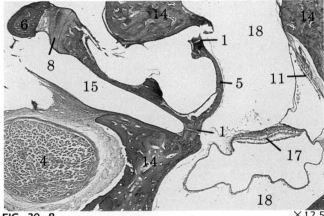

FIG. 20–8 ×12.5

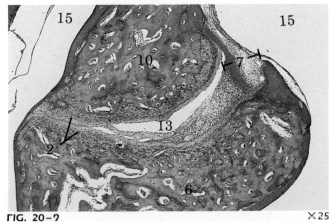

FIG. 20–9 ×25

FIG. 20–10 ×125

KEY	
1. Annular ligament	**10.** Malleus
2. Articular cartilage	**11.** Sacculus, macula of
3. External auditory meatus	**12.** Stapes, articular cartilage
4. Facial nerve	**13.** Synovial cavity
5. Footplate, stapes	**14.** Temporal bone, petrous
6. Incus	part
7. Joint capsule with elastic fibers	**15.** Tympanic cavity
	16. Tympanic membrane
8. Lenticular process, articular cartilage	**17.** Utriculus, macula of
	18. Vestibule
9. Ligament	

FIG. 20–6. Malleus and Tympanic Membrane, Puppy. The handle (manubrium) of the malleus is attached to the tympanic membrane.

FIG. 20–7. Tympanic Membrane, Puppy. Where the manubrium of the malleus is embedded in the tympanic membrane, the connective tissue of the tympanic membrane is thicker than elsewhere and blood vessels are abundant.

FIG. 20–8. Portion of Stapes and Incus, Puppy. The footplate of the stapes is attached to the oval window by an annular ligament (broken on one side in this section). The stapes articulates with the lenticular process of the incus.

FIG. 20–9. Joint, Malleus and Incus, Puppy. The head of the malleus articulates with the body of the incus in this synovial joint.

FIG. 20–10. Junction of Lenticular Process and Stapes, Puppy. The stapes articulates with the lenticular process of the incus.

FIG. 20–11   ×125

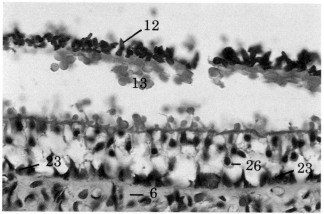

FIG. 20–12   ×250

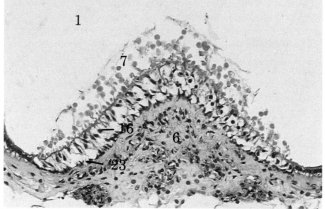

FIG. 20–13   ×125

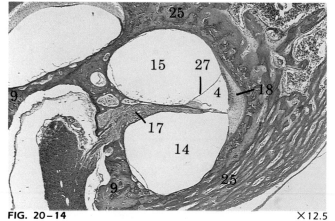

FIG. 20–14   ×12.5

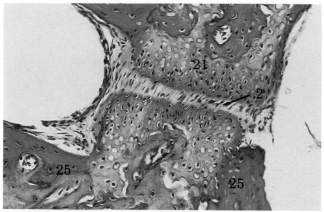

FIG. 20–15   ×62.5

KEY	
1. Ampulla, cavity	**15.** Scala vestibuli
2. Annular ligament	**16.** Sensory cell, nucleus
3. Basilar membrane	**17.** Spiral ganglion
4. Cochlear duct	**18.** Spiral ligament
5. Cochlear nerve	**19.** Spiral limbus
6. Connective tissue	**20.** Spiral tunnel
7. Cupula, portion of	**21.** Stapes, articular cartilage
8. Inner tunnel	**22.** Stria vascularis
9. Modiolus	**23.** Supporting cell, nucleus
10. Organ of Corti	**24.** Tectorial membrane
11. Osseous spiral lamina	**25.** Temporal bone, petrous
12. Otolith	part
13. Otolithic membrane	**26.** Type I cell
14. Scala tympani	**27.** Vestibular membrane

FIG. 20–11. Annular Ligament, Stapes, Puppy. The stapes is fastened to the circular cartilage of the oval window by the fibroelastic, annular ligament.

FIG. 20–12. Macula of Sacculus, Puppy. Otoliths are embedded in a gelatinous otolithic membrane, which lies upon an epithelium consisting of sensory and supporting cells. Chalice-like, Type I sensory cells and the basal nuclei of supporting cells are evident in this micrograph.

FIG. 20–13. Crista Ampullaris, Puppy. This ridge of sensory epithelium, supported by connective tissue, protrudes into the ampulla of a semicircular duct and is oriented at right angles to the long axis of the duct. The epithelium consists of sensory and supporting cells similar to those found in the maculae. A mass of gelatinous material, the cupula, covers the surface epithelium.

FIG. 20–14. Cochlea, Puppy. Cross section through a portion of the spiral cochlea.

FIG. 20–15. Cochlea, Puppy. Detail of the region of the cochlear duct (scala media, membranous cochlea).

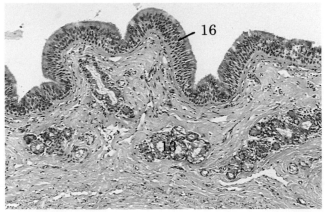

FIG. 20–16 ×62.5

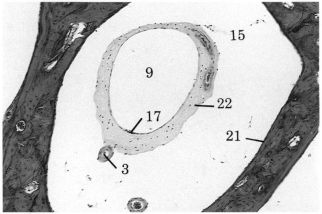

FIG. 20–17 ×62.5

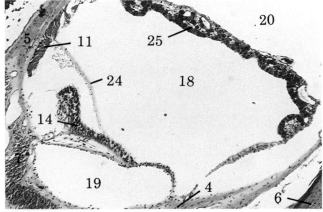

FIG. 20–18 ×62.5

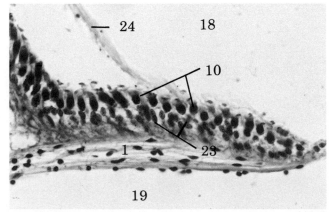

FIG. 20–19 ×250

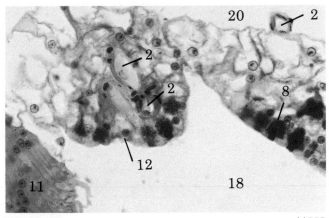

FIG. 20–20 ×250

KEY	
1. Basilar membrane	**13.** Mixed glands
2. Blood vessel of	**14.** Organ of Corti
connective base	**15.** Perilymphatic space
3. Capillary	**16.** Pseudostratified epithelium
4. Cartilaginous frame, caudal	**17.** Raphe
5. Cartilaginous frame, rostral	**18.** Scala media (cochlear duct)
6. Cochlea, bony wall	**19.** Scala tympani
7. Cochlear nerve	**20.** Scala vestibuli
8. Dark cell	**21.** Semicircular canal, wall
9. Endolymphatic space	**22.** Semicircular duct, wall
10. Hair cells	**23.** Supporting cells
11. Homogeneous cells	**24.** Tectorial membrane
12. Light cell	**25.** Tegmentum vasculosum

FIG. 20–16. Guttural Pouch, Horse. This diverticulum of the eustachian tube is lined by a ciliated, pseudostratified columnar epithelium with goblet cells. Mixed glands occur in the lamina propria.

FIG. 20–17. Semicircular Canal, x.s., Chicken. The semicircular canal is a part of the bony labyrinth. It contains the semicircular duct, a part of the membranous labyrinth. The duct is lined by a simple squamous epithelium except at the raphe, where cuboidal cells form the lining.

FIG. 20–18. Cochlea, x.s., Chicken, Masson's.

FIG. 20–19. Organ of Corti, Cochlea, x.s., Chicken, Masson's.

FIG. 20–20. Tegmentum Vasculosum, Cochlea, Chicken, Masson's. This thick membrane rests upon a thin connective base and possesses a highly folded epithelial surface with numerous vascular loops. The epithelium consists of light and dark cells. Dark cells have a constricted neck region that extends to the surface of the epithelium. Their basal portion contains the nucleus and is irregularly shaped. The cytoplasm is very dense. Light cells have a pale cytoplasm and surround the dark cells.

THE EAR **253**

BIBLIOGRAPHY

Adam, W.S., Calhoun, M.L., Smith, E.M., and Stinson, A.W.: Microscopic Anatomy of the Dog: A Photographic Atlas. Springfield, Illinois, Charles C Thomas, 1970.

Amann, R.P., Johnson, L., and Pickett, B.W.: Connection between the seminiferous tubules and the efferent ducts in the stallion. Am. J. Vet. Res., *38*:1571, 1977.

Amoroso, E.C.: Histology of the placenta. Br. Med. Bull., *17*:81, 1961.

Arey, L.B.: Human Histology. 4th Ed. Philadelphia, W.B. Saunders Company, 1974.

Banks, W.J.: Applied Veterinary Histology. 2nd Ed. Baltimore, Williams and Wilkins, 1986.

Björkman, N.H.: Fine structure of the fetal-maternal area of exchange in the epitheliochorial and endotheliochorial type of placentation. Acta Anat., *86*(Suppl. 1):1, 1973.

Bloom, W., and Fawcett, D.W.: A Textbook of Histology. 10th Ed. Philadelphia, W.B. Saunders Company, 1975.

Calhoun, M.L.: The microscopic anatomy of the digestive tract of Gallus domesticus. Iowa State Coll. J. Sci., 7:261, 1933.

Cole, H.H., and Cupps, P.T. (eds.): Reproduction in Domestic Animals. Vol. 1. New York, Academic Press, Inc., 1959.

Cole, H.H., and Cupps, P.T. (eds.): Reproduction in Domestic Animals. New York, Academic Press, Inc., 1969.

Czarnecki, C.M., and Hammer, R.F.: Auto-tutorial Laboratory Guide. Microscopic Anatomy of Domestic Animals. University of Minnesota, 1978.

Dellmann, H., and Brown, E.M.: Textbook of Veterinary Histology. 3rd Ed. Philadelphia, Lea & Febiger, 1987.

Delly, J.G., et al.: Photography Through the Microscope. 7th Ed. Rochester, Eastman Kodak Company, 1980.

Department of Anatomy: Histology Laboratory Manual (Microscopic Anatomy, VAN. 306). Iowa State University, 1987.

Di Fiore, M.S.H.: Atlas of Human Histology. 5th Ed. Philadelphia, Lea & Febiger, 1981.

Elias, H.: Comparison of duodenal glands in domestic animals. Am. J. Vet. Res., 8:311, 1947.

Evans, H.E., and Christensen, G.C.: Miller's Anatomy of the Dog. 2nd Ed. Philadelphia, W.B. Saunders Company, 1979.

Gartner, L.P., and Hiatt, J.L.: Atlas of Histology. Baltimore, Williams & Wilkins, 1987.

Geneser, F.: Color Atlas of Histology. Philadelphia, Lea & Febiger, 1989.

Gentle, M.J.: The lingual taste buds of Gallus Domesticus L. Brt. Poult. Sci., 12:245, 1971.

Getty, R.: Sisson and Grossman's The Anatomy of the Domestic Animals. Vol. 1. 5th Ed. Philadelphia, W.B. Saunders Company, 1975.

Getty, R.: Sisson and Grossman's The Anatomy of the Domestic Animals. Vol. 1. 5th Ed. Philadelphia, W.B. Saunders Company, 1975.

Ham, A.W., and Cormack, D.H.: Histology. 8th Ed. Philadelphia, J.B. Lippincott Company, 1979.

Hammersen, F.: Sabotta/Hammersen. Histology. A Color Atlas of Microscopic Anatomy. 3rd Ed. Baltimore, Urban & Schwarzenberg, 1985.

Hamre, C.J.: Origin and differentiation of heterophil, eosinophil and basophil leukocytes of chickens. Anat. Rec., 112:339, 1952.

Hodges, R.D.: The Histology of the Fowl. New York, Academic Press Inc., 1974.

Jain, N.C.: Schalm's Veterinary Hematology. 4th Ed. Philadelphia, Lea & Febiger, 1986.

Junqueira, L.C., and Carneiro, J.: Basic Histology. 2nd Ed. Los Altos, California, 1980.

Kelly, D.E., Wood, R.L., and Enders, A.C.: Bailey's Textbook of Microscopic Anatomy. 18th Ed. Baltimore, Williams & Wilkins, 1984.

Lawson, D.D., Nixon, G.S., Noble, H.W., and Weipers, W.L.: Dental anatomy and histology of the dog. Res. Vet. Sci., 1:201, 1960.

Leeson, T.S., and Leeson, C.R.: A Brief Atlas of Histology. Philadelphia, W.B. Saunders Company, 1979.

Lewis, H.B., and Rebar, A.H.: Bone Marrow Evaluation in Veterinary Practice. St. Louis, Ralston Purina, 1979.

Lindenmaier, P., and Kare, M.R.: The taste end-organs of the chicken. Poult. Sci., 38:545, 1959.

Lucas, A.M., and Jamroz, C.: Atlas of Avian Hematology. Washington, D.C., United States Department of Agriculture, 1961.

Lucas, A.M., and Stettenheim, P.R.: Avian Anatomy. Integument. Part I. Washington, D.C., United States Department of Agriculture, 1972.

Lucas, A.M., and Stettenheim, P.R.: Avian Anatomy. Integument. Part II. Washington, D.C., United States Department of Agriculture, 1972.

Melfi, R.C.: Permar's Oral Embryology and Microscopic Anatomy. 7th Ed. Philadelphia, Lea & Febiger, 1982.

Murphy, C.J.: Raptor ophthalmology. Compend. Contin. Educ. Pract. Vet., 9:241, 1987.

Natt, M.P., and Herrick, C.A.: Variation in the shape of the rodlike granules of the chicken heterophil leukocyte and its possible significance. Poult. Sci., 33:828, 1954.

Nickel, R., Schummer, A., Seiferle, E. (eds.): Anatomy of the Domestic Birds. Translated by W.G. Siller and P.A.L. Wight. New York, Springer-Verlag, 1977.

Olson, P.N., Behrendt, M.D., and Weiss, D.E.: Reproductive problems in the bitch: Finding answers through vaginal cytology. Vet. Med., 82:344, 1987.

Prince, J.H., Diesem, C.D., Eglitis, I., and Ruskell, G.L.: Anatomy and Histology of the Eye and Orbit in Domestic Animals. Springfield, Illinois, Charles C Thomas, 1960.

Rebar, A.H.: Handbook of Veterinary Cytology. St. Louis, Ralston Purina, 1980.

Reith, E.J., and Ross, M.H.: Atlas of Descriptive Histology. 3rd Ed. New York, Harper & Row, 1977.

Rich, L.J.: The Morphology of Canine and Feline Blood Cells, Including Equine References. St. Louis, Ralston Purina, 1976.

Ross, M.H., and Romrell, L.J.: Histology. 2nd Ed. Baltimore, Williams & Wilkins, 1989.

Samuel, C.A., Allen, W.R., and Steven, D.H.: Studies on the equine placenta. I. Development of the microcotyledons. J. Reprod. Fertil., 41:441, 1974.

Seely, J.C.: The harderian gland. Lab. Anim., 16:33, 1987.

Shackleford, J.M., and Wilborn, W.H.: Ultrastructure of bovine parotid glands. J. Morphol., 127:453, 1969.

Sloss, M.W.: The microscopic anatomy of the digestive tract of Sus scrofa domestica. Am. J. Vet. Res., 1:578, 1954.

Smith, R.F.: Microscopy and Photomicrography. A Practical Guide. New York, Appleton-Century-Crofts, 1982.

Strickland, J.H., and Calhoun, M.L.: The integumentary system of the cat. Am. J. Vet. Res., 24:1018, 1963.

Stump, J.E.: Anatomy of the normal equine foot, including microscopic features of the laminar region. J. Am. Vet. Med. Assoc., 151:1588, 1967.

Sturkie, P.D. (ed.): Avian Physiology. 3rd Ed. New York, Springer-Verlag, 1976.

Trautmann, A., and Fiebiger, J.: Fundamentals of the Histology of Domestic Animals. Translated and revised by R.E. Habel and E.L. Biberstein. Ithaca, N.Y., Comstock Publishing Associates, 1952.

Trautmann, A., and Fiebiger, J.: Fundamentals of the Histology of Domestic Animals. Translated and revised by R.E. Habel and E.L. Biberstein. Ithaca, N.Y., Comstock Publishing Associates, 1957.

Webb, A.J., and Calhoun, M.L.: The microscopic anatomy of the skin of mongrel dogs. Am. J. Vet. Res., 15:274, 1954.

Weiss, L.: The red pulp of the spleen: Structural basis of blood flow. Clin. Haematol., 12:375, 1983.

Weiss, L., and Greep, R.O.: Histology. 4th Ed. New York, McGraw-Hill, Inc., 1977.

Wheater, P.R., Burkitt, H.G., and Daniels, V.G.: Functional Histology. A Text and Colour Atlas. New York, Churchill Livingstone, 1979.

Nasal cavity, of chickens, 162–163, *171*
  of mammals, 161, *164*
Nasal concha, *164*
Nasal gland, *164*
Nasolabial gland, *85*
Nasopharynx, of mammals, 162, *165*
Neck, skin of, *87–89*
    of chickens, *103*
Nephron, of kidney, 151–153
Nerve, 45, *46–52*
Nerve fascicle, *50*
Nerve fiber layer, of eye, 233, *239–240, 245*
Nervous system, of chickens, 45, *51–52*
  of mammals, 45, *46–51*
Neuroglia cell, of pineal gland, 178, *182*
Neurohypophysis, of chickens, 179, *185–186*
  of mammals, 177, *180–181*
Neuromuscular spindle, *51, 171*
Neuron, 45, *48–52*
Neutrophil, as blood component, 28, *30–35*
  of bone marrow, *40*
  of connective tissue, *15*
  of vagina, 209, *224–225*
Neutrophilic band cell, of bone marrow, *39–40*
Neutrophilic metamyelocyte, of bone marrow, *40*
Neutrophilic myelocyte, of bone marrow, *39*
Nictitating membrane, of eye, 233–234, *240–241*
Nissl granule, of nervous system, *48–49*
Nonpigmented cell, of eye, 232, *237*
Nonpigmented epithelium, of eye, 232, *243–244*
Nonsinusal spleen, 66, *76–77*
Normoblast, of bone marrow, *38*
Nose, blood vessels of, *56, 59*
  connective tissue of, *16*
  membrane bone of, *23*
  sinus hair follicle of, *91*
  skin of, *82–83, 84–85*
  sweat gland of, *82–83, 92*
  See also Nasal cavity
Nuclear bag fiber, of nervous system, *51*
Nuclear chain fiber, of nervous system, *51*

Odontoblast, of tooth, *116*
Oil immersion, for blood smears, 27
Olfactory cell, 161, *164, 172*
Olfactory epithelium, 161, 163, *164, 172*
Omasum, 112, *125–126*
Oocyte, of ovary, 207–208, 210, *211, 225–226*
Optic disc, of eye, 233, *235, 239*
Optic nerve, of eye, 233, *235, 239, 245*
Ora ciliaris retinae, of eye, 233, *235, 238*
Orcein, connective tissue and, 13
  in histologic section preparation, 3
Organ of Corti, of inner ear, 248–249, *252–253*
Oropharynx, 112, *121–122*
Orthochromatic erythroblast, of bone marrow, 38, *39–40*
Os penis, 191, *199–200*
Osseous spiral lamina, of inner ear, 248, *252*
Ossicle, of middle ear, 247–248, *251*
Ossification center, of phalanx, *23*
Osteoblast, 21, *23–25*
  of bone marrow, 38, *39*
Osteoclast, 21, 23, *25*
  of bone marrow, 38, *39*
Osteocyte, 21, *23–26*
Osteoid, *23*
Otolith, of inner ear, 248, *252*
Otolithic membrane, of inner ear, 248, *22*
Outer enamel epithelium, *115–116*
Outer limiting membrane, of eye, *233*
Outer nuclear layer, of eye, 233, *239–240, 245*
Outer plexiform layer, of eye, 233, *239–240, 245*

Outer root sheath, of hair, 82, *88, 90–92*
Ovary, of chickens, 210, *225–226*
  of mammals, 207–208, *211–213*
Oviduct, of chickens, 210, *226–229*
  of mammals, 208, *213–215*
Oxyphilic cell, of parathyroid gland, 178

Pacinian corpuscle, of digital pad, *86*
  of mesentery, *51*
  of pancreas, 113
Palate, *117*
Palatine tonsil, 66, *69–70*
Palpebral conjunctiva, of eye, 233, *236–237, 240–242*
Pancreas, of chickens, 114, *150*
  of mammals, 113, *144–145*
    blood vessels of, *57*
    nerves of, *51*
Paneth cell, of duodenum, *133*
Papilla, of tongue, 111, *118–119*
Papillary duct, of kidney, 152, *156–157*
Papillary layer, dermal, 82, 86, *89–90, 105–106*
Parabasal cell, of vaginal epithelium, 209, *224–225*
Parabronchus, 163, *174–175*
Paraepiglottic tonsil, 66, *69*
Paraffin, in histologic section preparation, 1, 2, 3
Parafollicular cell, of thyroid, 178–179, *182*
Parasympathetic ganglion, *49*
Parathyroid gland, of chickens, 179, *187*
  of mammals, 178, *182–183*
Parenchyma, of pituitary gland, 178
  of spleen, 66–67, *75–78*
Parenchymal cell, of aortic body, *63*
  of endocrine glands, *177–179*
Parietal cell, of stomach, 112, *127–130*
Parietal pericardium, 54, *62*
Parietal pleura, *171*
Parietal prepuce, 191, *203*
Parotid gland, of mammals, *119–120*
Pars ciliaris retinae, of eye, 232, *235–236, 238*
Pars convoluta, of kidney, 151, *154*
Pars disseminata, of prostate gland, 190, *198–199*
Pars distalis, of pituitary gland, 177–179, *180–181, 185–186*
Pars intermedia, of pituitary gland, 178, *180–181*
Pars iridica retinae, of eye, 232, *235*
Pars nervosa, of pituitary gland, 178–179, *180–181, 185*
Pars radiata, of kidney, 151, *154, 156*
Pars tuberalis, of pituitary gland, 178–179, *180–181, 185–186*
Pecten, of eye, 234, *245*
Pectinate ligament, of eye, 232–234, *236–237, 240, 243–244*
Pelvic urethra, 191
Pelvis, renal, 151–152, *156–157*
Penicillus, of spleen, 66
Penile urethra, 191, *200–201*
Penis, 191, *199–202*
Periarterial lymphatic sheath, 66, *76*
Pericardial cavity, 54, *62*
Pericardium, 54, *62*
Perichondrium, of cartilage, 19, *20*
Perilobular collecting duct, of kidney, 153, *160*
Perilymphatic space, of ear, *253*
Perimetrium, of uterus, 208
Perimysium, of muscle, 41, *43–44*
Perineurium, *49–50*
Periodontal ligament, *116*
Periople, *100*
Perioplic dermis, of hoof, 99, *100–101*
Perioplic epidermis, of hoof, 99, *101*
Peritoneum, of testis, 189, 191
Perivitelline membrane, of ovary, 210, *226*
Permanent tooth, *115–116*
Pessulus, 163, *173–174*
Peyer's patch, 65, *68–69, 112*